Pharmacogenomics: From Basic Research to Clinical Implementation

Pharmacogenomics: From Basic Research to Clinical Implementation

Editor

Laura B. Scheinfeldt

MDPI • Basel • Beijing • Wuhan • Barcelona • Belgrade • Manchester • Tokyo • Cluj • Tianjin

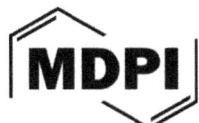

Editor
Laura B. Scheinfeldt
Director of Repository Science
Coriell Institute for Medical
Research
Camden
United States

Editorial Office
MDPI
St. Alban-Anlage 66
4052 Basel, Switzerland

This is a reprint of articles from the Special Issue published online in the open access journal *Journal of Personalized Medicine* (ISSN 2075-4426) (available at: www.mdpi.com/journal/jpm/special_issues/pharmacogenomics_basicresearch).

For citation purposes, cite each article independently as indicated on the article page online and as indicated below:

LastName, A.A.; LastName, B.B.; LastName, C.C. Article Title. *Journal Name* **Year**, *Volume Number*, Page Range.

ISBN 978-3-0365-2835-9 (Hbk)
ISBN 978-3-0365-2834-2 (PDF)

© 2022 by the authors. Articles in this book are Open Access and distributed under the Creative Commons Attribution (CC BY) license, which allows users to download, copy and build upon published articles, as long as the author and publisher are properly credited, which ensures maximum dissemination and a wider impact of our publications.

The book as a whole is distributed by MDPI under the terms and conditions of the Creative Commons license CC BY-NC-ND.

Contents

About the Editor vii

Laura B. Scheinfeldt
Pharmacogenomics: From Basic Research to Clinical Implementation
Reprinted from: *J. Pers. Med.* **2021**, *11*, 800, doi:10.3390/jpm11080800 1

Patrick Silva, David Jacobs, John Kriak, Asim Abu-Baker, George Udeani, Gabriel Neal and Kenneth Ramos
Implementation of Pharmacogenomics and Artificial Intelligence Tools for Chronic Disease Management in Primary Care Setting
Reprinted from: *J. Pers. Med.* **2021**, *11*, 443, doi:10.3390/jpm11060443 3

Pritmohinder S. Gill, Feliciano B. Yu, Patricia A. Porter-Gill, Bobby L. Boyanton, Judy C. Allen, Jason E. Farrar, Aravindhan Veerapandiyan, Parthak Prodhan, Kevin J. Bielamowicz, Elizabeth Sellars, Andrew Burrow, Joshua L. Kennedy, Jeffery L. Clothier, David L. Becton, Don Rule and G. Bradley Schaefer
Implementing Pharmacogenomics Testing: Single Center Experience at Arkansas Children's Hospital
Reprinted from: *J. Pers. Med.* **2021**, *11*, 394, doi:10.3390/jpm11050394 21

Fei Yee Lee, Farida Islahudin, Aina Yazrin Ali Nasiruddin, Abdul Halim Abdul Gafor, Hin-Seng Wong, Sunita Bavanandan, Shamin Mohd Saffian, Adyani Md Redzuan, Nurul Ain Mohd Tahir and Mohd Makmor-Bakry
Effects of CYP3A5 Polymorphism on Rapid Progression of Chronic Kidney Disease: A Prospective, Multicentre Study
Reprinted from: *J. Pers. Med.* **2021**, *11*, 252, doi:10.3390/jpm11040252 41

Jeeyun A. Kim, Rachel Ceccarelli and Christine Y. Lu
Pharmacogenomic Biomarkers in US FDA-Approved Drug Labels (2000–2020)
Reprinted from: *J. Pers. Med.* **2021**, *11*, 179, doi:10.3390/jpm11030179 55

Laura B. Scheinfeldt, Andrew Brangan, Dara M. Kusic, Sudhir Kumar and Neda Gharani
Common Treatment, Common Variant: Evolutionary Prediction of Functional Pharmacogenomic Variants
Reprinted from: *J. Pers. Med.* **2021**, *11*, 131, doi:10.3390/jpm11020131 69

Nayoung Han, Jung Mi Oh and In-Wha Kim
Combination of Genome-Wide Polymorphisms and Copy Number Variations of Pharmacogenes in Koreans
Reprinted from: *J. Pers. Med.* **2021**, *11*, 33, doi:10.3390/jpm11010033 83

Samantha Breaux, Francis Arthur Derek Desrosiers, Mauricio Neira, Sunita Sinha and Corey Nislow
Pharmacogenomics at the Point of Care: A Community Pharmacy Project in British Columbia
Reprinted from: *J. Pers. Med.* **2020**, *11*, 11, doi:10.3390/jpm11010011 95

Pauline Lanting, Evelien Drenth, Ludolf Boven, Amanda van Hoek, Annemiek Hijlkema, Ellen Poot, Gerben van der Vries, Robert Schoevers, Ernst Horwitz, Reinold Gans, Jos Kosterink, Mirjam Plantinga, Irene van Langen, Adelita Ranchor, Cisca Wijmenga, Lude Franke, Bob Wilffert and Rolf Sijmons
Practical Barriers and Facilitators Experienced by Patients, Pharmacists and Physicians to the Implementation of Pharmacogenomic Screening in Dutch Outpatient Hospital Care—An Explorative Pilot Study
Reprinted from: *J. Pers. Med.* **2020**, *10*, 293, doi:10.3390/jpm10040293 . . . . **113**

Amy L. Pasternak, Kristen M. Ward, Mohammad B. Ateya, Hae Mi Choe, Amy N. Thompson, John S. Clark and Vicki Ellingrod
Establishment of a Pharmacogenetics Service Focused on Optimizing Existing Pharmacogenetic Testing at a Large Academic Health Center
Reprinted from: *J. Pers. Med.* **2020**, *10*, 154, doi:10.3390/jpm10040154 . . . . **127**

Tara Schmidlen, Amy C. Sturm and Laura B. Scheinfeldt
Pharmacogenomic (PGx) Counseling: Exploring Participant Questions about PGx Test Results
Reprinted from: *J. Pers. Med.* **2020**, *10*, 29, doi:10.3390/jpm10020029 . . . . **137**

About the Editor

Laura B. Scheinfeldt

Laura Scheinfeldt, Ph.D., is the principal investigator of the National Institute of Neurological Disorders and Stroke (NINDS) Human Genetics Resource Center and the NHGRI Sample Repository for Human Genetic Research at the Coriell Institute for Medical Research.

The NINDS Human Genetics Resource Center at Coriell Institute receives blood samples and clinical data from individuals diagnosed with neurological disorders and stroke, as well as unaffected relatives and population controls and distributes DNA and cell lines to promote neurological disease research.

The NHGRI Sample Repository for Human Genetic Research distributes cell lines and DNA from 27 HapMap and 1000 Genomes Project population samples. These biospecimens are high-quality resources for the study of genetic and genomic variation in human populations living around the world.

Laura previously served as a research scientist in Coriell Institute's Coriell Personalized Medicine Collaborative (CPMC), a research study to evaluate the clinical utility of genetic data. In this role, Laura applied her background in population genetics to the participant-based initiative and supported the research and analysis goals of the study.

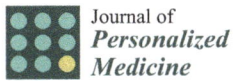

Editorial
Pharmacogenomics: From Basic Research to Clinical Implementation

Laura B. Scheinfeldt

Coriell Institute for Medical Research, Camden, NJ 08003, USA; lscheinfeldt@coriell.org

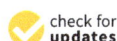

Citation: Scheinfeldt, L.B. Pharmacogenomics: From Basic Research to Clinical Implementation. *J. Pers. Med.* **2021**, *11*, 800. https://doi.org/10.3390/jpm11080800

Received: 12 August 2021
Accepted: 14 August 2021
Published: 17 August 2021

Publisher's Note: MDPI stays neutral with regard to jurisdictional claims in published maps and institutional affiliations.

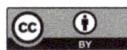

Copyright: © 2021 by the author. Licensee MDPI, Basel, Switzerland. This article is an open access article distributed under the terms and conditions of the Creative Commons Attribution (CC BY) license (https://creativecommons.org/licenses/by/4.0/).

The established contribution of genetic variation to drug response has the potential to improve drug efficacy and reduce drug toxicity [1]. The uptake of pharmacogenomics (PGx) in clinical care, however, has been relatively slow despite the documentation and validation of many known genetic determinants of drug response. This special issue, entitled "Pharmacogenomics: From Basic Research to Clinical Implementation," focuses on the current state of pharmacogenomics and the extensive translational process required for clinical implementation, including the characterization of functionally important PGx variation, the clinical interpretation of PGx variation, clinical PGx decision support, and the incorporation of PGx into clinical care.

Four of the special issue articles, Han et al. [2], Lee et al. [3], Scheinfeldt et al. [1], and Kim et al. [4] focus on the identification, characterization, and documentation of functionally important PGx variation. Kim et al. [4] conducted a longitudinal review of FDA-approved PGx drugs and FDA PGx drug labels. The authors identified a notable increase in PGx content between 2000 and 2020 but also note that the majority of these involved cancer treatment drug labels. This analysis demonstrates the need for more PGx support in non-cancer therapeutics. Han et al. [2] focused on the identification of pharmacogenetic single nucleotide polymorphisms (SNPs) and copy number variation (CNV) in the Korean Genome and Epidemiology Study, which included genome-wide SNP data collected from over 70,000 Korean Genome and Epidemiology Study participants and CNV data collected from 1000 study participants. The authors used their cohort data to confirm the clinical implications of important variants in several pharmacogenes, including *VKORC1*, *CYP2D6*, *CYP2C19*, and *TPMT*. Lee et al. [3] focused on the impact PGx variation at *CYP3A5* has on chronic kidney disease progression. This example demonstrates that PGx variation may impact disease treatment through drug response as well as through physiological effects in kidney that may exacerbate kidney disease. Scheinfeldt et al. [1] took a complementary in silico approach that leveraged the evolutionary history of the genes involved in drug response to predict functionally important pharmacovariants. Not only did they identify over 2000 new putative pharmacovariants, but they demonstrated that these pharmacovariants are common across worldwide communities.

Two of the special issue articles, Silva et al. [5] and Schmidlen et al. [6], focused on PGx clinical decision support. Silva et al. [5] leveraged a Clinical Semantic Network framework to apply a pharmacogenomic model to patient electronic medical record data. They validated this framework with a virtual case study and demonstrated that their approach can identify clinically significant drug–drug and drug–gene interactions. Given the increasingly complex challenges to integrating medical informatics data for clinical decision-making, this framework and others like it will be needed to support precision medication management. Schmidlen et al. [6] conducted a retrospective qualitative analysis of genetic counseling requests from participants in a personalized medicine research study and demonstrated the critical role that genetic counselors play in supporting providers in their communication of PGx results to patients and supporting patients in their understanding of PGx results.

Several of the studies included in this special issue focus more directly on the incorporation of PGx into clinical care. Gill et al. [7] focused on PGx implementation in pediatric care. Importantly, the authors described a framework in which PGx testing is incorporated into the EHR system being used by clinicians involved in the study (in this case, EPIC). Breaux et al. [8] presented an example of PGx implementation for mental health medications involving a collaborative framework of pharmacists and clinicians. The authors found that PGx-led medication changes added minimal short-term cost to patient care and emphasized potential long-term benefits, including improved dosing and reduced adverse drug reactions. Pasternak et al. [9] conducted a retrospective review of medical records and provided a detailed assessment of documented PGx testing. These authors used this review to develop several recommendations for improving clinical PGx testing, including the establishment of a clinical PGx consult service involving pharmacists and clinicians and the application of standardized CPIC terminology. Lanting et al. [10] also focused on challenges to clinical PGx implementation in a complementary prospective manner involving patients, physicians, and pharmacists. While patient and clinician attitudes toward PGx testing were typically positive, the authors documented a need for additional PGx education for clinicians and a clear determination of which clinicians should take primary responsibility for clinical PGx testing.

Taken together, this body of work builds upon the extensive information already known about contributions of genetic variation to drug response and describes important gaps in this knowledge as well as challenges to the clinical implementation of pharmacogenomics that remain to be addressed. Several examples of clinical PGx implementation in a variety of settings highlight areas of ongoing improvement and momentum toward more broad integration of PGx testing.

Funding: This research was funded by NHGRI, U41HG008736-05.

Institutional Review Board Statement: Not applicable.

Informed Consent Statement: Not applicable.

Data Availability Statement: Not applicable.

Conflicts of Interest: The author declares no conflict of interest.

References

1. Scheinfeldt, L.B.; Brangan, A.; Kusic, D.M.; Kumar, S.; Gharani, N. Common Treatment, Common Variant: Evolutionary Prediction of Functional Pharmacogenomic Variants. *J. Pers. Med.* **2021**, *11*, 131. [CrossRef] [PubMed]
2. Han, N.; Oh, J.M.; Kim, I.W. Combination of Genome-Wide Polymorphisms and Copy Number Variations of Pharmacogenes in Koreans. *J. Pers. Med.* **2021**, *11*, 33. [CrossRef] [PubMed]
3. Lee, F.Y.; Islahudin, F.; Ali Nasiruddin, A.Y.; Abdul Gafor, A.H.; Wong, H.S.; Bavanandan, S.; Mohd Saffian, S.; Md Redzuan, A.; Mohd Tahir, N.A.; Makmor-Bakry, M. Effects of CYP3A5 Polymorphism on Rapid Progression of Chronic Kidney Disease: A Prospective, Multicentre Study. *J. Pers. Med.* **2021**, *11*, 252. [CrossRef] [PubMed]
4. Kim, J.A.; Ceccarelli, R.; Lu, C.Y. Pharmacogenomic Biomarkers in US FDA-Approved Drug Labels (2000-2020). *J. Pers. Med.* **2021**, *11*, 179. [CrossRef] [PubMed]
5. Silva, P.; Jacobs, D.; Kriak, J.; Abu-Baker, A.; Udeani, G.; Neal, G.; Ramos, K. Implementation of Pharmacogenomics and Artificial Intelligence Tools for Chronic Disease Management in Primary Care Setting. *J. Pers. Med.* **2021**, *11*, 443. [CrossRef] [PubMed]
6. Schmidlen, T.; Sturm, A.C.; Scheinfeldt, L.B. Pharmacogenomic (PGx) Counseling: Exploring Participant Questions about PGx Test Results. *J. Pers. Med.* **2020**, *10*, 29. [CrossRef] [PubMed]
7. Gill, P.S.; Yu, F.B.; Porter-Gill, P.A.; Boyanton, B.L.; Allen, J.C.; Farrar, J.E.; Veerapandiyan, A.; Prodhan, P.; Bielamowicz, K.J.; Sellars, E.; et al. Implementing Pharmacogenomics Testing: Single Center Experience at Arkansas Children's Hospital. *J. Pers. Med.* **2021**, *11*, 394. [CrossRef] [PubMed]
8. Breaux, S.; Desrosiers, F.A.D.; Neira, M.; Sinha, S.; Nislow, C. Pharmacogenomics at the Point of Care: A Community Pharmacy Project in British Columbia. *J. Pers. Med.* **2020**, *11*, 11. [CrossRef] [PubMed]
9. Pasternak, A.L.; Ward, K.M.; Ateya, M.B.; Choe, H.M.; Thompson, A.N.; Clark, J.S.; Ellingrod, V. Establishment of a Pharmacogenetics Service Focused on Optimizing Existing Pharmacogenetic Testing at a Large Academic Health Center. *J. Pers. Med.* **2020**, *10*, 154. [CrossRef] [PubMed]
10. Lanting, P.; Drenth, E.; Boven, L.; van Hoek, A.; Hijlkema, A.; Poot, E.; van der Vries, G.; Schoevers, R.; Horwitz, E.; Gans, R.; et al. Practical Barriers and Facilitators Experienced by Patients, Pharmacists and Physicians to the Implementation of Pharmacogenomic Screening in Dutch Outpatient Hospital Care-An Explorative Pilot Study. *J. Pers. Med.* **2020**, *10*, 293. [CrossRef] [PubMed]

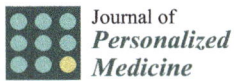

Article

Implementation of Pharmacogenomics and Artificial Intelligence Tools for Chronic Disease Management in Primary Care Setting

Patrick Silva [1], David Jacobs [2,*], John Kriak [2], Asim Abu-Baker [1], George Udeani [1], Gabriel Neal [1] and Kenneth Ramos [1,*]

1 Texas A&M Health Science Center, 8441 Riverside Pkwy, Bryan, TX 77807, USA; ricksilva@tamu.edu (P.S.); abu-baker@tamu.edu (A.A.-B.); udeani@tamu.edu (G.U.); gneal@tamu.edu (G.N.)
2 Goldblatt Systems, LLC., 5151 E. Broadway Blvd., Tucson, AZ 85711, USA; jkriak@molecdx.com
* Correspondence: djacobs@goldblattsystems.com (D.J.); kramos@tamu.edu (K.R.); Tel.: +1-520-382-5999 (D.J.); +1-713-677-7522 (K.R.)

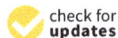

Citation: Silva, P.; Jacobs, D.; Kriak, J.; Abu-Baker, A.; Udeani, G.; Neal, G.; Ramos, K. Implementation of Pharmacogenomics and Artificial Intelligence Tools for Chronic Disease Management in Primary Care Setting. *J. Pers. Med.* **2021**, *11*, 443. https://doi.org/10.3390/jpm11060443

Academic Editor: Laura B. Scheinfeldt

Received: 31 March 2021
Accepted: 20 May 2021
Published: 21 May 2021

Publisher's Note: MDPI stays neutral with regard to jurisdictional claims in published maps and institutional affiliations.

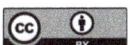

Copyright: © 2021 by the authors. Licensee MDPI, Basel, Switzerland. This article is an open access article distributed under the terms and conditions of the Creative Commons Attribution (CC BY) license (https://creativecommons.org/licenses/by/4.0/).

Abstract: Chronic disease management often requires use of multiple drug regimens that lead to polypharmacy challenges and suboptimal utilization of healthcare services. While the rising costs and healthcare utilization associated with polypharmacy and drug interactions have been well documented, effective tools to address these challenges remain elusive. Emerging evidence that proactive medication management, combined with pharmacogenomic testing, can lead to improved health outcomes and reduced cost burdens may help to address such gaps. In this report, we describe informatic and bioanalytic methodologies that integrate weak signals in symptoms and chief complaints with pharmacogenomic analysis of ~90 single nucleotide polymorphic variants, CYP2D6 copy number, and clinical pharmacokinetic profiles to monitor drug–gene pairs and drug–drug interactions for medications with significant pharmacogenomic profiles. The utility of the approach was validated in a virtual patient case showing detection of significant drug–gene and drug–drug interactions of clinical significance. This effort is being used to establish proof-of-concept for the creation of a regional database to track clinical outcomes in patients enrolled in a bioanalytically-informed medication management program. Our integrated informatic and bioanalytic platform can provide facile clinical decision support to inform and augment medication management in the primary care setting.

Keywords: pharmacogenomics; polypharmacy; chronic disease; medication management; electronic medical record; artificial intelligence

1. Introduction

The management of chronic diseases in the primary care setting often involves polypharmacy challenges that often drive considerable healthcare utilization and costs. While the term polypharmacy is used inconsistently in the literature [1], for the purposes of this report, we are making reference to clinical instances where five or more medications are used concurrently. Analysis of the Observational Health Data Sciences and Informatics data set has documented that 10% of diabetes, 24% of hypertension and 11% of depression patients followed a treatment pathway that was unique among 250 million cases [2], thus yielding a daunting number of permutations in drug combinations. This increasing armamentarium necessitates individualized care plans, a challenging task for primary care practitioners managing complex patient populations. OptumRx has estimated that polypharmacy affects about 15% of the US population and costs over $175 B per year [3]. As such, polypharmacy is believed to have increased healthcare cost burdens in recent years by ~30% [4]. Reduced adherence to drug therapy regimens and heightened incidence of adverse drug reactions (ADRs) represent major challenges for polypharmacy patients, including at-risk patients with multiple comorbid conditions.

An estimated 15 million people 65 years of age and older face a polypharmacy challenge, with nearly 50% of them using at least one unnecessary medication [5]. The prevalence of potential hepatic cytochrome (CYP) enzyme-mediated drug–drug interactions has been estimated to be as high as 80% [6], with elder adults considered to be more susceptible to problematic drug interactions due to declining levels of hepatic and renal functions [7]. In a recent report, 56% of a study population prescribed (es)citalopram showed underlying drug–drug and drug–gene interactions, which would be difficult for a practitioner to address absent of pharmacogenomic testing [8]. Further complicating the optimization of complex pharmacotherapies, individual variations in response to the same medication can fluctuate over three orders of magnitude [9]. These issues collectively contribute to over 2 million documented ADRs in the US and over 100,000 deaths [10]. Analysis of the genetic variation in response to drugs and ADRs has been enabled somewhat by the Pharmacogenomics Knowledge Base (PharmGKB), Pharmacogenomics Research Network (PGRN), and the Clinical Pharmacogenetics Implementation Consortium (CPIC) [11–13]. However, data linkages and documentation of the full diversity of clinical phenotypes associated with rare or emergent variants remain a significant hurdle. One of the largest pharmacogenomic targeted exome sequencing studies conducted to date [14] has shown that 96.2% of patients in a cohort of 5424 had CPIC Level A actionable variants, with half of the variants identified in the population identified as novel variants [15]. In a different but concordant report by Van Driest et al., 98% of the study population carried CPIC actionable variants [16].

ADRs are major drivers of healthcare utilization, and precision interventions designed to address these deficits provide tremendous opportunities for improved health outcomes and reduced costs. These challenges are especially prevalent among rural and socioeconomically disadvantaged populations, with most studies to date largely limited to retrospective observations and data mining. These approaches pose data linkage limitations that preclude longitudinal assessment of the natural history of polypharmacy and chronic disease progression at the individual level [17]. As such, robust studies of polypharmacy and the contribution of genetics to drug response have continued to be sparse.

Pharmacogenomics (PGx) is a discipline that focuses on a genome-wide assessment of how individual genes alone or in combination with other loci affect individual responses to drug treatment. PGx combines pharmacology (the science that focuses on the uses, effects, and modes of action of drugs) and genomics (the study of structure, function, evolution, and mapping of genomes) to develop effective, safe medication regimens tailored to an individual's genetic makeup [13]. PGx can aid in the prediction and stratification of who may benefit from a medication, who may not respond at all, and who may experience adverse reactions. Clinical use and reimbursement of pharmacogenomic testing remains challenging, largely due to a dearth of evidence supporting clinical utility and cost effectiveness. While clinical decision support is recognized [18] as a key component for the successful implementation of pharmacogenomic testing, widespread utilization of pharmacogenomic testing is not commonplace [19]. Pharmacogenomic-based studies can inform how single nucleotide polymorphisms (SNPs) and other variations in the human genome correlate with disease, drug response, and the occurrence of clinically significant phenotypes [20]. SNPs, the most common type of genetic variation found in humans and the most commonly tested variant affecting drug response [20], may be present between genes or within genes and their regulatory sequences. While most SNPs do not affect health, some may be linked to disease or help to predict an individual's response to a particular drug [20]. As such, SNP-based pharmacogenomic analysis can highlight specific targets and their impact on the subject's medication blood levels and response. Genomic and pharmacogenomic data combined with personal health and psychosocial data may be effectively used to support providers with treatment-related decisions in the management of chronic disease patients.

Here we present proof-of-concept for a clinical care protocol with the potential to predict and confirm a subject's response to their medication based on chief complaints and symptom functionality, specific medication-associated genomic data on receptors and transporters, and measurement of drug levels. Evidence is presented that a computational rendering of a patient's complaints and medications alone can be useful in the identification of symptoms with pharmacologic root-cause and that genotypes and pharmacokinetic information can be used computationally in a way that is practical for guiding prescribing choices in a primary care setting.

2. Materials and Methods

2.1. Clinical Environment and Process

A Texas A&M Interprofessional Pharmacogenomics (IPGx) Clinic is being established as part of the Texas A&M Family Medicine Program, a clinical practice serving diverse and underserved populations with chronic disease burden, including a high prevalence of polypharmacy.

A digital continuity of care document/file with the contents listed in Table 1 above is produced by the primary care electronic medical record for digital importation into the (Clinical Semantic Network) CSN (Figure 1, step 2). This represents the baseline information required for completion of the data analysis underlying the IPGx care model (Figure 1, step 3a). Basic medical and family history information is collected followed by a physical exam and collection of blood and/or buccal swabs for processing by a CAP-CLIA bioanalytic laboratory (Figure 1, step 3b). A medication management report citing complaints of potential pharmacological root causes and suggested alternative medications is provided to the referring physician (Figure 1, step 4). Patients are offered an opportunity to participate in a research registry underlying the IPGx database (Figure 1, step 5), and if opting into the registry, administered baseline validated quality of life questionnaires in digital format.

Table 1. Health Data Inputs into the Clinical Semantic Network to Interrogate for Symptoms and Complaints that Might have Pharmacological Root-Cause.

Input Datum
Progress Notes (6 months)
Complaints
Active problem list
Medical History
Family History
Social History
Vitals
Vaccination History
Patient encounters (10 years)
Medication and dosing
Diagnosis codes
Billing
Quality of life questionnaires (disease specific, digital)
Continuity of care documents
Procedural notes

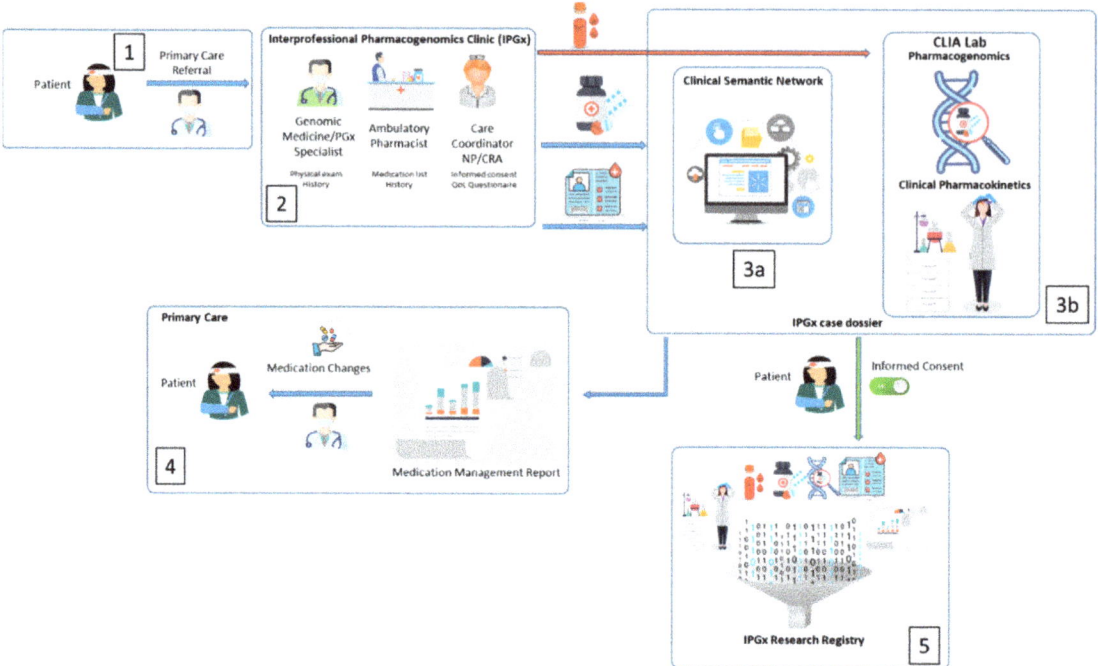

Figure 1. Interprofessional Pharmacogenomics (IPGx) Model. **1.** Referral of polypharmacy patient to the IPGx clinic. **2.** Interprofessional team collects relevant medical history with an emphasis on information related to chief complaints, which also includes a transition of care history from primary care to the IPGx. This information is analyzed using the Clinical Semantic Network to identify complaints of possible pharmacological root cause. **3a.** When warranted, pharmacogenomic profiling is performed. **3b.** When warranted, pharmacokinetic profiling is performed. **4.** A medication management report citing complaints of potential pharmacological root causes and suggested alternative medications or adjustments to drug regimen is provided to the referring physician. **5.** If patient chooses to give informed consent, all clinical data, bioanalytic data and biological specimens are entered into a pharmacogenomic research registry (clinical-genomic database).

2.2. Medical Record Analysis and the Clinical Semantic Network

The first piece of the artificial intelligence phase in the IPGx model is an analysis of symptoms residing in electronic medical records that might be indicative of suboptimal or problematic medication regimens. The Clinical Semantic Network (Goldblatt Systems, Inc., Tucson, AZ, USA [21] is a computable medical record that enables facile analysis of symptoms and complaints imported from the Texas A&M Primary Care medical record (eClinical Works), in an HL7 clinical document architecture (CDA, see Table 1 IPGx continuity of care (CoC) data). The IPGx CoC data in the CDA Clinical Document Architecture [22] includes chief complaints such as drug side effects and symptoms, known diagnoses, and medications prescribed. This information is exported from the electronic health record into the CSN to render case specific data computable by the CSN [21].

The CSN is built on a commercial grade software that is tiered from Oracle, DOM, Hibernate, and Java. It maps relational data to a domain model. The data structure is computationally tractable and configured to enable the application of AI in terms of predictive analytics.

2.3. Bioanalytic Phase

The bioanalytic phase of the IPGx model involves interrogation of specific and actionable pharmacogenomic targets (per CPIC guidelines) and confirmation of genotype impact on the subject's steady state blood levels of medication.

2.3.1. Clinical Pharmacogenomics

SNPs identified with genomic and pharmacogenomic analyses combined with personal health and psychosocial data may be used to develop a model for prediction of disease outcome as well as an aid to physicians with clinical management [23]. The Molecular Dx pharmacogenomic (PGx) assay targets an extensive list of medications and therapeutic symptoms. For low daily volume and fast turn-around time, the MolecularDx Comprehensive PGx panel is utilized (Table 2). Primers designed to amplify specific genetic variations (SNPs, insertions, deletions, multi-nucleotide polymorphisms) in genes coding for pharmacogenes or their regulatory elements are listed in Table 2.

Table 2. Drug Classes, Potentially Impacted Drugs, and Genes Texted in the MolecularDx Pharmacogenomics Platform as of March 2021.

Drug Class	Potentially Impacted Drugs	Gene(s) Tested
ADHD	Atomoxetine, Amphetamines, Dexmethylphendiate, Dextroamphetamine, Lisdexamfetamine, Methylphendiate Clonidine, Guanfacine	CYP2D6, COMT
Alzheimer's Disease	Donepezil, Galantamine Memantine	CYP2D6
Antiarrhythmics	Donepezil, Galantamine Memantine	CYP2D6
Anticancer Agents	Methotrexate, Belinostat, Erlotinib, Gefitinib, Nilotinib, Pazopanib, Azathioprine, Mercaptopurine, Thioguanine, Irinotecan, Irinotecan Liposomal	
Antidepressants, SSRIs/SNRI	Citalopram, Escitalopram, Desvenlafaxine, Duloxetine, Mirtazapine, Paroxetine, Sertraline, Venlafaxine	CYP2D6, CYP2C19
Antidepressants, Tricyclic	Amitriptyline, Clomipramine, Desipramine, Doxepin, Imipramine, Nortriptyline, Trimipramine Amoxapine, Fluoxetine, Fluvoxamine, Levomilnacipran, Maprotiline, Nefazodone, Protriptyline, Vilazodone, Vortioxetine	CYP2C9
Antidiabetics	Glimepiride, Glipizide, Glyburide, Tolbutamide, Chlorpropamide Nateglinide, Repaglinide	CYP2C9
Antiemetics	Ondansetron, Dolasetron, Metoclopramide, Palonosetron	CYP2D6
Antiepileptic	Phenytoin, Carbamazepine, Carbatrol, Eslicarbazepine, Ethosuximide, Ezogabine, Felbamate, Fosphenytoin, Gabapentin, Lacosamide, Lamotrigine, Levetiracetam, Oxcarbazepine, Perampanel, Pregabalin, Rufinamide, Tiagabine, Topiramate, Valproic Acid, Vigabatrin, Brivaracetam, Phenobarbital, Primidone, Zonisamide	CYP2C9
Antihyperlipidemic Agents	Atorvastatin, Fluvastatin, Lovastatin, Pravastatin, Pitavastatin, Simvastatin, Rosuvastatin	SLCO1B1, CYP3A4, CYP2C9
Antihypertensives	Carvedilol, Metoprolol, Irbesartan, Nebivolol, Propranolol, Timolol, Labetalol	CYP2D6, CYP2C9
Antiplatelets/Anticoagulants	Clopidogrel, Prasugrel, Ticagrelor, Warfarin, Vorapaxar, Apixaban, Dabigatran Etexilate, Edoxaban, Fondaparinux, Rivaroxaban	CYP2C19, CYP2C9, VKORC1, CYP3A5

Table 2. Cont.

Drug Class	Potentially Impacted Drugs	Gene(s) Tested
Antipsychotics	Aripiparazole, Haloperidol, Iloperidone, Paliperidone, Perphenazine, Pimozide, Risperidone, Thioridazine, Asenapine, Brexpiprazole, Chlorpromazine, Fluphenazine, Loxapine, Lurasidone, Pimavanserin, Quetiapine, Thiothixene, Trazodone, Trifluoperazine, Ziprasidone, Clozapine, Olanzapine, TetrabenazineOther Neurological Agents: Dextromethorphan/Quinidine, Flibanserin	CYP2D6, CYP1A2
Anxiety/Insomnia	Diazepam, Clobazam, Alprazolam, Clonazepam, Lorazepam, Oxazepam	CYP2C19
Acid Related Disorders	Dexlansoprazole, Esomeprazole, Lansoprazole, Omeprazole, Pantoprazole, Rabeprazole	CYP2C19
Cardiovascular	Angiotensin II Receptor Antagonists: Azilsartan, Candesartan, Eprosartan, Irbesartan, Losartan, Olmesartan, Telmisartan, Valsartan Antianginal Agents: Ranolazine Diuretics: Torsemide	
Huntington Disease	Tetrabenazine	CYP2D6
Immunosuppressants	Tacrolimus	CYP3A5
Infections	Antifungals: Voriconazole Anti-HIV Agents: Atazanavir Antimalarials: Proguanil	
Antifugals: Voriconazole	Carisoprodol, Tizanidine, Cyclobenzaprine, Metaxalone, Methocarbamol	CYP2C19, CYP1A2
Anti-HIV Agents: Atazanavir	Methadone	CYP2B6
Antimalarials: Proguanil	Codeine, Fentanyl, Hydrocodone, Morphine, Oxycodone, Tramadol, Alfentanil, Buprenorphine, Dihydrocodeine, Hydromorphone, Levorphanol, Meperidine, Oxymorphone, Sufentanil, Tapentadol, Methadone	CYP2D6, OPRM1
Other	Bupropion, Naltrexone	COMT, OPRM1, ANKK1/DRD2
Other Analgesics	Celecoxib, Flurbiprofen, Piroxicam, Diclofenac, Ibuprofen, Indomethacin, Ketoprofen, Ketorolac, Meloxicam, Nabumetone, Naproxen, Sulindac	CYP2C9
Pain	Fibromyalgia Agents: Milnacipran	
Rheumatology	Anti-Gout Agents: AllopurinolImmunomodulators: Apremilast, Leflunomide, Tofacitinib	
Urinary Incontinence	Antispasmodics: Tolterodine, Darifenacin, Fesoterodine, Mirabegron, Oxybutynin, Solifenacin, Trospium 5-Alpha Reductase Inhibitors: Dutasteride, Finasteride Alpha Blockers: Alfuzosin, Doxazosin, Silodosin, Tamsulosin, Terazosin Phosphodiesterase Inhibitors for Erectile Dysfunction: Avanafil, Sildenafil, Tadalafil, Vardenafil	CYP2D6

This technology uses TaqMan Genotyping Assays [24] to target 90 PGx-related SNPs plus CYP2D6 copy number. Genotyping is performed on the Applied Biosystems QuantStudio 12K Flex. For higher daily volume and lax turn-around time, a custom-designed SARS-CoV-2 research diversity array can be utilized. Whole blood with no centrifugation is extracted using QIAamp DNA Blood Mini Kit (Cat. # 51106) used on QiaCube. TaqMan Genotyper v1.6 software was used to make genotype calls. Calls are manually reviewed by two pharmacists with pharmacogenomic expertise and agreed upon before reporting.

2.3.2. Clinical Pharmacokinetics

Candidate pharmacologic symptoms coupled with genotypes that portend drug–drug and drug–gene interactions can be further validated by the measurement of steady state blood concentrations of the medications of interest. Under the IPGx protocol, target drugs corresponding to the drug–gene pairs in Table 2 and their metabolites are measured utilizing a validated liquid chromatography mass spectrometry assay. Such results were not entered into the virtual exercise presented in this report, but are available for use in clinical practice.

2.4. Synthesis and Reporting

The CSN deconstructs and enhances a medication identification procedure utilizing the medication's molecular weight, excretion pathways, ATC class, volume of distribution, bioavailability, elimination half-life, anticholinergic burden, steady state, and CYP_{450}, or transporter pathways. In this light, the CSN enabled the development of a polypharmacy report that can be utilized by a clinician at point of care to get a holistic, yet cogent snapshot of symptoms, complaints, diagnoses, and medications that might reflect drug–drug and drug–gene interactions. This function generates a medication management summary report that identifies high probability and actionability per CPIC guidelines of drug–gene and drug–drug interactions at the root cause for select symptoms. These relationships can ideally be confirmed by genotyping and/or clinical pharmacokinetic assays.

3. Results

3.1. Clinical Environment and Process

Polypharmacy patients and patients demonstrating symptoms and complaints that might be indicative of possible medication interactions are referred to the IPGx clinic for evaluation by the attending clinician (Figure 1, step 1). Patients are not required to consent to the registry to receive the bioanalytic workup and medication management care; registry participation is optional and not a condition of care. The program entails a process of stepwise progression of electronic medical record analysis toward pharmacokinetic ground truth to inform primary care practitioners. The first step consists of a clinically aware computational analysis such that entry of complaints into the patient's record, updates the rendering of complaints that match the known side effects (from First Data Bank) of drugs taken by the patient. The second step strengthens these associations if a pharmacokinetic model of the medications renders potential instances of pathway overload (Epocrates). Next, the CSN can further strengthen these associations by identification of pharmacogene variants of known clinical significance that are consistent with the list of candidate side-effects or pathway overload. Finally, pharmacokinetic data is incorporated to distinguish among and validate instances of drug–gene or drug–drug interactions.

3.2. Medical Record Analysis and the Clinical Semantic Network

The first step is a computational and semantic comparison of case history to the medications the patient is taking. This is powered by DrugBank [25], Epocrates [26], and Lexicomp [27] to tally the subset of symptoms that are present and known to occur as side effects of the medications the patient is taking. At a clinical informatics level, cough with fever might be connected/mapped to curated ontologies such as SNOMED (Systematized Nomenclature of Medicine [28]) about SARS-CoV-2, or pneumonia in a weighted fashion, by subject matter experts who then have the capability to markedly enhance this highly navigable information. A net result is that a SNOMED identification can be established with multiple attributes built into the CSN system. Other analogies in the CSN include instances when a chief complaint is entered such that the system knows which history of present illness questions should be used to interrogate. The technology works much in the same manner as Google can predict shopping preferences based on user actions.

For the purposes of this communication, we created a virtual patient with medication, pharmacogenomic, and side effect profiles that were aggregated drawing from previous experiences with a number of real-life clinical cases. The clinical characteristics assessed included:

- Number of side effects/complaints/diagnoses identified in the patient and believed to be related to his/her current medication regimen,
- Number of medications possibly contributing to the identified/diagnosed side effects,
- Number of drug metabolic pathways identified as being potentially overloaded,
- Number of drug metabolic pathways identified as borderline overloaded,
- Number of medications with pharmacogenomic profiles,
- Number of medications putting the patient at risk for serotonin syndrome,
- Number of medications putting the patient at risk for QT prolongation,
- Number of anticholinergic medications.

At this step, a side-effects dashboard is created by the CSN utilizing any drug in the First Databank to distill complaints that could be of pharmacological origin. Figure 2 provides a summary of selected computational clinical findings for the virtual patient which are also a rendering of the complaints from Table 1, that correspond to the subset of complaints that are also known side effects of the medications the patient is taking. Those side effects, as initially rendered prior to pharmacogenomic profiling, may not inherently be of pharmacological origin, or may arise due to drug–drug interactions, or as a result of drug–gene interactions. Pharmacogenomic testing and pharmacokinetic testing can reveal whether these complaints are rooted in drug–gene or drug–drug interactions. The CSN can be contrasted from step-and-fetch functionality of most electronic medical records by the interconnectivity of medical terms. Those medical terms are connected in a neural-like network of semantic associations that effectively represent knowledge and contextual awareness of potentially related data elements in a patient record. The network consists of nodes representing objects and arcs which describe the relationship between those objects. Semantic networks can categorize the objects in various forms and can link those objects making it particularly useful in an electronic health record which can utilize and act on computable data. Interconnecting a patient's clinical content (phenotypes) with this form of health care knowledge gives the data in these relationships actionable context. There is a pharmacokinetic modeling dimension in this analysis that examines the repertoire of medications a patient has been prescribed and that models these data based on known pathways for those medications to assess drug–drug interactions that might result from pathways that are excessively taxed by virtue of the combination of medications (Figure 3).

This dashboard can incorporate correlative associations (complaints-drug side effects) and bioanalytic associations (PGx genotypes and predicted or measured pharmacokinetic). As such, this computationally rendered dashboard provides useful insight on the potential root cause of complaints both before and after bioanalytic analysis is entered into the CSN case record.

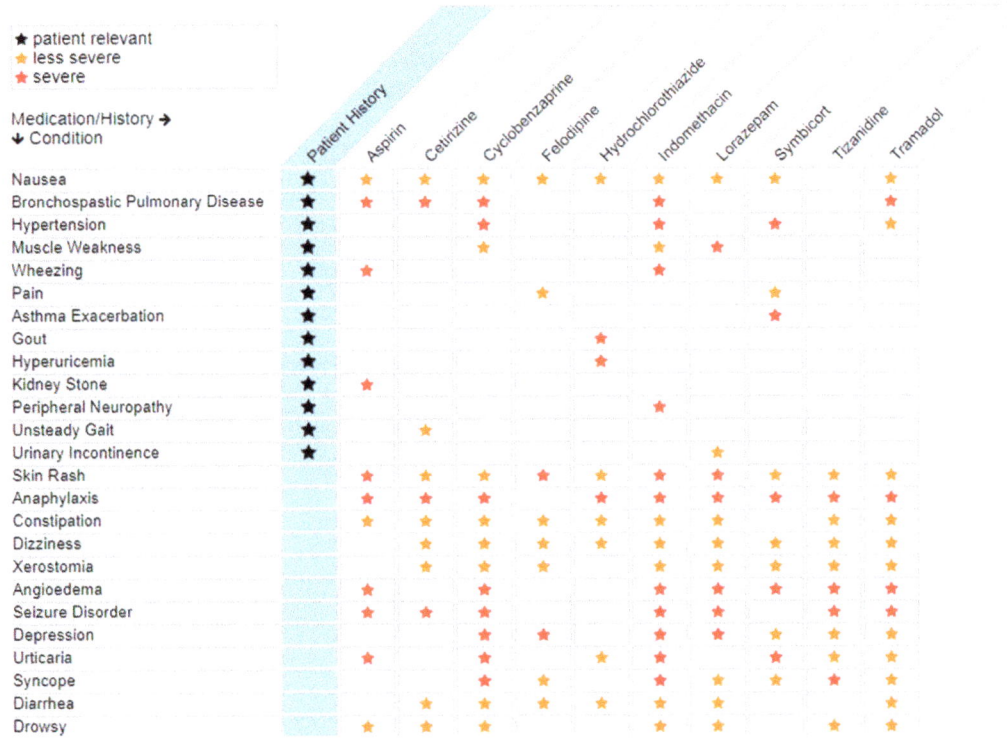

Figure 2. Side Effects Dashboard. List of symptoms indicating potential pharmacological origin.

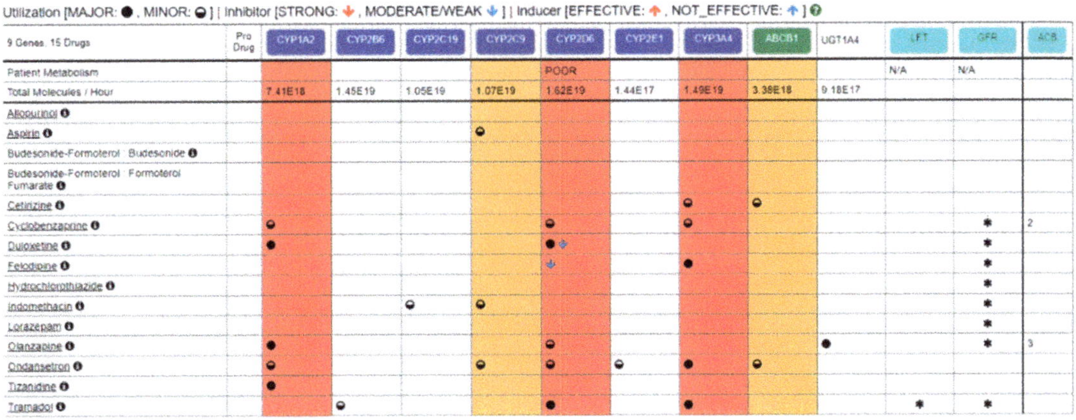

Figure 3. *Cont.*

↓ - Drug moderately inhibits the CYP or transport enzyme.
↑ - Drug moderately induces the CYP or transport enzyme.
⬇ - Drug strongly inhibits the CYP or transport enzyme Ki> 1
⬆ - Drug strongly induces the CYP or transport enzyme.
◐ - Drug is metabolized on CYP or transport enzyme.
● - Drug CYP or transport enzyme is a major metabolizer above 30%.
✱ - Denotes an occurrence.

Poor - patient is a poor metabolizer due to variant for CYP or transport enzyme
INT - patient is intermediate metabolizer due to variant for CYP or transport enzyme
ULT - patient is ultra-rapid metabolizer due to variant for CYP or transport enzyme
EXT - patient Extensive metabolizer due to variant for CYP or transport enzyme

Pro drug - a compound that, on administration, must undergo chemical conversion by metabolic processes before becoming an active pharmacological agent; a precursor of a drug. Any of various drugs that are administered in an inactive form and converted into active form by normal metabolic processes.

Key

CYP/Trans Column Yellow
- Two drugs with moderate or above utilization CYP or transport enzyme
- Patient is an intermediate metabolizer of CYP

CYP/Trans Column Orange
- Three or more drugs with moderate or above utilization CYP or transport enzyme
- Patient is an extensive or ultra-rapid metabolizer of CYP

Cyp/Trans Column Red
- Four or more drugs with moderate or above utilization CYP or transport enzyme
- Patient is a poor metabolizer of CYP or transport enzyme variant that impedes the enzyme

GFR Yellow - patient's last glomerular filtration rate value < 55
GFR Orange - patient's last glomerular filtration rate value < 44
GFR Red - patient's last glomerular filtration rate value < 30
LFT Yellow - patient's last Alanine Aminotransferase > 60
LFT Orange - orange patient's last Alanine Aminotransferase > 180
LFT Red - last Alanine Aminotransferase > 240

Figure 3. Medication and Pharmacokinetic Pathway Summary. The green rectangles are a few salient transporters, and the light blue box represents anticholinergic burden. The left most vertical column denotes the patient's medications. Vertically, the column beneath named alleles in red indicates that the respective pathway could be overloaded. Panel B Key.

3.3. Bioanalytics

Pharmacogenomics is used to assess the impact of individual pharmacogenomic variants on how subjects respond to their medication by evaluating specific medication receptor targets as well as transporter functionality [29]. The dashboard design incorporates Clinical Pharmacogenetics Implementation Consortium (CPIC) guidelines and the knowledgebases contained in PharmGKB and PharmVar to provide a cogent front-end presentation of case-relevant and actionable pharmacologic considerations for use by the clinician at point-of-care. The report reflects a comprehensive analysis of known pharmacogenomic knowledge through the filter of established consensus medical guidelines. For illustrative purposes, Table 3 presents a list of CYP2D6 haplotypes that the CSN is configured to dynamically incorporate into the rendering of the pharmacogenomic analysis. The CSN is capable of incorporating all variants of known clinical significance. The patient scope varies and is dynamically adjusted to the variants that are presented by the instrumentation. The CYP2D6 haplotype call is made from the core variants for each haplotype and all other variants are verified as constant relative to that haplotype so variants of unknown significance are not presented as normal.

Table 3. List of CYP2D6 alleles incorporated into the rendering of the Medication and Pharmacokinetic Pathway Summary in Figure 3.

CYP2D6 Haplotypes
* 2, * 3, * 4, * 5, * 6, * 7, * 8, * 9, * 10, * 11, * 12, * 14, * 15, * 17, * 19, * 20, * 21, * 22, * 23, * 24, * 25, * 27, * 28, * 29, * 30, * 31, * 32, * 33, * 34, * 35, * 36, * 37, * 38, * 39, * 40, * 41, * 42, * 43, * 44, * 45, * 46, * 47, * 48, * 49, * 50, * 51, * 52, * 53, * 54, * 55, , * 56, * 57, * 58, * 59, * 60, * 62, * 64, * 65, * 69, * 70, * 71, * 72, * 73, * 74, * 75, * 81, * 82, * 83, * 84, * 85, * 86, * 87, * 88, * 89, * 90, * 91, * 94, * 95, * 96, * 98, * 99, * 100, * 101, * 102, * 103, * 104, * 105, * 106, * 107, * 108, * 109, * 110, * 111, * 112, * 113, * 114, * 115, * 116, * 117, * 118, * 119, * 121, * 122, * 123, * 125, * 126, * 127, * 128, * 129, , * 130, * 131,* 132, * 133, * 134, * 135, * 136, * 137, * 138, * 139

*: alleles.

3.4. Virtual Patient A

Patient A is a 60-year-old African American female with a ten-year history of depression, schizophrenia, and chronic pain who is referred to the IPGx Clinic by her primary care physician for a polypharmacy consult. She began complaining of worsening shifts in her mood and increasing feelings of worthlessness and sadness for the past six-months. She stated that there have been to changes in her family life and that her work shifts had ended a year before. She lives with her husband of 30 years and has two pets. The patient stated that she does not understand why she feels sad all of the time and unable to enjoy life the way she used to after her depression, schizophrenia, and pain had been so well controlled with medications. She stated that her family commented that she is more "irritable" and "angry all the time". Upon further questioning, she noted that her physician had been making adjustments to her medications and prescribed cyclobenzaprine for rigidity and duloxetine for the worsening feelings of depression six months ago. She denies having any other medical problems at this time and any known allergies to medications. The patient reports taking duloxetine, tramadol, ondansetron, cyclobenzaprine, and olanzapine as prescribed, and denies using over the counter medications, herbal supplements, or illicit drugs. Her vital signs were all within normal limits and her physical examination was unremarkable. The patient consents to pharmacogenomic and pharmacokinetic testing and opts to join the pharmacogenomics registry. A blood sample is drawn and buccal swabs are collected for analysis. The patient returns to clinic after one month for follow up and discussion of findings. The results of the metabolic panel and blood cell counts were unremarkable. Pharmacogenomic testing is conducted and shows that the patient is a poor CYP2D6 metabolizer. Figure 2 presents screenshot depictions of side-effects—a listing of patient reported symptoms and complaints attributed to potential pharmacological root causes (denoted by black stars) compared to known side effects of the medications the patient has been prescribed (denoted by red and yellow stars, for moderate and severe side effects, respectively).

4. Discussion

4.1. Integration with Primary Care

The IPGx program has leveraged health care policy mandates calling for health data standardization protocols [30]. The transitioning of the IPGx CoC data set (Table 1) into the CSN is somewhat amenable to HL7 continuity of care data CDA formats. These data can be output in a readily computable format from most medical records, and have proven to be tractable and scalable in the IPGx model. The side effects table (Figure 2) for composite clinic case represented by patient A were compiled from a medical history, in the form of a CDA, composed of data enumerated in Table 1 that were extracted from a primary care electronic medical record (eClinical Works) from which patients are being referred for an ongoing pilot project digitally linking the IPGx with primary care. Future work will examine and confirm the utility of using CoC HL7 CDAs using data from other providers and health systems that refer patients to the IPGx clinic. Most current electronic medical record vendors will have standard capability to produce a CoC CDA similar or identical to the one used here. The return of results and medication management recommendations to primary care are a work-in-progress and currently presented in the form of a PDF report that can be appended to the electronic medical record at the referring primary care clinic. However, the CSN retains "clinical awareness" meaning that the semantic linkage between relevant threads in phenotypes->(complaints->potential side-effects)->genotypes->pharmacokinetic ground truth for a given patient are not lost. One existing constraint is that this functionality and the underlying data structures are unique to the CSN and not readily transferrable to any know electronic medical record beyond standard SNOWMED nomenclatures.

A current challenge in primary care environments with populations of polypharmacy and polydisease burden is managing the increased complexity of medication repertoires and standards of care that do not account for this emergent complexity. Some medical records have alerts for potential drug–drug interactions, but none of these computational tools are linked to what the patient is actually experiencing, and as such, they do little to distinguish among complaints caused by disease versus those potentially caused by medications. The status quo leaves the primary care with a dearth of tools to respond to these noisy considerations in an environment with personalized and precision strategies increasingly necessary to avoid ADRs.

4.2. Medical Record Analysis and the Clinical Semantic Network

Nausea and depression are symptoms and complaints that the CSN identified in the side effects table as potentially having a pharmacological root cause (Figure 2). The side effects table provides an emerging view of phenotypes that may have a pharmacologic root cause, based on First Data Bank side effects, and warrant further pharmacogenomic and pharmacokinetic analysis of a patient and their case. The combination of worsening symptoms and new medications in Patient's A dashboard suggests that these symptoms may result from overburdening of the CYP2D6 pathway, an oxidative drug metabolizing pathway utilized by 25% of medications, and a common nexus for ADRs in polypharmacy [31,32]. This assessment is consistent with the finding that many of the medications taken by Patient A (duloxetine, tramadol, ondansetron, cyclobenzaprine, and olanzapine) interact with the CYP2D6 metabolic pathway. Duloxetine is a recognized inhibitor of CYP2D6, thus potentially increasing circulating drug levels for agents such as tramadol that are metabolized by this pathway. Duloxetine, olanzapine, cyclobenzaprine, and ondansetron are also utilizers of CYP1A2, and may be collectively contributing to overload of this metabolic pathway (refer to Figure 3). Several of these agents also utilize the CYP3A2 and CYP3A4 pathways, thus compounding the level of taxation of several alternative oxidative metabolism pathways. In the top left header bar of Figure 3, the dashboard indicates there are 15 drugs, corresponding to 10 genes/pathways of interest in this patient's medication regimen and that two alternatives to ondansetron (granisetron, palonosetron) should be considered to offload CYP metabolic pathways and possibly improve the patient's symptoms and optimize response to drug therapy.

Electronic health record alerts, computerized order entry systems, and pharmaceutical box warnings are insufficient in helping physicians at point of care to identify critical drug–drug or drug–gene interactions that might result from polypharmacy [31]. In this case, CYP1A2, CYP2D6, and CYP3A4 may be overburdened (Figure 3) and perhaps overloaded to a point of significant clinical consequence. In this patient's case, the inclusion of drug–drug interactions in the assessment is complicated by a pre-existing history of dementia and chronic pain, disorders that can themselves present with symptoms of depression. We recognize that ordering a pharmacogenomic test is currently not within established clinical guidelines at this time. In fact, our research registry was established in order to generate clinically relevant evidence to support expanded use of pharmacogenomic testing in chronic disease management and polypharmacy. Again, the medical record analysis is simply an exercise in computational filtering of the symptoms with potential pharmacologic origins from the broader noise contained within the medical and complaint history—a tool that is likely useful in primary care even without deployment of a downstream bioanalytic program.

4.3. Bioanalytics

Patient A was designated as a poor metabolizer variant of CYP2D6 into the CSN to establish the utility of layering genotype information onto the pathway analysis dashboard and to incorporate this information in triangulating symptoms with pharmacological root cause to generate medication alternatives. A recent analysis of CYP2D6 genotypes in an Austrian population evaluated in a family practice setting revealed that the metabolizer status of patients taking medications metabolized by CYP2D6 [32] would be clinically actionable in 16% of cases. A 2016 report by Bush et al. focused on variation in 82 pharmacogenes in a cohort of 5000 clinical subjects, and CYP2D6 was identified among the most polymorphic gene present [15]. In their study, over 96% of subjects had one or more CPIC Level A actionable variant identified and more than a third had three or more actionable variants, suggesting that these variations may influence the clinical care of affected patients over their lifetime. In a similar study, Van Driest et al. [16] reported that the number of CYP2D6 variants is highest among African-Americans [15], as seen in Patient A. Accordingly, implementation of our informatic and bioanalytic platform would place critical information at the fingertips of primary care and ambulatory care pharmacy providers. Under the working premise of our virtual case, genotyping confirmed that Patient A had a CYP2D6* 17 variant of CYP2D6 that made her a poor metabolizer. To gain further insight and to validate the functional significance of the findings, a pharmacokinetic assay of CYP2D6 metabolized medications would be ordered to hyperlink steady state levels in the dashboard under the black circle with the letter "i" next to the drug name in the pathway analysis dashboard (Figure 3). This would be done to establish with certainty if the patient has elevated steady state levels of duloxetine and tramadol that not only overload CYP pathways, but may also be material contributors to the chief complaint profile and polypharmacy burden for the virtual patient.

Patient A is taking five medications that utilize a low functioning variant of CYP2D6: duloxetine, tramadol, ondansetron, cyclobenzaprine, and olanzapine. Virtual Patient A notes depression, which could be attributable to several medications this patient is using, including cyclobenzaprine and tramadol. Cyclobenzaprine, a medication that creates a high anticholinergic burden, can exacerbate depression, and could be contributing to CYP1A2, CYP2D6, and CYP3A4 overload. This medication is at the nexus of many of the issues confronting this patient and warrants consideration for alternative medications or supervised deprescribing. If nausea is persistent in the face of a CYP2D6 poor metabolizer with an already overloaded pathway, the system informs the clinician to consider to replace ondansetron with granisetron which lowers metabolic burden at CYP2D6.

This patient has an anticholinergic burden (ACB) score of 5, which is high [33] and could be contributing to adverse effects. Of note is the fact that ondansetron, tramadol, and duloxetine add serotonergic stress and the potential for QT prolongation in our virtual patient. In this instance, the dashboard was further annotated with predicted phenotypes associated with a known actionable variant of CYP2D6 (CYP2D6* 17) that is a poor metabolizer (Figure 3; pursuant to CPIC guidelines). This would augment a genotype annotated and refined computational rendering of a list of side effects with a likely pharmacological root cause. The decision support would identify tizanidine as a potentially less problematic alternative to cyclobenzaprine, or even deprescribing cyclobenzaprine and monitoring the patient. Further, the medications pathway dashboard identifies ondansetron as another potential contributor to CYP2D6 overload (but not depression directly per se) Another therapeutic option that emerges from this case is reconsidering tramadol. Tramadol is metabolized at CYP2D6. It can interact with duloxetine from a drug–drug interaction perspective. Tramadol can induce nausea. If it is clinically determined that Tramadol is required for pain management then a blood drug level is recommended to optimize dosage. If not, tapering and seeking an alternative is reasonable. In this case, stiff person syndrome is in the differential diagnosis due to the burdened serotonin system. In this case, the CSN identifies and presents complaints (depression) that might have pharmacologic root cause (serotonergic burden) likely due to a CYP2D6 variant rendering the patient a poor metabolizer of ondansetron and cyclobenzaprine. In our virtual case, drug–drug–gene interactions were identified electronically from historical clinical data and confirmed with a bioanalytic workup. Specific recommendations for alternative medications included in the final report may help resolve an otherwise disorderly and noisy interplay of polypharmacy, genetic variation, and history of present illness.

5. Conclusions

5.1. Challenges and Realities

The most obvious challenge with clinical roll-out of the IPGx model is that most of the bioanalytic methodologies described herein are not currently reimbursed by payers and disappointingly, out of reach for most primary care practices. The triggers for genotyping the patients in our test case were rather compelling cases with symptomatology that could with relative ease be attributed to pharmacological root causes: CYP2D6 overload, ACB, and drug–drug and drug–gene interactions. However, this practice is not currently a reimbursable use case for ordering pharmacogenomic testing or clinical pharmacokinetic assays. As such, the methodology described is currently impractical for implementation across the healthcare system due to reimbursement constraints for nearly all private and Medicare insurance policies. The IPGx registry program provides a strategy to measure the positive impact of medication management to deconvolute chronic disease and polypharmacy burdens in a clinically actionable manner and provide evidence of the value-based approach.

Haga and colleagues have published rich commentary [34–36], and some primary research, on clinical outcomes in populations in which pharmacogenomic testing has been implemented. The chicken-and-egg paradox to further outcomes research is the dearth of patients for whom pharmacogenomic testing is ordered because of a limited reimbursement landscape [37], and the data linkage challenges posed by efforts to document the public health impact of medication choices. Inherently, genotyping will likely continue to be viewed as having questionable clinical utility absent the grounding provided by measurements of actual drug levels and the clinical actionability that can be inferred when combining genotyping and patient chief complaints.

The evidence versus usage paradox described is the underlying rationale for creation of our IPGx registry. The goal is to collect evidence that these bioanalytic methods are cost effective and can improve outcomes in cases where chronic disease burden and polypharmacy are detrimental to health. Grant funding is often a key component of expanded pharmacogenomic testing beyond the narrow scope provided by the healthcare system in the US. The Vanderbilt University [18] and Duke University Health Systems [38] have robust, interprofessional clinical pharmacogenomic programs, but it is unclear the degree to which access to unreimbursed bioanalytical technology constrains the scope and scale of their efforts to study pharmacogenomic testing at scale, in a clinical setting.

5.2. Significance to ADRs

It has been reported that about 2/3 of ADRs are attributable to drug–drug interactions and about 1/3 to drug–gene interactions [39], so a diagnostic battery would ideally inform both of these endpoints. Indeed, the CSN medical record analysis process enables identification of clinically relevant, and inherently actionable, elevated drug levels and/or clinically relevant pharmacogenomic variants. The final medication management report produced by the CSN can reflect suspected medication effects, and provide grounding for both drug–drug and drug–gene interactions. In complex cases, the final report is refined by IPGx clinical staff through an interprofessional consultation among clinical pharmacists, the attending genomic medicine specialist, and the primary care physician to produce a report listing medication management considerations for the referring physician. Such recommendations might include alternative medications to reduce anticholinergic burden or load on specific cytochrome P450 pathways, or deprescribing. In essence, the IPGx platform distills vast electronic health record, genotype, and pharmacokinetic information into an informed, understandable, and actionable set of medication management considerations.

The workflows and reporting for the IPGx and the interface between IPGx and primary care were thoughtfully constructed. Disruptions of workflows or additional work can be a nonstarter for research in a primary care environment and the same holds true for piloting new care models. The upshot of the IPGx platform is that (1) the medical informatic analysis can reveal potential ADR signals in standard continuity of care information sets using the Clinical Semantic Network at the front end, and (2) can be complemented with the bioanalytical analysis from that patients' pharmacogenomic and clinical pharmacokinetic workup, at the back end of the IPGx encounter. The IPGx model can serve as a force multiplier for the primary care physician in managing their most complex cases driving healthcare utilization by "de-noising" dense medical histories and complementing the analysis with bioanalytic ground truth, to provide cogent actionable data to inform prescribing choices.

5.3. Bioanalytics and Future Directions

The IPGx registry has the potential to enroll individuals who possess variants of unknown significance and novel variants. The significant clinical annotation (phenotype) that accompanies each registry record is likely to provide insights on structure–function relationships inherent in emergent variants. Additionally, over time, accumulation of a meaningful number of cases with a given novel variant has utility as a de facto cohort for future research. In fact, we expect that the IPGx registry will be a channel to recruit subjects for future research looking into the nexus of chronic disease management, pharmacogenomics, and public health; to demonstrate the value of personalized medicine approaches on public health outcomes.

The genotyping profiles and informatics in the CSN are amenable to addition of HLA insigh, a functionality that is being considered for integration into the IPGx care model and the IPGx registry in the future. This addition has great potential to inform the clinical significance of emergent HLA variants.

Oncology is a specialty from which the care of a referred population might be augmented by the IPGx model. The primary care environment utilized for the present report is not a practical context in which to develop the IPGx care platform for oncology care. A number of complementary diagnostic and drug safety paradigms for cancer therapy will be the basis for future work.

5.4. Opportunities

Most pharmacogenomic testing finds its way into clinical practice in a bottom-up pathway, meaning that an individual variant (genotype) or drug–gene pair is implicated in an ADR (phenotype) that is observed in the population. At that time, clinical outcomes associated with testing use cases and interventions (i.e., CYP2C19 for clopidogrel) with respect to that variant must be studied in randomized controlled trials before a recommendation for clinical testing is adopted. This approach has proven to be challenging, even for one of the most advanced areas of pharmacogenomic testing, anticoagulant therapy [40]. It takes time for the justification (pilot studies of ancillary studies piggybacked on drug registration trials) to reach a critical threshold calling for a randomized controlled trial that might ultimately demonstrate the clinical utility of testing for a given drug–gene pair. The standard innovation pathway for a pharmacogenomic use case for a drug–gene pair, can take many years for an emergent drug–gene pair to achieve reimbursement and even longer for clinical adoption [41]. The lack of a large scale clinical-genomic databases to link genotypes and drug dispensing data with outcomes is recognized as a challenge in further advancing the field of pharmacogenomics [8]. By expanding the diversity of disease and populations receiving pharmacogenomic testing beyond those fitting in narrow, existing reimbursement paradigms, the IPGx platform has the potential to produce outcome evidence for emergent drug–gene pairs and clinical use cases for pharmacogenomic testing that is supported by phenotype outcomes before (i.e., complaints in the electronic health record) and after testing (steady-state drug levels). Use of the IPGx methodology presented here would allow clinicians to make inferences from symptoms and genotyping that are in turn informed by the grounding of clinical pharmacokinetic data. This approach may provide useful insights into potential phenoconversion, a limiting challenge in relying on pharmacogenetic testing alone for clinical decision-making [42]. The clinical-genomic database of the IPGx can become a resource to inform the clinical decision making of the referring physician, and accelerate guideline maturation cycles for emergent gene–drug pairs. In the IPGx program, the informed consent and data strategy enable a simplified portrayal of bioanalytic validation of symptoms and complaints that have a pharmacologic root cause. As such, the approach is practical and actionable for a primary care provider. At the same time, the process generates a rich corpus of longitudinally integrated biological, genomic, and clinical information that is highly valuable for supporting research, practice improvement, policy, and reimbursement.

Author Contributions: Conceptualization, K.R., P.S. and D.J.; methodology, K.R., D.J. and J.K.; software, D.J. and J.K.; validation, D.J., G.N., J.K., G.U., A.A.-B. and K.R.; formal analysis, D.J. and J.K.; investigation, D.J., J.K. and G.N.; resources, K.R., D.J.; data curation, D.J., J.K., P.S.; writing—original draft preparation, P.S. and K.R.; writing—review and editing, P.S., D.J., G.U., A.A.-B., G.N., J.K. and K.R.; visualization, D.J., J.K. and P.S.; supervision, K.R.; project administration, P.S., D.J.; funding acquisition, K.R. All authors have read and agreed to the published version of the manuscript.

Funding: This research received no external funding.

Institutional Review Board Statement: Not applicable.

Informed Consent Statement: Not applicable.

Data Availability Statement: Not applicable.

Acknowledgments: The authors wish to acknowledge the contributions of Jesus Palomo in manuscript editing and preparation.

Conflicts of Interest: The authors declare no conflict of interest. The funders had no role in the design of the study; in the collection, analyses, or interpretation of data; in the writing of the manuscript, or in the decision to publish the results.

References

1. Masnoon, N.; Shakib, S.; Kalisch-Ellett, L.; Caughey, G.E. What is polypharmacy? A systematic review of definitions. *BMC Geriatr.* **2017**, *17*, 230. [CrossRef]
2. Hripcsak, G.; Ryan, P.B.; Duke, J.D.; Shah, N.H.; Park, R.W.; Huser, V.; Suchard, M.A.; Schuemie, M.J.; DeFalco, F.J.; Perotte, A.; et al. Characterizing treatment pathways at scale using the OHDSI network. *Proc. Natl. Acad. Sci. USA* **2016**, *113*, 7329. [CrossRef]
3. Quinn, K.J.; Shah, N.H. A dataset quantifying polypharmacy in the United States. *Sci. Data* **2017**, *4*, 170167. [CrossRef]
4. Akazawa, M.; Imai, H.; Igarashi, A.; Tsutani, K. Potentially inappropriate medication use in elderly Japanese patients. *Am. J. Geriatr. Pharmacother.* **2010**, *8*, 146–160. [CrossRef]
5. Maher, R.L.; Hanlon, J.; Hajjar, E.R. Clinical consequences of polypharmacy in elderly. *Expert Opin. Drug Saf.* **2014**, *13*, 57–65. [CrossRef]
6. Mallet, L.; Spinewine, A.; Huang, A. The challenge of managing drug interactions in elderly people. *Lancet* **2007**, *370*, 185–191. [CrossRef]
7. Jennings, E.L.M.; Murphy, K.D.; Gallagher, P.; O'Mahony, D. In-hospital adverse drug reactions in older adults; prevalence, presentation and associated drugs—a systematic review and meta-analysis. *Age Ageing* **2020**, *49*, 948–958. [CrossRef] [PubMed]
8. Bahar, M.A.; Lanting, P.; Bos, J.H.J.; Sijmons, R.H.; Hak, E.; Wilffert, B. Impact of Drug-Gene-Interaction, Drug-Drug-Interaction, and Drug-Drug-Gene-Interaction on (es)Citalopram Therapy: The PharmLines Initiative. *J. Pers. Med.* **2020**, *10*, 256. [CrossRef]
9. Ingelman-Sundberg, M. Genetic variability in susceptibility and response to toxicants. *Toxicol. Lett.* **2001**, *120*, 259–268. [CrossRef]
10. Lazarou, J.; Pomeranz, B.H.; Corey, P.N. Incidence of adverse drug reactions in hospitalized patients: A meta-analysis of prospective studies. *JAMA* **1998**, *279*, 1200–1205. [CrossRef] [PubMed]

11. Relling, M.V.; Klein, T.E. CPIC: Clinical Pharmacogenetics Implementation Consortium of the Pharmacogenomics Research Network. *Clin. Pharmacol. Ther.* **2011**, *89*, 464–467. [CrossRef]
12. Caudle, K.E.; Klein, T.E.; Hoffman, J.M.; Muller, D.J.; Whirl-Carrillo, M.; Gong, L.; McDonagh, E.M.; Sangkuhl, K.; Thorn, C.F.; Schwab, M.; et al. Incorporation of pharmacogenomics into routine clinical practice: The Clinical Pharmacogenetics Implementation Consortium (CPIC) guideline development process. *Curr. Drug Metab.* **2014**, *15*, 209–217. [CrossRef] [PubMed]
13. Whirl-Carrillo, M.; McDonagh, E.M.; Hebert, J.M.; Gong, L.; Sangkuhl, K.; Thorn, C.F.; Altman, R.B.; Klein, T.E. Pharmacogenomics knowledge for personalized medicine. *Clin. Pharmacol. Ther.* **2012**, *92*, 414–417. [CrossRef]
14. Gordon, A.S.; Fulton, R.S.; Qin, X.; Mardis, E.R.; Nickerson, D.A.; Scherer, S. PGRNseq: A targeted capture sequencing panel for pharmacogenetic research and implementation. *Pharm. Genom.* **2016**, *26*, 161–168. [CrossRef]
15. Bush, W.S.; Crosslin, D.R.; Owusu-Obeng, A.; Wallace, J.; Almoguera, B.; Basford, M.A.; Bielinski, S.J.; Carrell, D.S.; Connolly, J.J.; Crawford, D.; et al. Genetic variation among 82 pharmacogenes: The PGRNseq data from the eMERGE network. *Clin. Pharm. Ther.* **2016**, *100*, 160–169. [CrossRef]
16. Van Driest, S.L.; Shi, Y.; Bowton, E.A.; Schildcrout, J.S.; Peterson, J.F.; Pulley, J.; Denny, J.C.; Roden, D.M. Clinically actionable genotypes among 10,000 patients with preemptive pharmacogenomic testing. *Clin. Pharm. Ther.* **2014**, *95*, 423–431. [CrossRef] [PubMed]
17. Khezrian, M.; McNeil, C.J.; Murray, A.D.; Myint, P.K. An overview of prevalence, determinants and health outcomes of polypharmacy. *Ther. Adv. Drug Saf.* **2020**, *11*, 2042098620933741. [CrossRef]
18. Pulley, J.M.; Denny, J.C.; Peterson, J.F.; Bernard, G.R.; Vnencak-Jones, C.L.; Ramirez, A.H.; Delaney, J.T.; Bowton, E.; Brothers, K.; Johnson, K.; et al. Operational Implementation of Prospective Genotyping for Personalized Medicine: The Design of the Vanderbilt PREDICT Project. *Clin. Pharmacol. Ther.* **2012**, *92*, 87–95. [CrossRef] [PubMed]
19. Roosan, D.; Hwang, A.; Roosan, M.R. Pharmacogenomics cascade testing (PhaCT): A novel approach for preemptive pharmacogenomics testing to optimize medication therapy. *Pharm. J.* **2021**, *21*, 1–7. [CrossRef]
20. Shastry, B.S. SNPs in disease gene mapping, medicinal drug development and evolution. *J. Hum. Genet.* **2007**, *52*, 871–880. [CrossRef] [PubMed]
21. Rahman, F.G.S.; Boyd, I.; Kriak, J.; Meyer, R.; Boyd, S. AI Based Health Signals Discovery Engine. In Proceedings of the SNOMED CT Expo, Kuala Lampur, Malaysia, 31 October–1 November 2019.
22. Dolin, R.H.; Alschuler, L.; Beebe, C.; Biron, P.V.; Boyer, S.L.; Essin, D.; Kimber, E.; Lincoln, T.; Mattison, J.E. The HL7 Clinical Document Architecture. *J. Am. Med. Inf. Assoc.* **2001**, *8*, 552–569. [CrossRef] [PubMed]
23. Brown-Johnson, C.G.; Safaeinili, N.; Baratta, J.; Palaniappan, L.; Mahoney, M.; Rosas, L.G.; Winget, M. Implementation outcomes of Humanwide: Integrated precision health in team-based family practice primary care. *BMC Fam. Pract.* **2021**, *22*, 28. [CrossRef] [PubMed]
24. TaqMan SNP Genotyping Assays. Available online: https://www.thermofisher.com/document-connect/document-connect.html?url=https%3A%2F%2Fassets.thermofisher.com%2FTFS-Assets%2FLSG%2Fmanuals%2Fcms_040597.pdf&title=VGFxTWFuJnJlZzsgU05QIEdlbm90eXBpbmcgQXNzYXlz (accessed on 20 May 2021).
25. Chang, H.W.; Chuang, L.Y.; Tsai, M.T.; Yang, C.H. The importance of integrating SNP and cheminformatics resources to pharmacogenomics. *Curr. Drug Metab.* **2012**, *13*, 991–999. [CrossRef]
26. McConachie, S.M.; Volgyi, D.; Moore, H.; Giuliano, C.A. Evaluation of adverse drug reaction formatting in drug information databases. *J. Med. Libr. Assoc.* **2020**, *108*, 598–604. [CrossRef]
27. Elovic, A.; Pourmand, A. Lexicomp App Review. *J. Digit. Imaging* **2020**, *33*, 17–20. [CrossRef] [PubMed]
28. Wang, Y.; Halper, M.; Wei, D.; Gu, H.; Perl, Y.; Xu, J.; Elhanan, G.; Chen, Y.; Spackman, K.A.; Case, J.T.; et al. Auditing complex concepts of SNOMED using a refined hierarchical abstraction network. *J. Biomed. Inform.* **2012**, *45*, 1–14. [CrossRef]
29. National Institute of General Medical Sciences 2011. Available online: https://www.nigms.nih.gov/education/fact-sheets/Pages/pharmacogenomics.aspx (accessed on 20 May 2021).
30. Saripalle, R.; Runyan, C.; Russell, M. Using HL7 FHIR to achieve interoperability in patient health record. *J. Biomed. Inform.* **2019**, *94*, 103188. [CrossRef] [PubMed]
31. Rutman, M.P.; Horn, J.R.; Newman, D.K.; Stefanacci, R.G. Overactive Bladder Prescribing Considerations: The Role of Polypharmacy, Anticholinergic Burden, and CYP2D6 Drug-Drug Interactions. *Clin. Drug Investig.* **2021**, *41*, 293–302. [CrossRef]
32. Kamenski, G.; Ayazseven, S.; Berndt, A.; Fink, W.; Kamenski, L.; Zehetmayer, S.; Pühringer, H. Clinical Relevance of CYP2D6 Polymorphisms in Patients of an Austrian Medical Practice: A Family Practice-Based Observational Study. *Drugs Real World Outcomes* **2020**, *7*, 63–73. [CrossRef] [PubMed]
33. Boustani, M.; Campbell, N.; Munger, S.; Maidment, I.; Fox, C. Impact of anticholinergics on the aging brain: A review and practical application. *Aging Health* **2008**, *4*, 311–320. [CrossRef]
34. Haga, S.B.; Allen LaPointe, N.M.; Moaddeb, J. Challenges to integrating pharmacogenetic testing into medication therapy management. *J. Manag. Care Spec. Pharm.* **2015**, *21*, 346–352. [CrossRef]
35. Haga, S.B.; Moaddeb, J. Comparison of delivery strategies for pharmacogenetic testing services. *Pharm. Genom.* **2014**, *24*, 139–145. [CrossRef] [PubMed]
36. Haga, S.B. Managing Increased Accessibility to Pharmacogenomic Data. *Clin. Pharmacol. Ther.* **2019**, *106*, 922–924. [CrossRef] [PubMed]
37. Hresko, A.; Haga, S.B. Insurance coverage policies for personalized medicine. *J. Pers. Med.* **2012**, *2*, 201–216. [CrossRef] [PubMed]

38. Haga, S.B. Integrating pharmacogenetic testing into primary care. *Expert Rev. Precis. Med. Drug Dev.* **2017**, *2*, 327–336. [CrossRef] [PubMed]
39. Verbeurgt, P.; Mamiya, T.; Oesterheld, J. How common are drug and gene interactions? Prevalence in a sample of 1143 patients with CYP2C9, CYP2C19 and CYP2D6 genotyping. *Pharmacogenomics* **2014**, *15*, 655–665. [CrossRef]
40. Raymond, J.; Imbert, L.; Cousin, T.; Duflot, T.; Varin, R.; Wils, J.; Lamoureux, F. Pharmacogenetics of Direct Oral Anticoagulants: A Systematic Review. *J. Pers. Med.* **2021**, *11*, 37. [CrossRef]
41. Heise, C.W.; Gallo, T.; Curry, S.C.; Woosley, R.L. Identification of populations likely to benefit from pharmacogenomic testing. *Pharm. Genom.* **2020**, *30*, 91–95. [CrossRef] [PubMed]
42. Shah, R.R.; Smith, R.L. Addressing phenoconversion: The Achilles' heel of personalized medicine. *Br. J. Clin. Pharm.* **2015**, *79*, 222–240. [CrossRef]

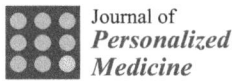

Article

Implementing Pharmacogenomics Testing: Single Center Experience at Arkansas Children's Hospital

Pritmohinder S. Gill [1,2,*,†], Feliciano B. Yu, Jr. [3,†], Patricia A. Porter-Gill [2], Bobby L. Boyanton, Jr. [4], Judy C. Allen [5], Jason E. Farrar [1,2,6], Aravindhan Veerapandiyan [2,7], Parthak Prodhan [2,8], Kevin J. Bielamowicz [1,2,6], Elizabeth Sellars [1,2,9], Andrew Burrow [1,2,9], Joshua L. Kennedy [1,2], Jeffery L. Clothier [10], David L. Becton [1,2,6], Don Rule [11] and G. Bradley Schaefer [1,2,12]

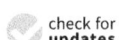

Citation: Gill, P.S.; Yu, F.B., Jr.; Porter-Gill, P.A.; Boyanton, B.L., Jr.; Allen, J.C.; Farrar, J.E.; Veerapandiyan, A.; Prodhan, P.; Bielamowicz, K.J.; Sellars, E.; et al. Implementing Pharmacogenomics Testing: Single Center Experience at Arkansas Children's Hospital. *J. Pers. Med.* 2021, *11*, 394. https://doi.org/10.3390/jpm11050394

Academic Editor: Laura B. Scheinfeldt

Received: 31 March 2021
Accepted: 6 May 2021
Published: 11 May 2021

Publisher's Note: MDPI stays neutral with regard to jurisdictional claims in published maps and institutional affiliations.

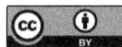

Copyright: © 2021 by the authors. Licensee MDPI, Basel, Switzerland. This article is an open access article distributed under the terms and conditions of the Creative Commons Attribution (CC BY) license (https://creativecommons.org/licenses/by/4.0/).

1. Department of Pediatrics, University of Arkansas for Medical Sciences, Little Rock, AR 72202, USA; JEFarrar@uams.edu (J.E.F.); KJBielamowicz2@uams.edu (K.J.B.); EASellars@uams.edu (E.S.); TABurrow@uams.edu (A.B.); KennedyJoshuaL@uams.edu (J.L.K.); BectonDavidL@uams.edu (D.L.B.); SchaeferGB@uams.edu (G.B.S.)
2. Arkansas Children's Research Institute, Little Rock, AR 72202, USA; PortergillPA@archildrens.org (P.A.P.-G.); AVeerapandiyan@uams.edu (A.V.); ProdhanParthak@uams.edu (P.P.)
3. Pediatrics and Biomedical Informatics, University of Arkansas for Medical Sciences, Little Rock, AR 72202, USA; Pele.Yu@archildrens.org
4. Departments of Pathology and Laboratory Medicine, University of Arkansas for Medical Sciences and Arkansas Children's Hospital, Little Rock, AR 72202, USA; bboyanton@uams.edu
5. Informatics, Arkansas Children's Hospital, 1 Children's Way #512-10, Little Rock, AR 72202, USA; AllenJC@archildrens.org
6. Pediatric Hematology/Oncology, Arkansas Children's Hospital, 1 Children's Way #512-10, Little Rock, AR 72202, USA
7. Pediatric Neurology, Arkansas Children's Hospital, 1 Children's Way, Little Rock, AR 72202, USA
8. Pediatric Cardiology, Arkansas Children's Hospital, Little Rock, AR 72202, USA
9. Section of Genetics and Metabolism, Arkansas Children's Hospital, Little Rock, AR 72202, USA
10. Psychiatry, College of Medicine, University of Arkansas for Medical Sciences, Little Rock, AR 72205, USA; JLClothier@uams.edu
11. Translational Software, Inc., TSI, Bellevue, WA 98005, USA; Don.rule@translationalsoftware.com
12. Arkansas Children's Hospital NW, Springdale, AR 72762, USA
* Correspondence: PSGill@uams.edu; Tel.: +1-(501)-364-1418; Fax: +1-(501)-364-3654
† These authors contributed equally to this work.

Abstract: Pharmacogenomics (PGx) is a growing field within precision medicine. Testing can help predict adverse events and sub-therapeutic response risks of certain medications. To date, the US FDA lists over 280 drugs which provide biomarker-based dosing guidance for adults and children. At Arkansas Children's Hospital (ACH), a clinical PGx laboratory-based test was developed and implemented to provide guidance on 66 pediatric medications for genotype-guided dosing. This PGx test consists of 174 single nucleotide polymorphisms (SNPs) targeting 23 clinically actionable PGx genes or gene variants. Individual genotypes are processed to provide per-gene discrete results in star-allele and phenotype format. These results are then integrated into EPIC-EHR. Genomic indicators built into EPIC-EHR provide the source for clinical decision support (CDS) for clinicians, providing genotype-guided dosing.

Keywords: pharmacogenomics (PGx); pediatrics; best practice alerts (BPAs); electronic health records (EHR); genomic indicators; clinical decision support (CDS); phenotype; genotype

1. Introduction

Adverse drug reactions (ADRs) are the fourth leading cause of death in the USA [1] and account for 135K deaths per year with an economic burden of over USD 136 billion [2,3]. A systematic review of prospective studies showed that 5.3% of hospital admissions were associated with ADRs [4]. These are alarming statistics that illustrate the potential of widespread pharmacogenomic profiling to help mitigate some of these ADRs. More broadly, medical practice is moving away from the concept of "one size fits all" medications [5], as drugs that help some patients will not work for others, and the same drug may have adverse effects in some patients (Figure 1).

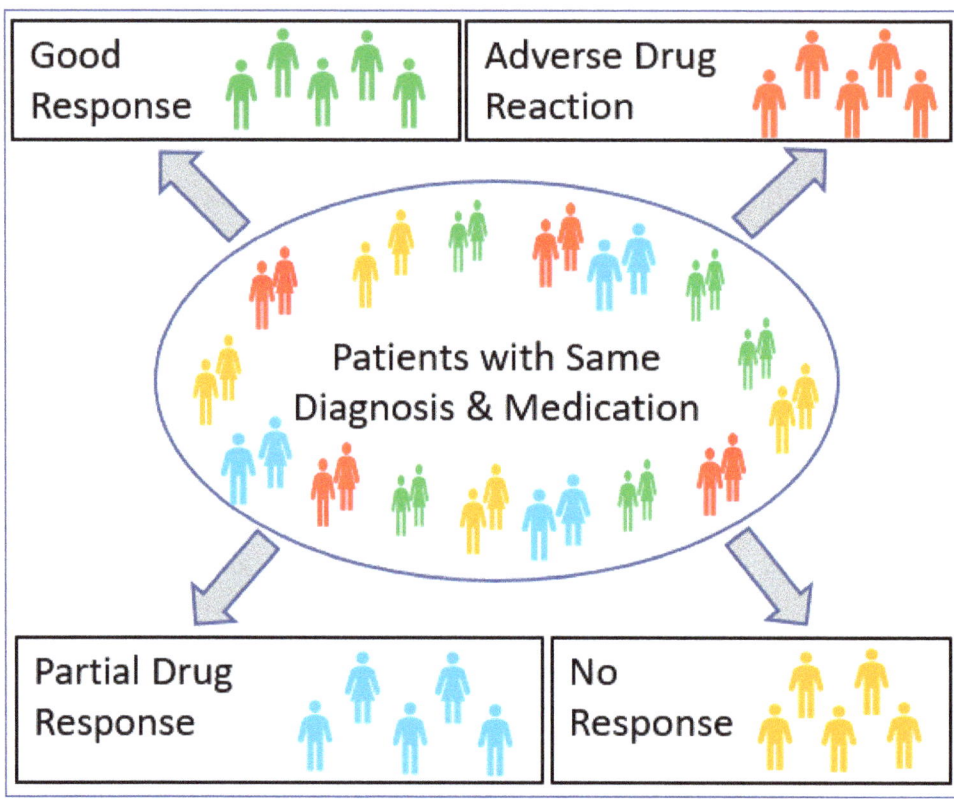

Figure 1. Pharmacogenomics and drug response in individuals with different genotypes.

Completion of the Human Genome Project [6], International HapMap Project [7], and the 1000 Genomes Project [8] showed the complex nature of underlying human genetic variations, which can determine and contribute to differential drug responses. Pharmacogenomics (PGx) looks at how heritable genetic differences affect individual response to drugs [1,9]. PGx broadly considers an individual's genetic makeup, lifestyle, and environmental factors to help design interventions that impact drug response and adverse effects. Getting therapeutic choices correct the first time is critical to a successful outcome of drug therapy. Advances in genetics and in our understanding of the potential of the human genome in the pathogenesis of disease and in the prediction of drug treatment effects have spawned a new approach to drug therapy called "genomic medicine". Genomic medicine has the potential to advance modern therapeutics (e.g., cancer and transplantation treatments) while presenting opportunities to extend value and safety through customized and individualized genotype-guided drug treatments; this is a fundamental premise of precision medicine. Although precision medicine is transforming clinical care for adult medicine, in pediatric medicine this process lags behind for many drugs with well-established pharmacogenetic associations and guidelines [10,11], because the ontogeny of drug metabolizing enzymes and transporters dictates drug response in children and adults.

The 10th Genomic Medicine meeting on "Research Directions in Pharmacogenomics" [12], outlined that success in PGx implementation has been largely through NIH-funded efforts, but recommended broadening these efforts by updating and annotating genomic data in existing electronic health records (EHRs), along with the development of robust "plug-in" modules to make these advances available to the medical practitioner and patient. A successful implementation of PGx in available EHRs requires providing timely information to clinicians in terms of discrete data results, clinical interpretation of phenotype and genotype data, and clinical decision support (CDS) on the PGx actionable variants at the point of care in Epic™ (Epic Systems Corporation, Wausau, WI, USA).

Arkansas Children's is a medium-large tertiary medical facility providing primary and comprehensive subspecialty care services to children, adolescents, and young adults throughout Arkansas though several campuses and an integrated clinical network of care. Since 2018, the health system has used EPIC (Wausau, WI, USA) as the primary EHR vendor. As dedicated pediatric providers, we believe it imperative that the promise of precision medicine become comprehensively integrated into the pediatric medical care models. With the quality of the current faculty's expertise, recent recruitment of several highly skilled medical professionals, and expansion of clinical research capabilities, Arkansas Children's is ideally positioned to quickly become a leader in the field of pediatric precision medicine. Here we describe our early approach to successful PGx implementation in this environment.

2. Materials and Methods

A small committee of individuals with expertise in toxicology and genetics convened to form the Precision Medicine (PM) group. Simultaneously, multiple items had to be addressed, including physician and patient family interest, proper instrumentation, genotyping panel design, evaluation of current medications prescribed at the ACH pharmacy, and comprehensive IT support, from genotype calling through EMR reporting and integration. Champion clinicians were enlisted, as well as EPIC support and an outside company to provide robust data interpretation and templated guidance for CDS. A clinical pharmacogenomics (PGx) program was established at Arkansas Children's Hospital to tailor the therapeutic care delivered to children using genomics. The following project details were reviewed by the Institutional Review Board (IRB) at the University of Arkansas for Medical Sciences (UAMS), Little Rock, Arkansas, which considered the project to be a development and implementation of an internal genetics panel at ACH for the purpose of improving local patient care that, as such, did not meet the regulatory definition of research or require IRB oversight (PI: Schaefer; IRB #-262792).

2.1. Adoption of PGx-Patient and Physician Interest Survey

A preliminary electronic survey in August–September 2018 at ACH was given to primary care physicians as well as patients' families to determine if there was an unmet need to provide PGx testing to improve drug prescribing practices.

2.2. Pharmacy Records Data Extraction

For the year 2018 all pharmacy records were evaluated to identify prescribing practices associated with drugs with extant pediatric pharmacogenomic guidance (Table 1) per clinically based guidelines from the U.S. FDA, Clinical Pharmacogenomics Implementation Consortium (CPIC), and the Dutch Pharmacogenetic Working Group (DPWG). Table 1 shows the relevant associated gene/s for the prescribed drugs.

Table 1. Prescriptions (in-patient and out-patient) filled at ACH Pharmacy in 2018.

Drug Name	Gene/s	Total	Drug Name	Gene/s	Total
Amikacin	MT-RNR1	6	Hydrocodone	CYP2D6	303
Amitriptyline	CYP2C19, CYP2D6	1382	Imipramine	CYP2C19, CYP2D6	190
Aripiprazole	CYP2D6	24	Mercaptopurine	TPMT, NUDT15	809
Atazanavir	UGT1A1	3	Neomycin	MT-RNR1	33
Atomoxetine	CYP2D6	59	Nortriptyline	CYP2D6	147
Azathioprine	TPMT, NUDT15	116	Ondansetron	CYP2D6	21,147
Celecoxib	CYP2C9	55	Oxybutynin	NA	795
Cisplatin	ACYP2	59	Oxycodone	CYP2D6	12,978
Citalopram	CYP2C19	21	Paroxetine	CYP2D6	5
Clomipramine	CYP2C19, CYP2D6	1	Phenytoin	CYP2C9	31
Clopidogrel	CYP2C19	16	Pimozide	CYP2D6	9
Doxepin	CYP2C19, CYP2D6	11	Salmeterol	ADRB2	224
Eltrombopag	F5	7	Sertraline	CYP2C19	271
Escitalopram	CYP2C19	46	Simvastatin	CYP3A4, SLCO1B1	24
Fluorouracil	DDYD	9	Tacrolimus	CYP3A5	463
Fluoxetine	CYP2D6	197	Thioguanine	TPMT, NUDT15	36
Fluvoxamine	CYP2D6	11	Tobramycin	MT-RNR1	61
Formoterol	ADRB2	995	Tramadol	CYP2D6	90
Fosphenytoin	CYP2C9	113	Vincristine	CEP72	1528
Gentamicin	MT-RNR1	258	Voriconazole	CYP2C19	31
			Warfarin	CYP2C9, VKORC1, CYP2C, DYP4F2	313

2.3. Selection and Generation of PGx Panel

The pediatric PGx test panel was designed to assess genes and gene variants with drug response that were targeted by the above prescribed drugs (Table 1) at ACH and were designated evidence level 1 with established evidence-based clinical guidelines.

2.3.1. Real-Time PCR Instrument and OpenArray® Panel Analytical Validation

The validation of QuantStudio™12K Flex Real-time PCR instrument (Thermo Fisher Scientific, Waltham, MA, USA) was performed in March 2020 by Thermo Fisher Scientific field application specialists. Review of Table 1 gave 23 gene/gene variants targeting 174 clinically actionable SNPs for pediatric genotype-guided drug dosing (Table 2). A Custom OpenArray® (www.thermofisher.com) was designed for the 174 SNPs PGx panel and validated by Thermo Fisher Scientific in September 2020.

Table 2. ACH pharmacogenomics (PGx) panel design summary highlighting gene, number of SNPs and SNP Rs#.

PGx 174 SNP Panel		
Gene	No. of SNPs	SNP rs#
ACYP2	1	rs1872328
CACNA1S	2	rs772226819, rs1800559
CEP72	1	rs924607
CYP2C	1	rs12777823
CYP2C19	12	rs12769205, rs12248560, rs17884712, rs72552267, rs4986893, rs56337013, rs72558186, rs6413438, rs58973490, rs41291556, rs28399504, rs4244285
CYP2C9	13	rs72558193, rs72558189, rs2256871, rs7900194, rs1799853, rs1057910, rs28371686, rs9332239, rs56165452, rs28371685, rs9332131, rs72558187, rs72558190
CYP2D6	42	rs730882170, rs28371710, rs1135822, rs267608319, rs28371696, rs267608279, rs16947, rs35742686, rs72549352, rs61736512adjC, rs61736512, rs148769737, rs148769737, rs267608297, rs267608313, rs28371706, rs1065852, rs1135840, rs3892097, rs769258, rs5030862, rs201377835, rs5030867, hCV32407220, rs72549349, rs5030656, rs72549351, rs72549353, rs28371717, rs72549356, rs5030655, rs774671100, rs1080985, rs59421388, rs72549348, rs28371725, rs72549346, rs72549347, rs1135823, rs5030865, rs5030865, rs730882251
CYP3A4	5	rs4986910, rs4987161, rs12721629, rs55785340, rs35599367
CYP3A5	3	rs776746, rs10264272, rs41303343
CYP4F2	1	rs2108622
DPYD	22	rs75017182, rs3918289, rs3918289, rs1801159, rs1801158, rs1801268, rs1801267, rs1801266, rs1801265, rs1801160, rs55886062, rs2297595, rs17376848, rs56038477, rs67376798, rs6670886, rs3918290, rs72549309, rs72549306, rs72549310, rs80081766, rs115232898
F2	1	rs1799963
F5	1	rs6025
G6PD	11	rs137852328, rs72554665, rs72554665, rs137852328, rs78478128, rs1050828, rs1050829, rs5030868, rs137852339, rs76723693, rs5030869
NUDT15	3	rs766023281, rs116855232, s186364861
RARG	1	rs2229774
RYR1	41	rs118192163, rs28933396, rs118192176, rs193922770, rs144336148, rs118192162, rs118192116, rs121918592, rs1801086, rs118192161, rs28933397, rs63749869, rs121918594, rs118192170, rs193922802, rs118192167, rs121918595, rs118192168, rs121918593, rs118192124, rs118192122, rs118192175, rs118192172, rs111888148, rs112563513, rs118192178, rs121918596, rs193922747, rs193922748, rs193922753, rs193922764, rs193922768, rs193922772, rs193922803, rs193922807, rs193922816, rs193922818, rs193922832, rs193922843, rs193922876, rs193922878
SLC28A3	1	rs7853758
SLCO1B1	1	rs4149056
TPMT	5	rs1142345, rs56161402, rs1800584, rs1800462, rs1800460
UGT1A1	3	rs4148323, rs35350960, rs887829
UGT1A6	1	rs17863783
VKORC1	1	rs9923231

SNP = single nucleotide polymorphism; CNV assays: *CYP2D6*—Hs00010001_cn (exon 9) and Hs04502391_cn (Intron 6); All alleles that are negative for above sequence variation were defaulted to *1 assignment.

2.3.2. PGx OpenArray® and CNV Assay Validation

The samples were loaded onto OpenArray® plate using the QuantStudio™12K Flex OpenArray AccuFill System. Detection and genotyping are performed on the QuantStudio™12K Flex system, which includes the QuantStudio Software v1.1.2 and TaqMan® Genotyper Software v1.3. For genotyping TaqMan® assays are used which consist of pre-optimized PCR primer pairs and two probes (FAM dye label and VIC dye label) for allelic discrimination (www.ThermoFisher.com). The complete test consists of 2 components; genotyping and copy number quantification. All genotyping and CNV assays identify alleles in human samples obtained from buccal swabs and blood samples, which are used to determine drug metabolism and specific disease condition risk factors. The copy number component consists of 2 TaqMan copy number assays for the *CYP2D6* gene (exon 9 and intron 2).

2.4. Build of Genomic Indicators in EPIC

One of the challenging aspects of implementing pharmacogenetics across systems is that there is no standardized nomenclature to draw upon. While simple star-allele labels have gained acceptance for diplotypes (combinations of haplotypes), there are a wide variety of ways to represent the complex structural variations inherent in the *CYP2D6* gene. Although normal, intermediate, and rapid metabolizer monikers have become common for phenotypes, the terms "poor" or "intermediate" metabolizer do not capture subtle variations in *CYP2C9* metabolism that are indicated in current CPIC guidelines. To provide a more granular view of metabolism, a growing number of recommendations are provided on the basis of the predicted activity score of the resulting enzyme. Even the labeling of individual single nucleotide polymorphisms (SNPs) will be different when test results are analyzed with different genome builds. To alleviate these issues, Translational Software, Inc. (TSI, Bellevue, WA 98005, USA) collaborated with EPIC (Wausau, WI, USA) to establish a numbering system that represents both the type of result that is reported as well as the specific result for genotypes, diplotypes, phenotypes, and activity scores for each allele/SNP on the ACH PGx Panel. These numbers become the basis for rules that determine which specific recommendations to provide to the clinician as best practice alerts (BPAs). In the example (Table 3) below, a clinician would be warned that PGx test results indicate an increased risk of adverse effects or therapeutic failure for Amitryptyline. The recommendation would be to consider an alternative medication or use therapeutic drug monitoring to guide Amitryptyline dose adjustments. The reason for that guidance is based upon the patient's *CYP2C19* and *CYP2D6* metabolizer test results, which show a poor metabolizer phenotype for *CYP2C19* with diplotypes (*2/*2, *2/*3, or *3/*3); and a rapid metabolizer phenotype for *CYP2D6* with diplotypes (*1/*1)xN, (*1/*2)xN, or (*2/*2)xN [13]. Note that Table 3 shows two distinct identifiers that are labeled and may result in different recommendations for other drugs.

Table 3. Example for Amitriptyline illustrates a numbering system designed and built in EPIC and showing the specific result for genotypes, diplotypes, phenotypes, and activity scores for each SNP on the ACH PGx panel.

ID	Title	Indicators	Ordinal Value	Meaning	Logic
882001281	Decreased Amitriptyline Exposure	87005959	1	Amitryptyline Prescribed	1 AND ((2 AND 3) OR (3 AND 4))
		873000170	2	*CYP2C19* Poor Metabolizer	
		873000181	3	*CYP2D6* Rapid Metabolizer	
		873001569	4	*CYP2C19* Poor Metabolizer	

3. Results

3.1. Pharmacogenomics Program at ACH

3.1.1. Patient and Physician Interest Survey

The preliminary survey of physicians and patients' families (*unpublished*) showed that 88% of patients' parents ($n = 49$) were interested in having their child's DNA used to guide medical diagnosis and drug therapy. By contrast, 81% of ACH physicians ($n = 206$) indicated an interest in some kind of warning of drug-gene interaction within a patient's EHR. It was determined that there was a clear interest by the stakeholders (clinicians and patient families) and the PM Group in the development and implementation of a PGx program at ACH that would be of high priority and allow us to provide personalized drug therapy to our patients at ACH.

3.1.2. ACH Pharmacy Records Review

A review of pharmacy records for the year 2018 showed that 42,877 prescriptions (in-patient and out-patient) were filled by the hospital (Table 1). The pediatric PGx test panel covers the most-prescribed medications at ACH and was coupled with pediatric clinical guidelines to improve patient care. For example, prescriptions of ondansetron were filled 21,147 times followed by oxycodone at 12,978 times. These commonly prescribed medications covered 11 medical specialties including anesthesia, cancer, cardiology, gastrointestinal, genetics, hematology, infectious diseases, neurology, pain, psychiatry and addiction, and transplantation (Table 4). The above-listed personalized medications were explored for their pharmacogenetic data and clinical annotations in the U.S. FDA, Clinical Pharmacogenomics Implementation Consortium (CPIC), and the Dutch Pharmacogenetic Working Group (DPWG) and PharmGKB [14–17]. Our search gave us 23 actionable PGx variants and their associated pathogenic variant single nucleotide polymorphisms (SNPs), for a total of 174 SNPs (Table 2), that have drug response phenotypes.

Table 4. ACH pharmacogenomics panel and drug-gene targets by pediatric therapeutic area. Bold drugs show only adult guidance.

Condition	Drug	Gene/s
Anesthesia	Desflurane	RYR1/CACNA1S
	Enflurane	RYR1/CACNA1S
	Halothane	RYR1/CACNA1S
	Isoflurane	RYR1/CACNA1S
	Sevoflurane	RYR1/CACNA1S
	Succinycholine	RYR1/CACNA1S
Cancer	Azathioprine	TPMT/NUDT15
	Capecitabine	DPYD
	Cisplatin	ACYP2
	Daunorubicin	RARG/UGT1A6/SLC28A3
	Doxorubicin	RARG/UGT1A6/SLC28A3
	Fluorouracil	DPYD
	Mercaptopurine	TPMT/NUDT15
	Rasburicase	G6PD
	Thioguanine	TPMT/NUDT15
	Vincristine	CEP72
Cardiovascular	Clopidogrel	CYP2C19
	Propranolol	CYP2D6
	Simvastatin	CYP3A4/SLCO1B1
	Warfarin	CYP2C9/VKORC1/CYP2C/CYP4F2

Table 4. *Cont.*

Condition	Drug	Gene/s
Gastrointestinal (GI)	Dexlanosoprazole	CYP2C19
	Esomeprazole	CYP2C19
	Lansoprazole	CYP2C19
	Omeprazole	CYP2C19
	Ondansetron	CYP2D6
	Pantoprazole	CYP2C19
	Rabeprazole	CYP2C19
Gaucher Disease	Eliglustat	CYP2D6
Hematology	Eltrombopag	F5
Infectious Disease	Atazanavir	UGT1A1
	Chloroquine	G6PD
	Dapsone	G6PD
	Nitrofurantoin	G6PD
	Primaquine	G6PD
	Proguanil	CYP2c19
	Quinine	G6PD
	Sulfamethoxazole	G6PD
	Tafenoquine	G6PD
	Voriconazole	CYP2C19
Neurology	Fosphenytoin	CYP2C9
	Phenytoin	CYP2C9
Pain	Celecoxib	CYP2C9
	Codeine	CYP2D6
	Hydrocodone	CYP2D6
	Ibuprofen	CYP2C9
	Meloxicam	CYP2C9
	Oxycodone	CYP2D6
	Tramadol	CYP2D6
Psychiatry and Addiction Medicine	Amitriptyline	CYP2C19/CYP2D6
	Aripiprazole	CYP2D6
	Atomoxetine	CYP2D6
	Citalopram	CYP2C19
	Clomipramine	CYP2C19/CYP2D6
	Desipramine	CYP2D6
	Doxepin	CYP2C19/CYP2D6
	Escitalopram	CYP2C19
	Fluoxetine	CYP2D6
	Fluvoxamine	CYP2D6
	Iloperidone	CYP2D6
	Imipramine	CYP2C19/CYP2D6
	Nortriptyline	CYP2D6
	Paroxetine	CYP2D6
	Pimozide	CYP2D6
	Sertraline	CYP2C19
	Trimipramine	CYP2C19/CYP2D6
Transplantation	Tacrolimus	CYP3A5

3.1.3. PGx Assay Performance

Laboratory developed tests (LDTs) [18,19] including PGx testing, are developed and implemented to fulfill the unmet medical needs of an institution and the patient population it serves, when such laboratory-based testing is not commercially available. Although LDTs do not necessarily require approval from the FDA, laboratories must, at minimum, adhere to regulations set forth by the Clinical Laboratory Improvement Amendments of 1988 (CLIA'88) [20]. Thus, it is essential to thoroughly validate the performance of a laboratory method and establish standard operating procedures prior to implementing the test for clinical purposes.

The ACH PGx test was designed for a high-throughput laboratory that can process hundreds of samples across a large number of targets. For analytical validation, we used 24 Coriell samples and 10 different plasmid pools. Details could be sent to the reader upon request for critical components of the validation of this qualitative genotyping test, establishing the DNA sample concentration dynamic range, reproducibility, accuracy of genotyping, and copy number variation (CNV). Briefly, the dynamic range of tested DNA sample concentrations was between 3.13 ng/µL and 25 ng/µL. For CNV, good results were obtained for a final concentration between 10 ng/reaction (5 ng/µL) and 5 ng/reaction (2.5 ng/µL). Accuracy of genotyping and CNV results were 99.97% and 95.55%, respectively. Overall genotyping and CNV reproducibility were 99.52% and 99.26%, respectively. Finally, verification of the PGx test's ability to correctly detect polymorphisms was assessed using a mixed pool of samples (plasmid pool controls from Coriell (Camden, NJ, USA) and volunteer human samples (blood and buccal DNA)); all test results were specific to their intended SNP target. In addition, we performed bi-directional sequencing of volunteer DNA samples and thereby confirmed genotype data generated from the OpenArray PGx test (Table 2).

3.1.4. Integrating PGx into EHR with CDS

A significant impediment to the adoption of pharmacogenetics has been an inability to incorporate real-time physician education, CDS, and active ordering of PGx-directed genetic testing into the physician's normal workflow in EPIC. Under the guidance of ACH, EPIC collaborated with Translational Software, Inc. (TSI) to import TSI's rule set and curated recommendations into best practice advisories (BPAs). With this content enabled, physicians are prompted to consider PGx testing as per pre-alerts (Figure 2A,B) that are triggered by prescription orders of PGx relevant drugs.

When physicians order the PGx test in EPIC, there is an option to select drug-gene pair from the listed conditions (for example, cancer, cardiovascular, etc.) (Figure 2A); the system then prompts the physician to obtain genetic consent from the patient/family member and also to obtain PGx test pre-authorization (Figure 2B). If the pre-authorization is not available, then the patient blood sample can only be processed for DNA extraction. When the pre-authorization is received, the DNA sample is automatically placed for PGx panel runs in the molecular pathology laboratory at ACH. SNP data is reviewed by a molecular pathologist, then sent to TSI via a secured cloud platform using HL7/SFTP interphase. When SNP data results are completed, they are processed by TSI's cloud-based platform to provide a summary report as well as discrete test results that are submitted to EPIC's Advanced Genomic Module (Figure 3). The summary report provides the ordering physician an overview of the implications of the genetic test for the patient, and the test results in the Advanced Genomic Module provide data in a computable format that enables perpetual use of the test results within the EHR system. Once the test results are received, subsequent medication orders are evaluated on the basis of the rule set that is integrated into EPIC using component codes for gene, genotype, and phenotype of interest provided by the ACH-IT PGx group. When there are potential PGx implications for medication orders prepared by the physician, best practice advisories (BPAs) that provide evidence-based recommendations, including the clinical guidelines of the U.S. FDA, CPIC, and DPWG, are triggered.

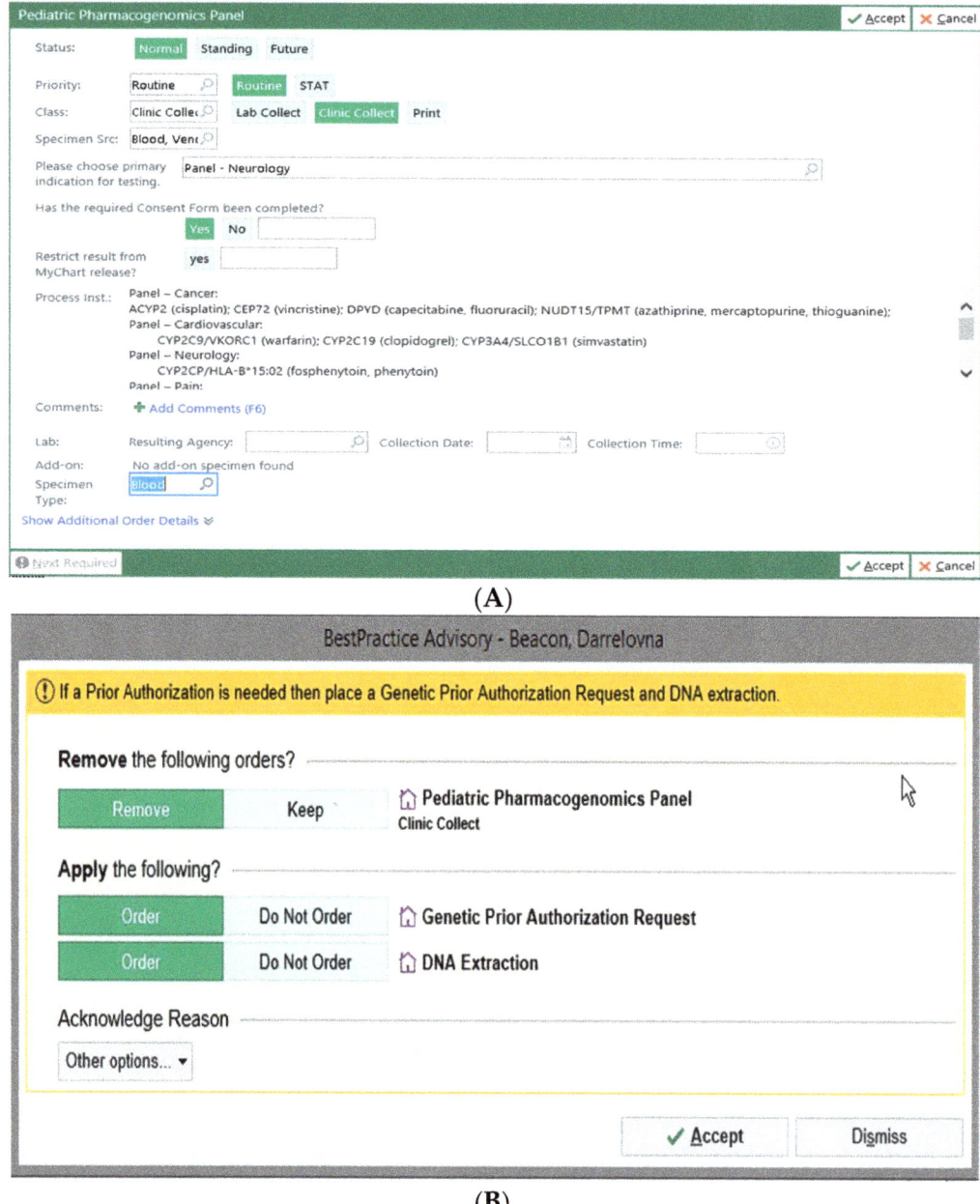

Figure 2. Placing an order for PGx test in ACH EPIC (**A**,**B**).

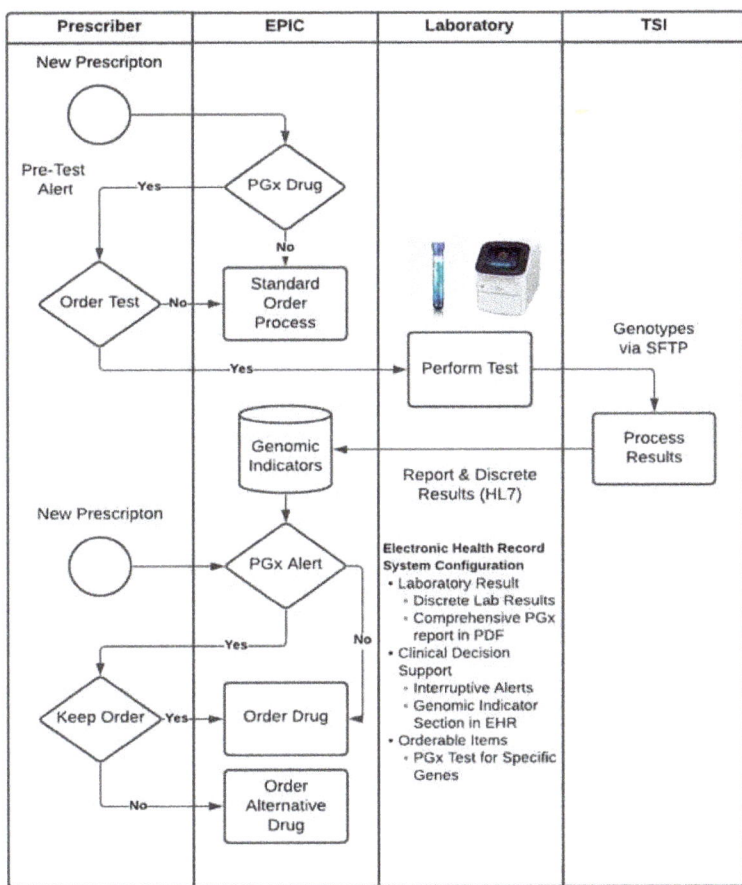

Figure 3. Implementation of pharmacogenomic workflow at ACH. The clinician can order the PGx test in EPIC; genomic indicators in EPIC were built with respective clinical decision supports (CDS). Physicians can receive discrete laboratory results, comprehensive PGx report, and BPAs.

The specific drug-gene pairs that are the focus of the alerts are high-risk PGx actionable genotypes (Figure 4A–C) and has been carefully chosen to avoid "alert fatigue" on the part of clinicians. The early implementation strategy at ACH is to focus on a handful of subspecialties that are either highly receptive to (e.g., genetics) or familiar with using PGx on some limited basis (e.g., oncology, neurology, and cardiology) to build out the process and scrutinize the BPAs. The goal is to grow to high-volume primary care clinics. BPAs may be passive or interruptive and may be configured to suggest alternative medication orders and enable the clinician to indicate why they are maintaining the current order.

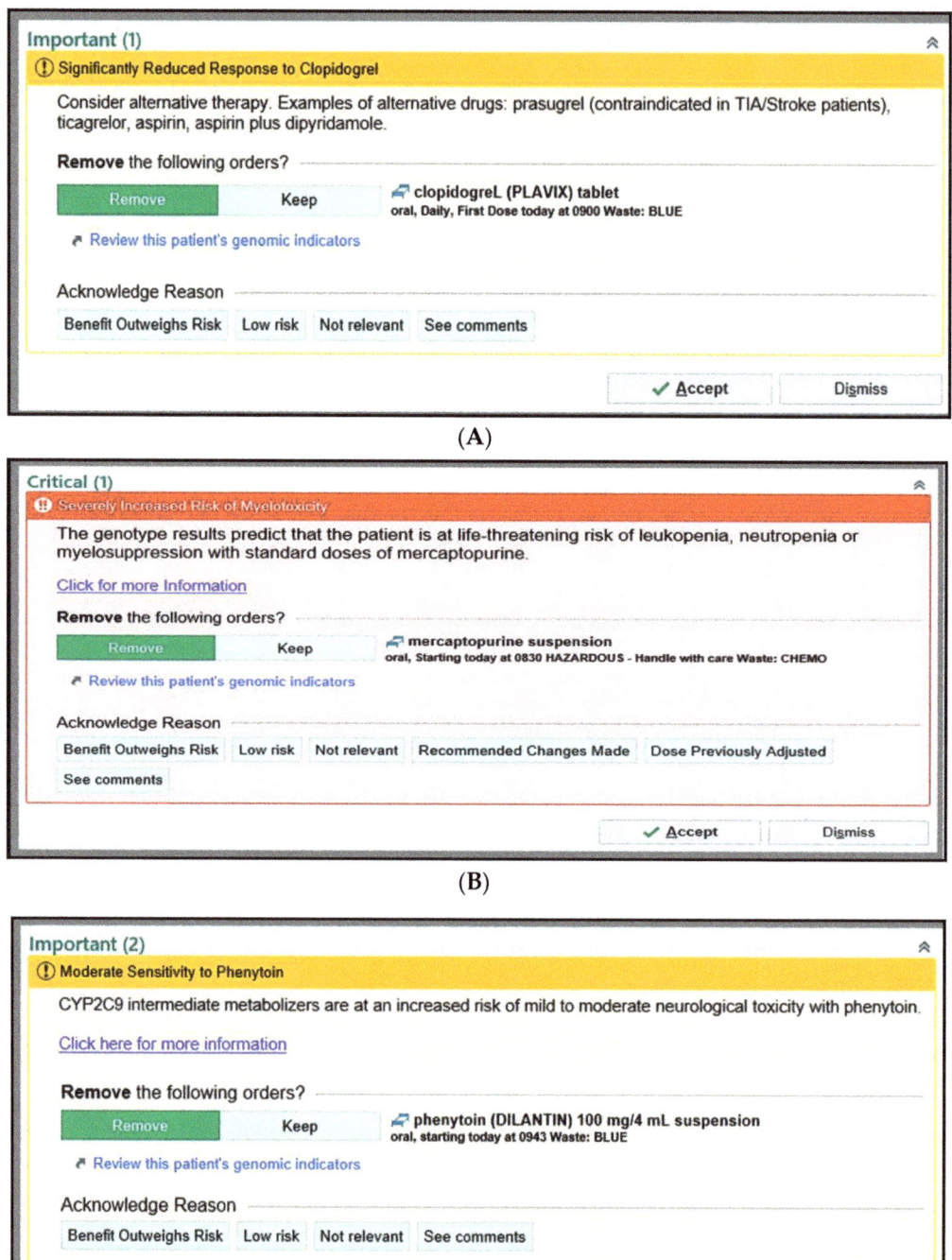

Figure 4. Best practice alerts (BPAs) for high risk PGx actionable genotypes with clinical decision support (CDS) for clinicians in EPIC (EPIC © 2021 Epic Systems Corporation): (**A**) clopidogrel, (**B**) mercaptopurine and (**C**) phenytoin.

3.1.5. Examples of BPAs in EPIC

We initially identified a small group of champion physicians for PGx implementation, including those with either a strong intrinsic interest in PGx (e.g., genetics) or who were thought to be most easily capable of incorporating PGx into their clinical practice work flows. Champion physicians for cardiovascular, neurology, hematology, and oncology were identified, and internal group meetings with the respective physician teams arranged. These clinicians reviewed and in some cases adjusted the BPA language to best fit local standards and practice in the EPIC-based EHR for genotype-guided therapy. Below are examples of interruptive BPAs for clopidogrel, thiopurine, and phenytoin (Figure 4A–C) (EPIC © 2021 Epic Systems Corporation). As mentioned earlier, we established a numbering system (Table 3) that provides CDSs for specific discrete results for 174 SNPs targeting 66 pediatric drugs on the ACH PGx Panel. The alert provides a tab where clinician can review a patient's full list of genomic indicators. Below are some examples of BPAs that will be invoked in EPIC for high-risk PGx actionable genotypes, when clinicians receive genotype-guided recommendations for a particular pediatric medication:

Clopidogrel-*CYP2C19*

A patient with a poor metabolizer phenotype for *CYP2C19* could have diplotypes as *2/*2, *2/*3 or *3/*3 [21]. BPA as shown in Figure 4A will be triggered, letting the physician know that the phenotype and genotype results for *CYP2C19* show significantly reduced response to clopidogrel and consider antiplatelet agents (prasugrel, ticagrelor) as a therapy alternative.

Thiopurine-*TPMT/NUDT15*

If a patient has a poor metabolizer status for *TPMT* with diplotypes (*3A/*3A, *2/*3A, *3A/*3C, *3C/*4, *2/*3C, *3A/*4) and normal metabolizer for *NUDT15* (*1/*1) [22], the BPA for mercaptopurine shown in Figure 4B will trigger. This alerts the physician that the patient has increased risk for myelotoxicity and that the genotype results predict life-threatening risk of leukopenia, neutropenia, and myelosuppression with standard doses of mercaptopurine.

Phenytoin-*CYP2C9*

If the discrete result shows a patient has intermediate metabolizer status for *CYP2C9* phenotype, with associated diplotypes *1/*2, *1/*3 or *2/*2 [23], then the alert in Figure 4C will trigger, showing that patients with *CYP2C9* intermediate phenotype and taking phenytoin are at increased risk of mild to moderate neurological toxicity.

In addition, to complement the EHR-intrinsic features of the return of PGx results to physicians through lab review modules and BPAs, we also formulated a comprehensive PGx report as a PDF document (Figure 3) showing details on current patient medications, risk management, potentially impacted medications, dosing guidance on drug-gene interactions, drug-drug interactions and test details. Supplementary Figure S1 displays a mock report for an patient on Clopidogrel and Codeine. This PGx report shows the clinician the *CYP2C19* and *CYP2D6* metabolizer status and dosing recommendations for adults as well as pediatric patients (Figure S1). Supplementary Figure S2 on the other hand, provides the clinician with a broader examination and understanding of the 23 PGx genes along with their genotype and phenotype status.

At ACH, we have implemented a pediatric personalized medicine program in PGx with ACH-IT focused on data management that is tied directly with electronic health records (EHRs) to alert physicians about drug-gene information that could aid in drug treatment decisions.

4. Discussion

Pediatric adverse drug reactions (ADRs) are a significant health concern [24,25], and clinical implementation of pharmacogenomics (PGx) may see the earliest and broadest use in clinical practice for improving patient care [26]. Pediatric drug studies were instrumental in adding dosing and risk information to the labelling of 80 pediatric drugs [27]. Ontogeny controls the pharmacokinetics and pharmacodynamics of drug response [28,29] and is the key to understanding the variability of drug efficacy/toxicity in neonates, adolescents, and adults. The cytochrome P-450 family of enzymes undergoes substantial ontogenic changes. For example, enzyme activity for *CYP2C19*, *CYP2C9*, *CYP3A4*, and *CYP2D6* until birth is low, but reaches adult levels in the first few weeks or months after birth [30]. Similarly, for *TPMT*, genetic polymorphism is a significant factor responsible for serious ADRs (myelosuppression) in patients treated with thiopurines, and *TPMT* activity is higher in infants and children than in adults when normalized for genotype [31]. Health care systems are slowly beginning to implement PGx tests that are at the forefront of moving precision medicine/genomic medicine to a new level, but there is still an urgent unmet need in pediatrics to refine and develop precision actionable PGx guidance through cutting-edge clinical research.

4.1. Clinical Utility of Pharmacogenomics

The majority of pharmacogenomic marker associations are based on the progress made in understanding the clinically actionable PGx variants in adult patient populations [15,16,32,33]. Codeine is a prodrug dependent on *CYP2D6* activation, and a majority of PGx guidance for it comes from adult studies [10,34]. Black box warnings on codeine were applied in 2013 and 2017 for children younger than 12 years of age [34], as PGx evidence showed codeine can cause respiratory depression and death. For drug-gene interaction, several drugs now available target PGx variants for which pediatric clinical guidelines are recommended [34]. The PGx test at ACH consists of 174 variant alleles in 23 pharmacogenes (Table 2) and can give guidance on 66 of the most commonly prescribed pediatric drugs. The list of personalized medications in recent years that have pharmacogenomic guidance has increased to 286 [35]. A clinician has the ability to look at a patient's genetic profile to determine if the treatment options will benefit the patient. Consortia such as CPIC and DPWG provide pharmacogenomic-based evidence guidelines for drug-gene pairs, along with data on frequency of polymorphisms in ethnic groups and their allele functionality status.

4.2. PGx Programs at Other Pediatric Medical Centers

Precision medicine (PM) is more common in adult medicine. Because children are our future, it is imperative that PM be integrated into ACH's method of clinical care. Assessing the pediatric patient as an individual will provide the best and most effective medical treatments.

At the beginning of the evolution of PGx at ACH, our group evaluated PM groups at other US and Canadian pediatric hospitals, along with their pharmacogenomic testing capabilities. We found that very few offer in-house PGx testing for children. Some pediatric hospitals offer PGx testing, but it is out-sourced to institutions such as OneOme (Minneapolis, MN, USA), ARUP (Salt Lake City, UT, USA), Gene by Gene (Houston, TX, USA), and RPRD (Milwaukee, WI, USA). In situations such as this, the interpretation of the PGx test is left to the out-sourced testing company. In some cases, in-house staff are necessary to give the interpretation data a second look, and to manually import the PGx test results into their hospital's electronic health record (EHR) system. These out-sourced PGx tests are not always pediatric specific, and adult drug:gene assays are included in the results. In addition, interpretations of the PGx results are not populated in the patients' EHRs as discrete information. The reader is advised to examine the CPIC implementation website for the institutes and commercial entities that utilize CPIC guidelines for PGx testing (https://cpicpgx.org/implementation/, accessed on 1 March 2021).

It is financially beneficial that ACH can offer PGx testing for its pediatric patients, and that all assays on the PGx panel have pediatric guidelines. Our PM group has one doctor of pharmacy that can interact with providers at any time to offer education and clinical information support. Our testing facility is housed within the Department of Pathology and Laboratory Medicine, which conforms to all regulations mandated by CLIA '88, the College of American Pathologists, and the American Association of Blood Banks. The accuracy of all analytical data is verified by a board-certified molecular pathologist, then sent to a third party for final genotype-phenotype interpretation. St. Jude's and Cincinnati Children's offer excellent PGx testing services comparable to the testing at ACH. For a PGx test to be successful, it requires complete patient drug coverage, easy ordering by providers, a quick turnaround time for interpreted results, and all easily available in the patient EHR.

4.3. EHR-Based Clinical Decision Support Systems (CDSS)

Pediatric hospitals have begun integrating PGx CDSS in their EHRs. The level of integration includes real-time at the point of care PGx treatment guidelines and dosing recommendations, ranging from interruptive alerts suggesting treatment recommendations to providing guidance to the presence of a specific PGx variant for a specific medication [11,36,37]. Some institutions leverage the use of machine learning and natural language processing to extract triggers for CDSS [38], and others have incorporated the patient consent process into the CDS workflow [36]. More importantly, institutions have established CDSS governance structures to help guide the implementation of PGx CDSS [11,36,37].

4.4. Challenges and Barriers to PGx Implementation

An extensive review of ongoing clinical pharmacogenomics implementation programs at various hospitals and institutions highlighted several adoption and implementation barriers for us to overcome, including scientific, information technology (IT), lack of education of clinical staff and patients, test reimbursement, PGx clinical decision support (CDS), lack of clinician adoption, and data storage for clinical research [12,39–42].

4.4.1. Education of Future Clinicians on PGx

A recent survey [43] of medical schools about perceptions on adding pharmacogenomics instruction to the medical curricula found that physicians and health care workers do not possess appropriate knowledge of PGx. A more recent work also illustrated the point that pharmacists and clinicians can gain understanding of PGx through education [44]. There is an urgent need to incorporate the PGx curriculum in medical school education, so the next generation of physicians can incorporate personalized therapies for their patients' wellbeing into their routine clinical practice.

In addition, much has been evaluated about the role of pharmacists in PGx. In a recent study, 35% (339 out of 978) of last-year pharmacy students across eight east coast college's felt that pharmacogenomics is a useful tool for pharmacists, yet only 40% of these same students considered it to be an important part of their training [45]. There was varying exposure to pharmacogenomics training, although many understood the clinical importance of PGx. At ACH, the plan is to focus on subspecialties that are knowledgeable of PGx and then expand to other subspecialties by building BPAs and educating clinical staff.

4.4.2. Consent/Parent Awareness

An important component of PGx testing at ACH is the informed consent process. With this in mind, it is crucial that the family be aware that the testing is offered and ordered, as appropriate. Parents/Guardians and/or patients must be given complete information about the risks and benefits of this testing and be given the opportunity to ask questions before providing informed consent. As with other genetic testing consent procedures, this should occur in an area that allows the patient and/or their parents and guardians to focus on the information presented without overt distractions. Empowering parents/guardians and patients as crucial members of the care team provides the opportunity for them to advocate for their health as future need arises.

4.4.3. Cost of PGx Test

The configuration of the OpenArray® (www.Thermofisher.com) TaqMan SNP-based genotyping PGx panel can accommodate a maximum of 16 samples per run; of these, two are dedicated to quality control. Therefore, a maximum of 14 patient samples can be performed on a single open-array chip. Fixed-cost test components include all reagents needed to extract and purify genomic DNA and perform analytical testing (USD 170 per patient sample), and the interpretative report generated by Translational Software Inc. (USD 35 per patient sample). Variable cost test components include technical labor (9 h at USD 30 per hour) and the OpenArray® chip (USD 720). More specifically, the variable cost of technical labor ranges from USD 270 (1 patient sample per run) to USD 19 (14 patient samples per run). Likewise, the variable cost of the OpenArray® chip ranges from USD 720 (1 patient sample per run) to USD 51 (14 samples per run). Using a blended fixed and variable cost matrix calculation, the total cost to perform the open array pharmacogenomics panel ranges from USD 1195 (1 patient plus 2 controls) to USD 276 (14 patients plus 2 controls).

4.4.4. Test Reimbursement

For billing purposes, each gene on the SNP-based genotyping pharmacogenomics test is paired with the corresponding AMA-approved CPT code as follows: *CYP2C19* (81225), *CYP2D6* (81226), *CYP2C9* (81227), *CYP3A4* (81230), *CYP3A5* (81231), *F2* (81240), *F5* (81241), *G6PD* (81247), *NUDT15* (81306), *SLCO1B1* (81328), *TPMT* (81335), *UGT1A1* (81350), and *VKORC1* (81355). CPT code 81479 is used for the following genes that currently lack AMA-approved CPT codes: *ACYP2*, *CEP72*, *CYP2C*, *CYP4F2*, *RARG*, *SLC6A4*, *SLC28A3*, *RYR1*, and *CACNA1S*. From 21 September 2020 to 12 March 2021, a total of 29 tests had been ordered. At this time, we do not have sufficient data to understand reimbursement based upon patient insurance (Medicaid, private insurance, etc.).

4.5. Integration of PGx Test Results into EPIC

Integration of PGx data into the EHR must ensure that the information related to the drug-gene pair maintains analytical validity, as well as the clinical utility of the test [46]. Currently, clinically relevant genetic results are often considered very similar to laboratory results, where the genetic report and raw genetic data are stored outside of the EHR [47]. Standards in implementing, storing, and transmitting genetic information across EHR systems have been poorly adopted. When it contains properly integrated PGx data, an EHR should be able to support timely access to genomic information at the point of care, trigger clinical decision support mechanisms, and facilitate ordering tests and tracking their results as well as notifying patients and families [48]. A recent survey of multidisciplinary healthcare providers found that 71.3% were slightly or not at all familiar with PGx, which suggests additional education and electronic resources are needed for pediatric PGx examples [49].

We performed a pharmacogenomics knowledge-assessment survey of prescribers at Arkansas Children's prior to the launch of PGx testing to help tailor our educational program [50]. The survey showed that prescribing clinicians are interested in the opportunity to provide PGx testing to their patients at ACH. Prescribers recognized the need for additional information about PGx and welcomed eLearning and specialty-specific educational sessions as alternative means of education. In addition, clinicians were concerned about cost, turnaround time, and efficacy of the test. Of note, a representative sample of younger clinicians (resident house staff) responded to the survey, perhaps presenting as a marker for their readiness to consider PGx as part of their routine decision-making process.

5. Conclusions

Pharmacogenomics (PGx) can help prevent ADRs and improve drug efficacy by enabling the physician to optimize drug dosage and avoid prescribing medications with adverse reactions due to the patient's genetic makeup. At ACH, PGx testing was successfully implemented with EPIC-based clinical decision support (CDS) for 66 pediatric drugs based upon genotype analysis of 174 single nucleotide polymorphisms (SNPs) targeting 23 actionable PGx gene variants. The clinicians receive discrete results for genotype-guided therapy in EPIC-based EHR. Although laboratory turnaround times are relatively short, it is not unusual for a patient's medication list to change in the time between when a test is ordered and the report is generated. To make the final PGx report more accurate, an application is in development under EPIC's App Orchard program that will allow the reporting engine to query the patient's medication list using EPIC's implementation of the Fast Health Interoperability Resource (FHIR) and an application programming interface (API). Efforts are underway to educate providers on how to order and incorporate these data into standard practice. We hope to provide cutting-edge technology and knowledge to a pediatric population that is often forgotten, but we know this starts with understanding the data and educating team members.

Pharmacogenomics is fast becoming a mainstay for the delivery of 21st century healthcare. Arkansas Children's clinicians are open to learning more about the promise of PGx for genotype-guided dosing and are eager to utilize this process to improve the quality of pediatric clinical care.

Supplementary Materials: The following are available online at https://www.mdpi.com/article/10.3390/jpm11050394/s1, Figure S1: Mock comprehensive PGx report shows patient on drugs Clopidogrel and Codeine. Figure S2: PGx test details provide information on gene, genotype, phenotype, and alleles tested.

Author Contributions: Conceptualization for study and PGx panel: P.S.G., F.B.Y.J., D.L.B., and G.B.S.; funding acquisition—G.B.S., P.S.G., and D.L.B.; supervision—P.S.G., D.L.B., G.B.S., P.A.P.-G., and F.B.Y.J.; methodology—QuantStudio™12K Flex system and OpenArray® PGx panel validation and standard operating protocols (SOPs): P.A.P.-G., F.B.Y.J., B.L.B.J., P.S.G., and J.C.A.; validations—EPIC built modules and drug-gene pair alerts: J.C.A., P.A.P.-G., F.B.Y.J., D.R., J.E.F., A.V., P.P., K.J.B., E.S., A.B., D.L.B., G.B.S., J.L.K., J.L.C., and B.L.B.J.; writing of manuscript: P.S.G., F.B.Y.J., P.A.P.-G., B.L.B.J., D.R., J.E.F., J.C.A., P.P., A.B., K.J.B., E.S., D.L.B., A.V., J.L.K., J.L.C., and G.B.S. All authors have read and agreed to the published version of the manuscript.

Funding: We gratefully acknowledge support from the Arkansas Children's Research Institute (ACRI) and the Arkansas Children's Foundation, Little Rock, Arkansas.

Institutional Review Board Statement: The study was conducted according to the guidelines of the Declaration of Helsinki, and approved by Institutional Review Board of the University of Arkansas for Medical Sciences (IRB# 262792). Ethical review and approval were waived, as it was determined that this project is NOT human subject research as defined in 45 CFR 46.102, and therefore it does not fall under the jurisdiction of the IRB review process.

Informed Consent Statement: Written Informed consent was obtained from all subjects involved in the study for PGx panel validation.

Data Availability Statement: PGx panel validation data are available on request.

Acknowledgments: The authors would like to thank Arkansas Children's Research Institute (ACRI) and Arkansas Children's Foundation, Little Rock, Arkansas for their support during all stages of the project. The PGx program at ACH was founded with generous philanthropic support from two donors with a strong personal interest in contributing to the startup of a Precision Medicine Group at ACRI.

Conflicts of Interest: D.R. is primary shareholder in Translational Software, Inc. (TSI). All other authors reported no conflict of interest.

References

1. Nebert, D.W. Pharmacogenetics and pharmacogenomics: Why is this relevant to the clinical geneticist? *Clin. Genet.* **1999**, *56*, 247–258. [CrossRef]
2. Sunshine, J.E.; Meo, N.; Kassebaum, N.J.; Collison, M.L.; Mokdad, A.H.; Naghavi, M. Association of Adverse Effects of Medical Treatment with Mortality in the United States: A Secondary Analysis of the Global Burden of Diseases, Injuries, and Risk Factors Study. *JAMA Netw. Open* **2019**, *2*, e187041. [CrossRef]
3. U.S. FDA. Preventable Adverse Drug Reactions: A Focus on Drug Interactions. Available online: https://www.fda.gov/drugs/drug-interactions-labeling/preventable-adverse-drug-reactions-focus-drug-interactions (accessed on 1 March 2021).
4. Kongkaew, C.; Noyce, P.R.; Ashcroft, D.M. Hospital admissions associated with adverse drug reactions: A systematic review of prospective observational studies. *Ann. Pharmacother.* **2008**, *42*, 1017–1025. [CrossRef]

5. Giacomini, K.M.; Yee, S.W.; Ratain, M.J.; Weinshilboum, R.M.; Kamatani, N.; Nakamura, Y. Pharmacogenomics and patient care: One size does not fit all. *Sci. Transl. Med.* **2012**, *4*, 153ps18. [CrossRef] [PubMed]
6. Lander, E.S.; Linton, L.M.; Birren, B.; Nusbaum, C.; Zody, M.C.; Baldwin, J.; Devon, K.; Dewar, K.; Doyle, M.; FitzHugh, W.; et al. Initial sequencing and analysis of the human genome. *Nature* **2001**, *409*, 860–921.
7. International HapMap Consortium. A second generation human haplotype map of over 3.1 million SNPs. *Nature* **2007**, *449*, 851. [CrossRef]
8. 1000 Genomes Project Consortium. A global reference for human genetic variation. *Nature* **2015**, *526*, 68–74. [CrossRef]
9. Pirmohamed, M. Pharmacogenetics and pharmacogenomics. *Br. J. Clin. Pharmacol.* **2001**, *52*, 345–347. [CrossRef]
10. Van Driest, S.L.; McGregor, T.L. Pharmacogenetics in clinical pediatrics: Challenges and strategies. *Personal. Med.* **2013**, *10*, 661–671. [CrossRef]
11. Ramsey, L.B.; Prows, C.A.; Zhang, K.; Saldana, S.N.; Sorter, M.T.; Pestian, J.P.; Wenstrup, R.J.; Vinks, A.A.; Glauser, T.A. Implementation of pharmacogenetics at Cincinnati Children's hospital medical center: Lessons learned over 14 years of personalizing medicine. *Clin. Pharmacol. Ther.* **2019**, *105*, 49–52. [CrossRef]
12. NHGRI. *The National Human Genome Research Institute (NHGRI) Sponsored Its 10th Genomic Medicine Meeting—Genomic Medicine X*; NHGRI: Silver Spring, MD, USA, 2017. Available online: https://www.genome.gov/27568408/genomic-medicine-x-research-directions-in-pharmacogenomics-implementation (accessed on 1 March 2021).
13. Hicks, J.K.; Sangkuhl, K.J.J.; Swen, J.J.; Ellingrod, V.L.; Muller, D.J.; Shimoda, K.; Bishop, J.R.; Kharasch, E.D.; Skaar, T.C.; Gaedigk, A.; et al. Clinical pharmacogenetics implementation consortium guideline (CPIC) for CYP2D6 and CYP2C19 genotypes and dosing of tricyclic antidepressants: 2016 update. *Clin. Pharmacol. Ther.* **2017**, *102*, 37–44. [CrossRef]
14. U.S. FDA. Available online: https://www.fda.gov/medical-devices/precision-medicine/table-pharmacogenetic-associations (accessed on 1 March 2021).
15. CPIC. Available online: https://cpicpgx.org/guidelines/ (accessed on 1 March 2021).
16. DPWG. Available online: https://upgx.eu/guidelines/ (accessed on 1 March 2021).
17. PharmGKB. Available online: http://www.pharmgkb.org (accessed on 1 March 2021).
18. Gatter, K. FDA oversight of laboratory-developed tests: Where are we now? *Arch. Pathol. Lab. Med.* **2017**, *141*, 746–748. [CrossRef] [PubMed]
19. Genzen, J.R.; Mohlman, J.S.; Lynch, J.L.; Squires, M.E.; Weiss, R.L. Laboratory-Developed Tests: A Legislative and Regulatory Review. *Clin. Chem.* **2017**, *63*, 1575–1584. [CrossRef] [PubMed]
20. CLIA'88. Available online: https://www.govinfo.gov/content/pkg/STATUTE-102/pdf/STATUTE-102-Pg2903.pdf (accessed on 1 March 2021).
21. Scott, S.A.; Sangkuhl, K.C.M.; Stein, C.M.; Hulot, J.-S.; Roden, D.M.; Klein, T.E.; Sabatine, M.S.; Johnson, J.A.; Shuldiner, A.R. Clinical Pharmacogenetics Implementation Consortium guidelines for CYP2C19 genotype and clopidogrel therapy. *Clin. Pharmacol. Ther.* **2013**, *94*, 317–323. [CrossRef]
22. Relling, M.V.; Schwab, M.; Whirl-Carrillo, M.; Suarez-Kurtz, G.; Pui, C.-H.; Stein, C.M.; Moyer, A.M.; Evans, W.E.; Klein, T.E.; Antillon-Klussmann, F.G.; et al. Clinical Pharmacogenetics Implementation Consortium Guideline for Thiopurine Dosing Based on TPMT and NUDT15 Genotypes: 2018 Update. *Clin. Pharmacol. Ther.* **2019**, *105*, 1095–1105. [CrossRef]
23. Karnes, J.H.; Rettie, A.E.; Somogyi, A.A.; Huddart, R.; Fohner, A.E.; Formea, C.M.; Ta, M.L.M.; Llerna, A.; Whirl-Carrillo, M.; Klein, T.E.; et al. Clinical Pharmacogenetics Implementation Consortium (CPIC) Guideline for CYP2C9 and HLA-B Genotypes and Phenytoin Dosing: 2020 Update. *Clin. Pharmacol. Ther.* **2021**, *109*, 302–309. [CrossRef] [PubMed]
24. O'Kane, D.J.; Weinshilboum, R.M.; Moyer, T.P. Pharmacogenomics and reducing the frequency of adverse drug events. *Pharmacogenomics* **2003**, *4*, 1–4. [CrossRef]
25. Elzagallaai, A.A.; Greff, M.; Rieder, M.J. Adverse Drug Reactions in Children: The Double-Edged Sword of Therapeutics. *Clin. Pharmacol. Ther.* **2017**, *101*, 725–735. [CrossRef]
26. Weinshilboum, R.M.; Wang, L. Pharmacogenomics: Precision Medicine and Drug Response. *Mayo Clin. Proc.* **2017**, *92*, 1711–1722. [CrossRef]
27. U.S. FDA. Available online: https://www.fda.gov/drugs/information-consumers-and-patients-drugs/drug-research-and-children (accessed on 1 March 2021).
28. Hines, R. The ontogeny of drug metabolism enzymes and implications for adverse drug events. *Pharmacol. Ther.* **2008**, *118*, 250–267. [CrossRef]
29. Ramsey, L.B.; Namerow, L.B.; Bishop, J.R.; Hicks, J.K.; Bousman, C.; Croarkin, P.E.; Mathews, C.A.; Van Driest, S.L.; Strawn, J.R. Thoughtful Clinical Use of Pharmacogenetics in Child and Adolescent Psychopharmacology. *J. Am. Acad. Child Adolesc. Psychiatry* **2020**. [CrossRef] [PubMed]
30. De Wildt, S.N.; Tibboel, D.; Leeder, J.S. Drug metabolism for the paediatrician. *Arch. Dis. Child.* **2014**, *99*, 1137–1142. [CrossRef]
31. Serpe, L.; Calvo, P.L.; Muntoni, E.; D'Antico, S.; Giaccone, M.; Avagnina, A.; Baldi, M.; Barbera, C.; Curti, F.; Pera, A.; et al. Thiopurine S-methyltransferase pharmacogenetics in a large-scale healthy Italian-Caucasian population: Differences in enzyme activity. *Pharmacogenomics* **2009**, *10*, 1753–1765. [CrossRef] [PubMed]
32. Bielinski, S.J.; Olson, J.E.; Pathak, J.; Weinshilboum, R.M.; Wang, L.; Lyke, K.J.; Ryu, E.; Targonski, P.V.; Van Norstrand, M.D.; Hathcock, M.A.; et al. Preemptive genotyping for personalized medicine: Design of the right drug, right dose, right time-using genomic data to individualize treatment protocol. *Mayo Clin. Proc.* **2014**, *89*, 25–33. [CrossRef]

33. Van Driest, S.L.; Shi, Y.; Bowton, E.A.; Schildcrout, J.S.; Peterson, J.F.; Pulley, J.; Denny, J.C.; Roden, D.M. Clinically actionable genotypes among 10,000 patients with preemptive pharmacogenomic testing. *Clin. Pharmacol. Ther.* **2014**, *95*, 423–431. [CrossRef] [PubMed]
34. Ramsey, L.B.; Brown, J.T.; Vear, S.I.; Bishop, J.R.; Van Driest, S.L. Gene-Based Dose Optimization in Children. *Annu. Rev. Pharmacol. Toxicol.* **2020**, *60*, 311–331. [CrossRef] [PubMed]
35. Personalized Medicine Coalition. Available online: http://www.personalizedmedicinecoalition.org/News/Press_Releases/New_Personalized_Medicine_Report_Shows_RecordSetting_Growth_to_286_in_Number_of_Personalized_Medicines_Available_Documents_Challenges_in_Regulation_Reimbursement_Clinical_Adoption (accessed on 1 March 2021).
36. Hoffman, J.M.; Haidar, C.E.; Wilkinson, M.R.; Crews, K.R.; Baker, D.K.; Kornegay, N.M.; Yang, W.; Pui, C.H.; Reiss, U.M.; Gaur, A.H.; et al. PG4KDS: A Model for the Clinical Implementation of Pre-emptive Pharmacogenetics. *Am. J. Med. Genet. Part C Semin. Med. Genet.* **2014**, *1*, 45–55. [CrossRef]
37. Pulley, J.M.; Denny, J.C.; Peterson, J.F.; Bernard, G.R.; Vnencak-Jones, C.L.; Ramirez, A.H.; Delaney, J.T.; Bowton, E.; Brothers, K.; Johnson, K.; et al. Operational Implementation of Prospective Genotyping for Personalized Medicine: The Design of the Vanderbilt PREDICT Project. *Clin. Pharmacol. Ther.* **2012**, *1*, 87–95. [CrossRef]
38. Gregornik, D.; Salyakina, D.; Brown, M.; Roiko, S.; Ramos, K. Pediatric pharmacogenomics: Challenges and opportunities: On behalf of the Sanford Children's Genomic Medicine Consortium. *Pharm. J.* **2021**, *21*, 8–19. [CrossRef]
39. Dunnenberger, H.M.; Biszewski, M.; Bell, G.C.; Sereika, A.; May, H.; Johnson, S.G.; Hulick, P.J.; Khandekar, J. Implementation of a multidisciplinary pharmacogenomics clinic in a community health system. *Am. J. Health Syst. Pharm.* **2016**, *73*, 1956–1966. [CrossRef]
40. Haga, S.B. Pharmacogenomic Testing in Pediatrics: Navigating the Ethical, Social, And Legal Challenges. *Pharmgenomics Pers. Med.* **2019**, *12*, 273–285. [CrossRef] [PubMed]
41. Giri, J.; Moyer, A.M.; Bielinski, S.J.; Caraballo, P.J. Concepts Driving Pharmacogenomics Implementation into Everyday Healthcare. *Pharmgenomics Pers. Med.* **2019**, *12*, 305–318. [CrossRef] [PubMed]
42. Cicali, E.J.; Weitzel, K.W.; Elsey, A.R.; Orlando, F.A.; Vinson, M.; Mosley, S.; Smith, D.M.; Davis, R.; Drum, L.; Estores, D.; et al. Challenges and lessons learned from clinical pharmacogenetic implementation of multiple gene-drug pairs across ambulatory care settings. *Genet. Med.* **2019**, *21*, 2264–2274. [CrossRef] [PubMed]
43. Basyouni, D.; Shatnawi, A. Pharmacogenomics Instruction Depth, Extent, and Perception in US Medical Curricula. *J. Med. Educ. Curric. Dev.* **2020**, *7*. [CrossRef] [PubMed]
44. Guy, J.W.; Patel, I.; Oestreich, J.H. Clinical Application and Educational Training for Pharmacogenomics. *Pharmacy* **2020**, *8*, 163. [CrossRef] [PubMed]
45. Coriolan, S.; Arikawe, N.; Arden Moscati, A.; Zhou, L.; Dyn, S.; Donmez, S.; Garba, A.; Falbaum, S.; Loewy, Z.; Lull, M.; et al. Pharmacy students' attitudes and perceptions toward pharmacogenomics education. *Am. J. Health Syst. Pharm.* **2019**, *76*, 836–845. [CrossRef]
46. Lose, E.J. The emerging role of primary care in genetics. *Curr. Opin. Pediatr.* **2008**, *20*, 634–638. [CrossRef]
47. Green, E.D.; Guyer, M.S. Charting a course for genomic medicine from base pairs to bedside. *Nature* **2011**, *470*, 204–213. [CrossRef] [PubMed]
48. Schrijver, I.; Aziz, N.; Farkas, D.H.; Furtado, M.; Gonzalez, A.F.; Greiner, T.C.; Grody, W.W.; Hambuch, T.; Kalman, L.; Kant, J.A.; et al. Opportunities and challenges associated with clinical diagnostic genome sequencing: A report of the Association for Molecular Pathology. *J. Mol. Diagn.* **2012**, *14*, 525–540. [CrossRef]
49. Liko, I.; Lee, Y.M.; Stutzman, D.L.; Blackmer, A.B.; Deininger, K.M.; Reynolds, A.M.; Aquilante, C.L. Providers' perspectives on the clinical utility of pharmacogenomic testing in pediatric patients. *Pharmacogenomics* **2021**, *22*, 263–274. [CrossRef]
50. Porter-Gill, P.A.; Gill, P.; Schaefer, G.B.; Allen, J.; Boyanton, B.L.; Yu, F. Arkansas Physicians' Interests and learning opportunities with Pharmacogenomics. *J. Ark. Med. Soc.* **2021**, in press.

Article

Effects of CYP3A5 Polymorphism on Rapid Progression of Chronic Kidney Disease: A Prospective, Multicentre Study

Fei Yee Lee [1,2], Farida Islahudin [1,*], Aina Yazrin Ali Nasiruddin [1,3], Abdul Halim Abdul Gafor [4], Hin-Seng Wong [2,5], Sunita Bavanandan [6], Shamin Mohd Saffian [1], Adyani Md Redzuan [1], Nurul Ain Mohd Tahir [1] and Mohd Makmor-Bakry [1]

1. Centre for Quality Management of Medicines, Faculty of Pharmacy, Universiti Kebangsaan Malaysia, Kuala Lumpur 50300, Malaysia; feiyee7890@gmail.com (F.Y.L.); aina@cyberjaya.edu.my (A.Y.A.N.); shamin@ukm.edu.my (S.M.S.); adyani@ukm.edu.my (A.M.R.); nurulainmt@ukm.edu.my (N.A.M.T.); mohdclinpharm@ukm.edu.my (M.M.-B.)
2. Clinical Research Centre, Hospital Selayang, Ministry of Health Malaysia, Batu Caves, Selangor 60800, Malaysia; hinseng@gmail.com
3. Faculty of Pharmacy, University of Cyberjaya, Cyberjaya 63000, Malaysia
4. Nephrology Unit, Department of Medicine, Universiti Kebangsaan Malaysia Medical Centre, Kuala Lumpur 56000, Malaysia; halimgafor@gmail.com
5. Nephrology Department, Hospital Selayang, Ministry of Health Malaysia, Batu Caves, Selangor 60800, Malaysia
6. Nephrology Department, Hospital Kuala Lumpur, Ministry of Health Malaysia, Kuala Lumpur 50586, Malaysia; sbavanandan@gmail.com
* Correspondence: faridaislahudin@ukm.edu.my; Tel.: +60-392-897-971

Abstract: Personalised medicine is potentially useful to delay the progression of chronic kidney disease (CKD). The aim of this study was to determine the effects of CYP3A5 polymorphism in rapid CKD progression. This multicentre, observational, prospective cohort study was performed among adult CKD patients ($\geq$18 years) with estimated glomerular filtration rate (eGFR) $\geq$30 mL/min/1.73 m^2, who had $\geq$4 outpatient, non-emergency eGFR values during the three-year study period. The blood samples collected were analysed for *CYP3A5*3* polymorphism. Rapid CKD progression was defined as eGFR decline of >5 mL/min/1.73 m^2/year. Multiple logistic regression was then performed to identify the factors associated with rapid CKD progression. A total of 124 subjects consented to participate. The distribution of the genotypes adhered to the Hardy–Weinberg equilibrium (X^2 = 0.237, p = 0.626). After adjusting for potential confounding factors via multiple logistic regression, the factors associated with rapid CKD progression were *CYP3A5*3/*3* polymorphism (adjusted Odds Ratio [aOR] 4.190, 95% confidence interval [CI]: 1.268, 13.852), adjustments to antihypertensives, young age, dyslipidaemia, smoking and use of traditional/complementary medicine. CKD patients should be monitored closely for possible factors associated with rapid CKD progression to optimise clinical outcomes. The *CYP3A5*3/*3* genotype could potentially be screened among CKD patients to offer more individualised management among these patients.

Keywords: pharmacogenomics; clinical translation; chronic kidney disease; CYP3A5; polymorphism; progression

1. Introduction

Chronic kidney disease (CKD) is a rising public health problem with an alarming increasing trend [1]. During management of CKD patients, optimal control is important to delay disease progression [2]. The control of progression among CKD patients is very often reliant on various pharmacological treatments, such as antihypertensives and antidiabetic drugs, to manage complications associated with kidney failure. However, pharmacotherapy requires close monitoring in order to delay rapid progression of CKD. Rapid progression of CKD is associated with poorer clinical outcomes, including cardiovascular events and death, irrespective of renal function [3]. Recently, optimising management has been focused on personalised treatment, involving identification of interpatient variability, as well as optimisation of treatment effectiveness and safety based on pharmacogenetic data [4].

Pharmacogenetic differences in the cytochrome P (CYP) 450 system have been of interest, as CYP450 enzymes metabolise more than 80% of all prescribed drugs [5]. One of the most common CYP450 enzymes among Asians is the CYP3A5, in which the single nucleotide polymorphisms (SNP) were found in 65.7–71.3% of the Asian population [6]. Genetic polymorphism of CYP3A5 affects the quantity of the functioning enzyme, which then potentially affects the metabolism of various drugs [7]. Interindividual variations of the *CYP3A5* gene expression occur with the presence of the *CYP3A5*3* allele, which causes a replacement of adenine (A) by a guanine (G), at position 6986 of the intron 3, creating a cryptic splice site that causes a premature stop codon, leading to the absence of the CYP3A5 protein [7,8]. Thus, individuals with the *CYP3A5*3* allele tend to express a lesser amount of CYP3A5 enzyme [7]. Despite the highly polymorphic nature of *CYP3A5* gene with variants from *CYP3A5*1* to *CYP3A5*9*, *CYP3A5*3* polymorphism (rs776746, RefSeq NG_007938.2:g.12083A>G) is the most commonly reported CYP3A5 polymorphism in almost all populations [6].

Potentially, the *CYP3A5*3* polymorphism could affect both antihypertensive management as well as blood pressure control [8–12]. Approximately 90% of CKD patients are treated with antihypertensive agents, of which pharmacogenetics have been shown to influence outcomes [13]. Interestingly, *CYP3A5*3* polymorphism has been found to be associated with variability in blood pressure response to several calcium-channel blockers, such as amlodipine [8], felodipine [9], diltiazem [10] and verapamil [11,12]. In contrast, the influence of *CYP3A5*3* pharmacogenetics was found to be lacking towards first-line antihypertensives for CKD, namely angiotensin converting enzyme inhibitor (ACEI) and angiotensin II blocker (ARB) [6]. Apart from the potential influence on drug-metabolising properties, the polymorphism of the *CYP3A5* gene has also been studied previously for its role in blood pressure control [8]. In animals, CYP3A5 enzymes have been shown to convert cortisol to 6β-hydroxycortisol, followed by promotion of post-renal proximal tubular sodium reabsorption, water retention and elevation of blood pressure [8].

Hypertension is a known consequence, as well as a cause, of CKD. Studies have shown that CKD progression is notably accelerated when blood pressure is sustainably high [3]. CYP3A5 activity may be related to the pathogenesis of CKD progression, through reduction of the renin-angiotensin-aldosterone system (RAAS) activity [14]. The CYP3A5 enzyme may reduce RAAS activity by converting corticosterone to 6β-hydroxycorticosterone instead of aldosterone, which subsequently reduces the aldosterone-induced RAAS activity [8]. This is also supported by the findings of a recent study involving CKD patients that showed 20-hydroxyeicosatetraenoic (HETE) acid, a product of CYP enzyme, is a predictor of CKD progression [15].

The possible link of CYP3A5 activity with blood pressure control, drug-metabolising activity of CYP3A5 and CKD progression have highlighted the potential role of CYP3A5 pharmacogenetics in optimising therapeutic management. Therapeutic outcomes could be better if monitoring based on CYP3A5-polymorphism status could be conducted, to adjust for the unexpected effects of medications driven by the SNP. The association between *CYP3A5*3* polymorphism and antihypertensive medication, blood pressure control and CKD progression show marked differences in results reported from different ethnicities and geographical locations [8]. Asians have been reported to exhibit faster CKD progression than Caucasians, which was not found to be related to their demographic and clinical characteristics, as well as their laboratory parameters [16]. Therefore, it is increasingly important to investigate genetic factors among this population, to identify potential factors that may contribute to the risk of rapid CKD progression. The impact of CYP3A5 polymorphism in Asians might be more profound than other CYP enzymes, given its higher prevalence than other CYP enzymes [6]. Therefore, the aim of this research was to determine the effects of *CYP3A5*3* genetic polymorphisms in rapid CKD progression among an Asian population of CKD patients with routine nephrology care.

2. Materials and Methods

2.1. Study Design

This multicentre, observational, prospective cohort study was performed among adult CKD patients (aged $\geq$ 18 years), with an estimated glomerular filtration rate (eGFR) of 30 mL/min/1.73 m^2 and above [3], in three tertiary hospitals with specialist nephrology clinics in Malaysia. The study was approved by the Medical Research Ethics Committee, Malaysia (KKM.NIHSEC.P19-2320(11))and the Universiti Kebangsaan Malaysia Research Ethic Committee (UKM PPI/111/8/JEP-2020-048). This study was conducted in compliance with ethical principles outlined in the Declaration of Helsinki and the Malaysian Good Clinical Practice Guidelines. The study report follows the Strengthening the Reporting Of Pharmacogenetic Studies (STROPS) guidelines [17].

Potentially eligible patients were identified via pre-screening from patient clinic lists and data from medical records. Patients were then recruited by the investigators during clinic visits from March 2020 until September 2020. Written informed consent was obtained from every subject prior to participation in this study. Patients with at least four outpatient visits and non-emergency eGFR values during the three-year study period were recruited, to ensure sufficient information was available to estimate the risk of CKD progression [18]. Patients who were pregnant, lactating, had incomplete medication regimen or without routine nephrology care were excluded.

2.2. Data Collection

After informed consent was obtained from subjects, each participant was assigned a unique subject identification number. Subjects' names were kept on a password-protected database. Demographic data, clinical information, laboratory data and medication characteristics for each subject from January 2018 to December 2020 were collected from the medical records from the respective institutions. Demographic data that were collected were age, sex and ethnicity.

The clinical information included the primary cause of CKD, co-morbidities, obesity (defined as body mass index (BMI) of 30 kg/m^2 and above), smoking status and blood pressure level, measured during clinic visits. The laboratory data collected were serum creatinine, albuminuria/proteinuria status and haemoglobin level during the study period.

Medication profiles of the subjects, adherence to medications and the use of traditional or complementary medicine (TCM) were compiled from the electronic medical record and prescription data, as well as from a structured interview with the subjects on their medication-taking behaviour, conducted by two investigators using a standardised questionnaire [2]. The data on the number of adjustments to antihypertensives (changes in dosage, frequency, timing or cessation, or commencement of new antihypertensives) were collected.

2.3. Study Definitions

Patients' renal function were quantified via eGFR calculated using the CKD Epidemiology Collaboration (CKD-EPI) equation. The CKD and albuminuria classification was based on the Kidney Disease: Improving Global Outcomes Workgroup (KDIGO) 2012 guidelines [18]. The definitions for each category are detailed in Table 1.

Patients' renal function were quantified via eGFR calculated using the CKD-EPI equation, using outpatient, non-emergency serum creatinine values [3]. Emergency serum creatinine values were defined as serum creatinine values obtained during visits to an emergency department. These values were excluded to avoid interference of transiently elevated serum creatinine values, due to acute illness or acute kidney injury (AKI) rather than actual CKD progression. The rapid progression of CKD was defined as a sustained decline in eGFR of more than 5 mL/min/1.73 m^2/year, in line with the KDIGO CKD guidelines [18] (Table 1). AKI was detected using the KDIGO guideline criteria from the serum creatinine values, as well as information about AKI episodes that occurred in other healthcare institutions and were documented in the subjects' medical records.

Table 1. Terminologies and their definitions. pertaining to the study.

Terminology		Definition
Classification of CKD [18]	Stage 1	Normal or elevated GFR, with GFR of 90 mL/min/1.73 m² and above
	Stage 2	Mildly decreased GFR of 60–89 mL/min/1.73 m²
	Stage 3a	Mild to moderately decreased GFR of 45–59 mL/min/1.73 m²
	Stage 3b	Moderately to severely decreased GFR of 30–44 mL/min/1.73 m²
	Stage 4	Severely decreased GFR of 15–29 mL/min/1.73 m²
	Stage 5	Low eGFR of less than 15 mL/min/1.73 m²
Albuminuria categorisation [18]	A1	Protein-to-creatinine ratio (PCR) of less than 15 mg/mmol and below or negative to trace from urine protein reagent strip
	A2	PCR of 15–50 mg/mmol or trace to + from urine protein reagent strip
	A3	PCR of more than 50 mg/mmol, or greater than + from urine protein reagent strip
Progression of CKD	Rapid CKD progression	Sustained decline in eGFR of more than 5 mL/min/1.73 m²/year [18], based on the rate of annual eGFR change using linear regression model to identify the eGFR slope using the eGFR collected during the study period [3]
Types of non-adherence [19]	Initiation phase	Medication is not taken by patient at all
	Implementation phase	A dose is missed, omitted or an extra dose taken
	Persistence phase	The medication is ceased without the instruction of prescriber
Others	TCM consumption	The use of therapies not included in the treatment and medicines prescribed by hospitals or health clinics, such as the use of herbs (or botanicals), as well as over-the-counter nutritional and dietary supplements, based on patient recall [20]

Routine nephrology care was defined as documentation of ambulatory nephrology care by a nephrologist in the medical records for at least 5 years [21].

Adjustments to antihypertensives included changes in dosage, frequency and timing, as well as cessation or commencement of new antihypertensives [20].

Adherence to medications was considered to be poor if there was a discrepancy between the prescribers' order and actual medication taken [19], based on documentations in medical records and patient recall (Table 1).

Consumption of TCM was defined as the use of treatment and medicines not prescribed from hospitals or health clinics, such as the use of herbs (or botanicals), as well as over-the-counter nutritional and dietary supplements, based on patient recall [20].

2.4. Sample Size

Prior data indicate that the proportion of the *CYP3A5*3/*3* genetic polymorphism status is 0.437 [6] and the population size of eligible patients was 180. If the Type I error probability and precision are 0.05 and 0.05, the sample size is 124 samples [22].

2.5. Detection of CYP3A5*3 Gene Polymorphism

Genomic DNA was extracted from blood samples using a DNeasy® Blood and Tissue extraction kit (Qiagen, Hilden, Germany). The extracted genomic DNA was then analysed for purity and measured for concentration through OPTIZEN NanoQ spectrophotometer (Kaia Bio-Ingenieria, Daejeon, Korea), in which the 260/280 absorption ratio between 1.70 to 1.99 was considered to be DNA with sufficient purity without contamination during the extraction process [23]. The extracted genomic DNA was stored at −80 °C until use.

The intron 3 of the CYP3A5 gene encompassing the rs776746 (RefSeq NG_007938.2: g.12083A>G) polymorphism was amplified by the primers 5′-CAGCAAGAGTCTCACA CAGG-3′ (Forward) and 5′-TACCACCCAGCTTAACGAAT-3′ (Reverse) (IDT DNA, Singapore) and TopTaq Mastermix Kit (Qiagen, Hilden, Germany) using the Arktik™ Thermal Cycler (Thermo Fisher Scientific, Finland). The polymerase chain reaction (PCR) products were examined by gel electrophoresis to ensure the quality of PCR products through Invitrogen™ 2% E-Gel™ Agarose Gels with SYBR Safe™ (Thermo Fisher Scientific, Kiryat Shmona, Israel) for 26 min, in which the PCR products were segregated by size and captured using the E-Gel® Safe Imager™ Realtime Transilluminator (Life Technologies, Kiryat Shmona, Israel) [24]. The PCR product was then purified by a commercialised PCR purification kit (Applied Biosystems, UK) as a precondition for DNA Sanger sequencing. Purified DNA fragments were analysed using the BigDye® Terminator version 3.1 cycle sequencing kit, which were run on a 96-capillary 3730xl DNA Analyzer at First BASE Laboratories Sdn. Bhd., Malaysia (developed by Applied Biosystem, USA, and produced by Thermo Fisher Scientific). The laboratory personnel were blinded, such that they were unable to distinguish samples with or without rapid CKD progression. The DNA sequences of the SNP results were transcribed using Sequence Scanner version 2.0 software (Applied Biosystems) and checked with the reference sequences in the Basic Local Alignment Search Tool (BLAST) program to confirm the presence of the polymorphism [25].

2.6. Statistical Analysis

All statistics were performed using IBM Statistical Package for Social Science for Windows version 23 (IBM Corp, Armonk, NY, USA). The results are presented as frequencies and percentages for categorical data, mean ± standard deviation (SD) for normally distributed numerical data, or as median (range) for non-normally distributed numerical data, based on the inspection of histograms. Adherence of the genotype groups to the Hardy-Weinberg equilibrium (HWE) assumption was examined. Expected percentages for each genotype group were calculated based on the Hardy-Weinberg equation using the allele frequencies ($p^2 + 2pq + q^2 = 1$). Chi-square test was then used to compare the allele and genotype distribution found with the predicted distribution. The observed genotype distribution was considered to be consistent with the assumptions of HWE if the p-value > 0.05 [24]. An independent T-test was used to compare the normally distributed numerical data between two groups, while the Mann-Whitney U test was used to compare the non-normally distributed numerical data between two groups. One-way ANOVA test was used to analyse normally distributed numerical data for comparison of more than two groups. Pearson's Chi-square test for independence was used to study the association between categorical data and categorical data, while Fisher's exact test was used if assumptions of Pearson's Chi-square test for independence were not met.

To investigate the relationship between CYP3A5 polymorphism and rapid CKD progression among the study population, linear regression was first performed using outpatient, non-emergency serum creatinine values over 3 years, to quantify the eGFR slope of each subject to identify subjects with rapid CKD progression [3]. Multiple logistic regression was then applied to identify the factors associated with rapid CKD progression, as the assumptions to perform a linear regression were not met. A simple logistic regression was performed with each independent variable, to determine factors at a level of significance of $p \leq 0.05$ [26]. A multiple stepwise logistic regression was then performed with all factors with $p < 0.25$, in which variables with $p \leq 0.05$ were considered as factors associated with rapid progression of CKD, followed by an examination of multicollinearity and interaction between these factors, by a Variance Inflation Factor (VIF) of 5 and above defined as presence of multicollinearity [27]. The Hosmer-Lemeshow goodness-of-fit test, classification tables and area under the receiving operator characteristic (ROC) curve were used to investigate any misrepresentation of data [26].

3. Results

3.1. Demographic and Clinical Characteristics

From 180 potentially eligible patients, a total of 124 subjects were included, with an average age of 52.2 ± 15.7 years, equal distribution of sex (n = 62, 50.0%) and predominantly Malay ethnicity (n = 71, 57.3%) (Table 2). Twenty-nine of the 124 subjects (23.4%) were found to have rapid CKD progression. The median eGFR decline per year for rapid CKD progressors was 6.0 mL/min/1.73 m²/year (range: −5.06 to −32.65 mL/min/1.73 m²/year). For non-rapid CKD progressors, the median eGFR decline per year was 0.86 mL/min/1.73 m²/year (range: −4.98 to 8.86 mL/min/1.73 m²/year).

Table 2. Demographic and clinical characteristics of subjects.

Characteristics	Non-Rapid CKD Progression (n = 95)	Rapid CKD Progression (n = 29)	Total (n = 124)
Age, mean (SD)	53.2 (15.4)	49.0 (16.2)	52.2 (15.7)
Ethnicity, n (%)			
Malay ethnicity, n (%)	55 (57.9)	16 (55.2)	71 (57.3)
Others, n (%)	40 (42.1)	13 (44.8)	53 (42.7)
Male sex, n (%)	46 (48.4)	16 (55.2)	62 (50.0)
CYP3A5 polymorphism, n (%)			
*1/*1	58 (61.1)	15 (51.7)	73 (58.9)
*1/*3	33 (34.7)	10 (34.5)	43 (34.7)
*3/*3	4 (4.2)	4 (13.8)	8 (6.5)
Stage of CKD, n (%)			
1	28 (29.5)	7 (24.1)	35 (28.2)
2	15 (15.8)	7 (24.1)	22 (17.7)
3a	17 (17.9)	6 (20.7)	23 (18.5)
3b	35 (36.8)	9 (31.0)	44 (35.5)
Baseline albuminuria status, n (%)			
A1	41 (43.2)	8 (27.6)	49 (39.5)
A2	17 (17.9)	7 (24.1)	24 (19.4)
A3	35 (36.8)	13 (44.8)	48 (38.7)
Missing	2 (2.1)	1 (3.4)	3 (2.4)
Baseline systolic blood pressure, mmHg, mean (SD)	133.0 (16.7)	135.2 (19.3)	133.6 (17.3)
CVD, n (%)	13 (13.7)	6 (20.7)	19 (15.3)
CCF, n (%)	6 (6.3)	1 (3.4)	7 (5.6)
Diabetes, n (%)	32 (33.7)	11 (37.9)	43 (34.7)
Dyslipidaemia, n (%)	60 (63.2)	22 (75.9)	82 (66.1)
Episode of AKI, n (%)	8 (8.4)	6 (20.7)	14 (11.3)
Gout, n (%)	23 (24.2)	6 (20.7)	29 (23.4)
Obesity (BMI > 30 kg/m²), n (%)	12 (12.6)	6 (20.7)	18 (14.5)
Anaemia, n (%)	36 (37.9)	13 (44.8)	49 (39.5)
Smoking status, n (%)			
Non-smoker	88 (92.6)	23 (79.3)	111 (89.5)
Ex-smoker	4 (4.2)	2 (6.9)	6 (4.8)
Currently smoking	3 (3.2)	4 (13.8)	7 (5.6)
Uncontrolled hypertension, n (%)	71 (77.2)	23 (79.3)	94 (77.7)
Adjustments to antihypertensives, median (range)	1 (0–15)	3 (0–19)	2 (0–19)
Poor medication adherence, n (%)	37 (38.9)	13 (44.8)	50 (40.3)
Use of calcium channel blockers, n (%)	55 (57.9)	20 (69.0)	75 (60.5)
Cessation of RAAS blockade, n (%)	6 (6.3)	3 (10.3)	9 (7.3)
Use of TCM, n (%)	10 (10.5)	6 (20.7)	16 (12.9)

AKI, acute kidney injury; BMI, body mass index; CCF, congestive cardiac failure; CKD, chronic kidney disease, CVD, cardiovascular disease; eGFR, estimated glomerular filtration rate; SD, standard deviation; TCM, traditional/complementary medicine.

Subjects with rapid CKD progression had a median of 3 (range: 0–19) adjustments to antihypertensives throughout the study period, which was significantly higher than subjects without rapid CKD progression, with a median of 1 (range: 0–15) adjustment ($p = 0.001$). Cessation of RAAS blockade occurred in 6 (6.3%) patients without rapid CKD progression and 3 (10.3%) patients with rapid CKD progression. TCM use was reported among 6 (20.7%) subjects with rapid CKD progression and 10 (10.5%) subjects without rapid CKD progression.

3.2. Allele and Genotype Analysis

Each participant's genotype was analysed to detect the presence of *CYP3A5*3* (rs776746, RefSeq NG_007938.2:g.12083A>G) polymorphism, and was compared with the rate of eGFR decline. The proportion of *CYP3A5*3* allele was found to be 23.8% ($n = 59$), while the proportion of the wildtype allele was 76.2% ($n = 189$). Meanwhile, the distribution of *CYP3A5*3* allele for each ethnic group was 19.7% ($n = 28$), 30.7% ($n = 27$) and 22.2% ($n = 4$) for Malay, Chinese and Indians, respectively. The distribution of the genotypes fulfilled the assumptions and predicted distribution from the Hardy-Weinberg equation ($X^2 = 0.237$, $p = 0.626$) [24].

The baseline eGFR did not differ significantly with variants of CYP3A5 allele ($p = 0.731$) nor genotypes ($p = 0.438$) (Table 3). By the end of the study period, the average eGFR among subjects with the *CYP3A5*3/*3* genotype of 45.7 ± 20.9 mL/min/1.73 m² was significantly lower than subjects with *CYP3A5*1/*1* genotype (58.2 ± 32.6 mL/min/1.73 m²) or *CYP3A5*1/*3* genotype (63.3 ± 34.7 mL/min/1.73 m²) ($p = 0.030$); while there was no statistically significant difference between subjects in terms of the allelic frequency ($p = 0.862$). Baseline albuminuria status did not differ significantly with variants of CYP3A5 allele ($p = 1.000$) nor genotype ($p = 0.487$). By the end of the study period, the distribution of albuminuria status was significantly different by allele ($p = 0.007$), as well as by genotype ($p = 0.029$) (Table 3). From the perspective of genotype, subjects with *CYP3A5*1/*1* genotype had a decline in the number of A3 albuminuria status by the end of the study period, from 28 (38.4%) to 22 (30.1%). Subjects with *CYP3A5*1/*3* genotype had more A3 albuminuria status by the end of the study period, from 15 (34.9%) to 21 (48.8%), while subjects with *CYP3A5*3/*3* genotype had the highest proportion of patients with A3 albuminuria category at baseline and at the end of the study period ($n = 4$, 50%). The number of patients with *CYP3A5*1* allele in A1 category declined from 74 (39.2%) to 62 (32.8%) by the end of the study period. For subjects with *CYP3A5*3* allele, A3 category patients increased from 23 (39.0%) to 29 (49.2%) by the end of the study period.

Twenty-nine (23.4%) subjects had rapid CKD progression, with 4 (13.8%) having the *CYP3A5*3/*3* genotype. From the remaining 95 patients without rapid CKD progression, 4 (4.2%) patients had *CYP3A5*3/*3* genotype, while 4 (13.8%) patients with rapid CKD progression had *CYP3A5*3/*3* genotype.

3.3. Factors Associated with Rapid CKD Progression

Table 4 shows the factors associated with rapid CKD progression. The simple logistic regression showed that adjustments to antihypertensives, *CYP3A5*3/*3* polymorphism, previous episode of AKI, smoking and use of TCM were factors associated with rapid CKD progression, with a significance level of $p < 0.05$. After adjusting for potential confounding factors with $p < 0.25$ using multiple logistic regression, the factors associated with rapid CKD progression were adjustments to antihypertensives (adjusted Odds Ratio [aOR] 1.172, 95% confidence interval [CI]: 1.055, 1.301), *CYP3A5*3/*3* polymorphism (aOR 4.190, 95% CI: 1.268, 13.852), young age (aOR 0.963, 95% CI: 0.937, 0.989), dyslipidaemia (aOR 2.317, 95% CI: 1.030, 5.211), smoking (aOR 7.126, 95% CI: 2.144, 23.685) and use of TCM (aOR 2.684, 95% CI: 1.045, 6.891) (Table 5).

Table 3. Renal function stratified by allele and genotype distribution.

Variables	Allele (n = 248)			Genotype (n = 124)			
	CYP3A5*1 (Wildtype)	CYP3A5*3 (Variant)	p-Value	Homozygous Wild Type (*1/*1)	Heterozygous (*1/*3)	Homozygous (*3/*3)	p-Value
Baseline eGFR, mL/min/1.73 m², mean (SD)	66.5 (33.0)	64.9 (32.0)	0.731 [a]	66.1 (32.9)	68.0 (33.5)	56.5 (25.8)	0.438 [c]
eGFR at 3 years, mL/min/1.73 m², mean (SD)	59.4 (33.1)	58.5 (32.5)	0.862 [a]	58.2 (32.6)	63.3 (34.7)	45.7 (20.9)	0.030 [d]
Baseline albuminuria status, n (%)							
A1	74 (39.2)	24 (40.7)		29 (39.7)	16 (37.2)	4 (50.0)	
A2	37 (19.6)	12 (20.3)	1.000 [b]	13 (17.8)	12 (27.9)	-	0.487 [e]
A3	72 (38.1)	23 (39.0)		28 (38.4)	15 (34.9)	4 (50.0)	
Missing	6 (3.2)	-		3 (4.1)	-	-	
Albuminuria category at 3 years, n (%)							
A1	62 (32.8)	22 (37.3)		24 (32.9)	14 (32.6)	4 (50.0)	
A2	61 (32.3)	7 (11.9)	0.007 [b]	27 (37.0)	7 (16.3)	-	0.029 [e]
A3	65 (34.4)	29 (49.2)		22 (30.1)	21 (48.8)	4 (50.0)	
Missing	1 (0.5)	1 (1.7)		-	1 (2.3)	-	

[a] Independent T-Test; [b] Chi-square Test; [c] ANOVA test; [d] Welch's ANOVA test as the variances were unequal; [e] Fisher's exact test.

Table 4. Factors associated with rapid CKD progression (simple logistic regression).

Variables (Reference)	b	Odds Ratio (95% CI)	p-Value
Adjustments to antihypertensives	0.176	1.192 (1.086, 1.309)	<0.001
Age, years	−0.017	0.983 (0.964, 1.002)	0.074
Anaemia of Hb < 13 g/dL (No anaemia)	0.286	1.332 (0.735, 2.414)	0.345
Baseline eGFR, mL/min/1.73 m²	0.003	1.003 (0.994, 1.012)	0.583
Baseline albuminuria status (A1)			
A2	0.747	2.110 (0.928, 4.797)	0.075
A3	0.644	1.904 (0.946, 3.832)	0.071
Baseline systolic blood pressure, mmHg	0.009	1.009 (0.992, 1.026)	0.303
CYP3A5*3 (CYP3A5*1) allele	0.492	1.635 (0.850, 3.148)	0.141
Cardiovascular disease (No cardiovascular disease)	0.498	1.645 (0.771, 3.512)	0.198
Congestive cardiac failure (No Congestive cardiac failure)	−0.635	0.530 (0.115, 2.439)	0.415
CYP3A5 polymorphism (CYP3A5*1/*1)			
*1/*3	0.158	1.172 (0.617, 2.225)	0.628
*3/*3	1.352	3.867 (1.341, 11.150)	0.012
Diabetes (No diabetes)	0.185	1.203 (0.654, 2.214)	0.552
Dyslipidaemia (No dyslipidaemia)	0.606	1.833 (0.938, 3.582)	0.076
Ethnicity (Malay) Others	0.111	1.117 (0.618, 2.020)	0.714
Gout (Absence of gout)	−0.203	0.817 (0.399, 1.672)	0.817
Male sex (Female sex)	0.271	1.311 (0.726, 2.366)	0.369
Obesity (No obesity)	0.590	1.804 (0.839, 3.882)	0.131

Table 4. Cont.

Variables (Reference)	b	Odds Ratio (95% CI)	p-Value
Occurrence of AKI (No AKI)	1.043	2.837 (1.255, 6.415)	0.012
Poor medication adherence (Good adherence)	0.242	1.274 (0.703, 2.307)	0.425
Smoking status (Non-smoker)			
Former smoker	0.649	1.913 (0.552, 6.633)	0.307
Current smoker	1.630	5.101 (1.686, 15.435)	0.004
Use of TCM (Did not use TCM)	0.796	2.217 (1.010, 4.868)	0.047
Use of calcium channel blockers (Did not use calcium channel blockers)	0.480	1.616 (0.864, 3.024)	0.133
Cessation of RAAS blockade (None)	0.537	1.712 (0.613, 4.782)	0.305
Uncontrolled hypertension (None)	0.126	1.134 (0.550, 2.335)	0.733

Table 5. Factors associated with rapid CKD progression (multiple logistic regression).

Variables (Reference)	b	Adjusted Odds Ratio (95% CI)	p-Value [a]
Age, years	−0.038	0.963 (0.937, 0.989)	0.013
Adjustments to antihypertensives	0.158	1.172 (1.055, 1.301)	0.003
CYP3A5 polymorphism (CYP3A5*1/*1)			
*1/*3	0.052	1.053 (0.509, 2.181)	0.889
*3/*3	1.433	4.190 (1.268, 13.852)	0.019
Dyslipidaemia (No dyslipidaemia)	0.840	2.317 (1.030, 5.211)	0.042
Smoking status (Non-smoker)			
Former smoker	1.016	2.763 (0.717, 10.650)	0.140
Current smoker	1.964	7.126 (2.144, 23.685)	0.001
Use of TCM (Did not use TCM)	0.987	2.684 (1.045, 6.891)	0.040

[a] Stepwise multiple logistic regression model was applied. Multicollinearity and interaction terms were checked and not found. Hosmer-Lemeshow test ($p = 0.352$), classification table (overall correctly classified percentage = 79.0%) and area under the ROC curve (77.4%) were applied to check the model fit.

4. Discussion

Rapid progression of CKD occurred in approximately a fifth of our study population with mild-to-moderate CKD within a span of three years. To the best of our ability and knowledge, this is the first study describing the link between CYP3A5 polymorphism and rapid CKD progression. As the HWE assumptions were not violated, systematic error was likely absent in the genotyping assays. After adjusting for potential confounding factors, CYP3A5*3/*3 genotype, adjustments to antihypertensives, young age, dyslipidaemia, smoking and use of TCM were found to be factors associated with rapid CKD progression.

Our study supports previous reports [15,28] that have demonstrated that CYP3A5 polymorphism may be associated with factors of CKD progression. CYP3A5 is not only a drug metabolising enzyme present in the liver, it is also present in the kidneys and might have important physiological functions [7]. The CYP3A5*3 allele is associated with less expression of the CYP3A5 enzyme in the kidneys of healthy human adults compared to the wildtype, CYP3A5*1 [28]. The diminished CYP3A5 activity from the CYP3A5*3/*3 polymorphism reduces the protection against aldosterone-induced active sodium transport in the kidneys, as less intrarenal conversion of the corticosterone into 6β-hydroxycorticosterone occurs [8]. Less inhibition of RAAS, which is related to glomerular hyperfiltration, exacerbates damage to the kidneys. This is supported by our finding that a greater proportion of subjects with CYP3A5*3/*3 genotype had category A3 albuminuria by the end of the study period, than those with CYP3A5*1/*1 or CYP3A5*3/*3 genotype, in line with findings from a previous study in which proteinuria was found to be an indicator of structural kidney damage [3]. Furthermore, maximal doses of ACEI or ARB did not improve renal function among patients with aldosterone excess [29], while CKD patients with aldosterone excess were reported to have accelerated progression of CKD [29].

Another possible mechanism for the effect of *CYP3A5*3/*3* genotype on rapid CKD progression is the elevation of 20-HETE production. The arachidonic acid-derived metabolites of CYP3A5 enzyme are 19-HETE and 6β-hydroxycortisol [30]. The *CYP3A5*3* polymorphism results in a reduced expression of CYP3A5 enzymes, which in turn reduces the formation of 19-HETE [30]. This may lead to an increased availability of the arachidonic acid precursor for greater production of 20-HETE. The increase of 20-HETE has been shown to increase renal vasoconstriction and peripheral vascular resistance, as 20-HETE is a potent vasoconstrictor that mediates angiotensin II-related renal effects in the proximal tubule and thick ascending limb of the loop of Henle [30]. In addition, a higher level of 20-HETE was recently identified as an independent predictor of CKD progression [15]. This demonstrates the need for more studies to be conducted to elucidate the mechanism of association between *CYP3A5*3* polymorphism and rapid CKD progression. Genotyping may be beneficial to identify CKD patients with *CYP3A5*3/*3* genotype for closer monitoring, given the association found between *CYP3A5*3/*3* genotype and accelerated CKD progression.

There was a significant association between antihypertensive adjustments and rapid CKD progression found in the current work. During early progression, first-line RAAS inhibitors may have been stopped once patients presented with a rapidly deteriorating eGFR, which could account for part of the medication adjustments [31]. On the other hand, genetic predisposition may also account for frequent medication adjustments. Pharmacokinetic properties of CYP3A5 substrate drugs are known to differ according to CYP3A5 polymorphism [8]. In particular, calcium channel blocker antihypertensives, such as amlodipine [8], felodipine [9], diltiazem [10] and verapamil [11,12] have been reported to be affected by CYP3A5 polymorphism, with blood pressure responses varying according to their CYP3A5 polymorphism status [8,11,12]. However, the complexity of genetic effects are evident as metabolism of CYP3A5 substrates among individuals who are CYP3A5 non-expressors (those expressing *CYP3A5*3/*3* genotype) have been reported to be carried out by the CYP3A4 enzyme, which is more prone to inductions and inhibitions by concurrent drugs [5]. These genetic effects may have led to the need for frequent medication adjustments for optimum outcome, as observed in the current work, supporting the need for closer monitoring of antihypertensive management.

Younger age and dyslipidaemia were also found to be associated with rapid CKD progression, in line with findings from previous studies on rapid CKD progression [32,33]. It is believed that the CKD aetiology is different in older patients, with more aggressive disease found among younger patients, while in adults some decline of eGFR is believed to occur as part of aging, rather than from deteriorating CKD [34]. On the other hand, in CKD patients, lipoproteins are oxidised, especially the small dense high-density lipoprotein cholesterol (LDL) particles, intermediate-density lipoproteins and chylomicron remnants [35]. Accumulation of these oxidised LDL, intermediate-density lipoproteins and chylomicron remnants accelerates systemic inflammation, through stimulating release of proinflammatory cytokines and chemokines from monocytes and macrophages [35]. The subsequent systemic inflammation and oxidative stress is believed to cause eGFR decline and CKD progression [35].

Smoking was also found to be associated with a higher risk of CKD progression, similar to previous work [36]. The potential mechanisms of smoking-associated CKD progression include smoking-induced hypoxic injury [36], myointimal hyperplasia of intrarenal arterioles [37] and adverse effects on intrarenal hemodynamics, through nicotine-induced release of angiotensin II [36]. This leads to increased activation of RAAS, as well as increased glomerular hypertension, which could potentially accelerate the progression of CKD. The study finding suggests that smoking cessation is an important component to preserve the kidney function of CKD patients who are currently smoking.

The association between TCM and CKD progression in Asian countries has been inconsistent to date [1,38]. A few studies have reported no association between TCM and CKD progression [38,39]. This may be due to the relatively short follow-up period that might not capture renal damage in the long term [38]. On the other hand, the lack of association has also been attributed to TCM that was prescribed by board-certified physicians and produced by pharmaceutical companies, which had certified manufacturing practices [39]. In the current work, we found a significant association between rapid CKD progression and TCM consumption, of which the TCM was used without the supervision of a registered practitioner or pharmacist. It was noted that many reported the use of TCM with unknown ingredients and quality. Most worrying is that some TCM, most often involving the use of herbal remedies popular among Asians, have been shown to contain nephrotoxic ingredients [40]. However, very often CKD patients report the use of TCM due to the lack of conventional medications that cure CKD, as well as the desire to see immediate improvement in their disease condition [40]. As there is no cure for CKD in conventional medicine, some patients might be inclined to use TCM, owing to their cultural beliefs and social influences [40]. Therefore, TCM use for CKD should be monitored closely for mitigation efforts in preventing rapid CKD progression.

There were a few limitations to our findings. Firstly, the findings of the study have limited applicability to advanced CKD patients with Stage 4 and above, in which the majority of these patients were shown to exhibit non-linear CKD progression [32]. In addition, the report of TCM use might be subject to recall bias at the time of interview. The potential effects of such bias were reduced by incorporating the report of TCM use from medical records. The lack of identification of TCM also provides fewer specific details of which moieties were nephrotoxic to the patients. Furthermore, the effects of other potential genes were not studied. As CYP3A4 and CYP3A5 enzymes have some overlapping in substrate specificity, the complete loss of metabolic activity with the *CYP3A5*3* allele might pronounce the impact of genetic variation in CYP3A4 expression among these patients [5]. Therefore, further work involving genetic variants of CYP3A4 polymorphism could possibly improve the current findings. The study might be limited by the absence of direct measurement in the expression level or activities of CYP3A5. Future studies could be designed to investigate the activity of CYP3A5 with renal function through usage of endogenous markers, such as 4β-hydroxycholesterol. More studies could be conducted to investigate other outcomes, such as initiation of renal replacement therapy, heart failure and mortality, as well as CKD progression over a longer period of time.

5. Conclusions

In conclusion, CKD must be monitored closely to reduce the risk of rapid progression. This could potentially mean monitoring of patient genetics, as the *CYP3A5*3/*3* genotype was found to be associated with accelerated CKD progression after adjusting for possible confounding factors. CKD patients with such characteristics, as well as those requiring antihypertensive adjustments, young age, dyslipidaemia, smokers and TCM users, may also benefit from intensified monitoring and care to reduce the propensity of developing adverse clinical outcomes. Most importantly, our findings suggest a potentially important role of CYP3A5 polymorphism in the pathogenesis of accelerated CKD progression. A personalised management approach could therefore be potentially useful for CKD patients based on genotyping data.

Author Contributions: Conceptualization: F.Y.L., F.I.; methodology: F.Y.L., F.I., software: F.Y.L.; validation: F.I.; formal analysis: F.Y.L., F.I.; investigation: F.Y.L., A.Y.A.N.; resources: A.H.A.G., H.-S.W., S.B.; data curation: F.Y.L., F.I., A.Y.A.N.; writing—original draft preparation: F.Y.L., F.I.; writing—review and editing: F.Y.L., F.I., A.Y.A.N., A.H.A.G., H.-S.W., S.B., S.M.S., A.M.R., N.A.M.T., M.M.-B. visualization: F.Y.L.; supervision: F.I., A.H.A.G., H.-S.W., S.B., N.A.M.T., M.M.-B.; project administration: F.I.; funding acquisition: F.I., M.M.-B., A.M.R., S.M.S. All authors have read and agreed to the published version of the manuscript.

Funding: The study received financial support from the Fundamental Research Grants Scheme by the Ministry of Higher Education of Malaysia (FRGS/1/2019/SKK09/UKM/02/2).

Institutional Review Board Statement: The study protocol was registered with the National Medical Research Register, Malaysia, under the protocol number NMRR-19-3424-51773, and was approved by the Medical Research Ethics Committee, Malaysia (KKM.NIHSEC.P19-2320(11))and the Universiti Kebangsaan Malaysia Research Ethic Committee (UKM PPI/111/8/JEP-2020-048). This study was conducted in compliance with ethical principles outlined in the Declaration of Helsinki and Malaysian Good Clinical Practice Guideline.

Informed Consent Statement: Informed consent was obtained from all subjects involved in the study.

Data Availability Statement: Authors do not have permission to share the data. The data underlying the results presented in the study are available upon request from corresponding author (faridaislahudin@ukm.edu.my) for researchers who meet the criteria for access to confidential data.

Acknowledgments: We would like to thank the Universiti Kebangsaan Malaysia in approving the conduct of this study, as well as Director General of Health Malaysia for his permission to publish this article.

Conflicts of Interest: The authors declare no conflict of interest. The funders had no role in the design of the study; in the collection, analyses, or interpretation of data; in the writing of the manuscript, or in the decision to publish the results.

References

1. Saminathan, T.A.; Hooi, L.S.; Mohd Yusoff, M.F.; Ong, L.M.; Bavanandan, S.; Rodzlan Hasani, W.S.; Tan, E.Z.Z.; Wong, I.; Rifin, H.M.; Robert, T.G.; et al. Prevalence of chronic kidney disease and its associated factors in Malaysia; Findings from a nationwide population-based cross-sectional study. *BMC Nephrol.* **2020**, *21*, 344. [CrossRef] [PubMed]
2. Islahudin, F.; Lee, F.Y.; Tengku Abd Kadir, T.N.I.; Abdullah, M.Z.; Makmor-Bakry, M. Continuous medication monitoring: A clinical model to predict adherence to medications among chronic kidney disease patients. *Res. Soc. Adm. Pharm.* **2021**. [CrossRef]
3. Go, A.S.; Yang, J.; Tan, T.C.; Cabrera, C.S.; Stefansson, B.V.; Greasley, P.J.; Ordonez, J.D.; Kaiser Permanente Northern California CKD Outcomes Study. Contemporary rates and predictors of fast progression of chronic kidney disease in adults with and without diabetes mellitus. *BMC Nephrol.* **2018**, *19*, 146. [CrossRef]
4. Adams, S.M.; Crisamore, K.R.; Empey, P.E. Clinical pharmacogenomics. *Clin. J. Am. Soc. Nephrol.* **2018**, *13*, 1561. [CrossRef] [PubMed]
5. Zanger, U.M.; Schwab, M. Cytochrome P450 enzymes in drug metabolism: Regulation of gene expression, enzyme activities, and impact of genetic variation. *Pharmacol. Ther.* **2013**, *138*, 103–141. [CrossRef] [PubMed]
6. Dorji, P.W.; Tshering, G.; Na-Bangchang, K. CYP2C9, CYP2C19, CYP2D6 and CYP3A5 polymorphisms in South-East and East Asian populations: A systematic review. *J. Clin. Pharm. Ther.* **2019**, *44*, 508–524. [CrossRef]
7. Kuehl, P.; Zhang, J.; Lin, Y.; Lamba, J.; Assem, M.; Schuetz, J.; Watkins, P.B.; Daly, A.; Wrighton, S.A.; Hall, S.D.; et al. Sequence diversity in CYP3A promoters and characterization of the genetic basis of polymorphic CYP3A5 expression. *Nat. Genet.* **2001**, *27*, 383–391. [CrossRef]
8. Zhang, Y.P.; Zuo, X.C.; Huang, Z.J.; Cai, J.J.; Wen, J.; Duan, D.D.; Yuan, H. CYP3A5 polymorphism, amlodipine and hypertension. *J. Hum. Hypertens.* **2014**, *28*, 145–149. [CrossRef]
9. Xiang, Q.; Li, C.; Zhao, X.; Cui, Y.M. The influence of CYP3A5*3 and BCRPC421A genetic polymorphisms on the pharmacokinetics of felodipine in healthy Chinese volunteers. *J. Clin. Pharm. Ther.* **2017**, *42*, 345–349. [CrossRef] [PubMed]
10. Zhou, L.-Y.; Zuo, X.-C.; Chen, K.; Wang, J.-L.; Chen, Q.-J.; Zhou, Y.-N.; Yuan, H.; Ma, Y.; Zhu, L.-J.; Peng, Y.-X.; et al. Significant impacts of CYP3A4*1G and CYP3A5*3 genetic polymorphisms on the pharmacokinetics of diltiazem and its main metabolites in Chinese adult kidney transplant patients. *J. Clin. Pharm. Ther.* **2016**, *41*, 341–347. [CrossRef]
11. Jin, Y.; Wang, Y.H.; Miao, J.; Li, L.; Kovacs, R.J.; Marunde, R.; Hamman, M.A.; Philips, S.; Hilligoss, J.; Hall, S.D. Cytochrome P450 3A5 genotype is associated with verapamil response in healthy subjects. *Clin. Pharmacol. Ther.* **2007**, *82*, 579–585. [CrossRef] [PubMed]
12. Langaee, T.Y.; Gong, Y.; Yarandi, H.N.; Katz, D.A.; Cooper-DeHoff, R.M.; Pepine, C.J.; Johnson, J.A. Association of CYP3A5 polymorphisms with hypertension and antihypertensive response to verapamil. *Clin. Pharmacol. Ther.* **2007**, *81*, 386–391. [CrossRef]
13. Schmidt, I.M.; Hübner, S.; Nadal, J.; Titze, S.; Schmid, M.; Bärthlein, B.; Schlieper, G.; Dienemann, T.; Schultheiss, U.T.; Meiselbach, H.; et al. Patterns of medication use and the burden of polypharmacy in patients with chronic kidney disease: The German Chronic Kidney Disease study. *Clin. Kidney J.* **2019**, *12*, 663–672. [CrossRef] [PubMed]

14. Rüster, C.; Wolf, G. Renin-Angiotensin-aldosterone system and progression of renal disease. *J. Am. Soc. Nephrol.* **2006**, *17*, 2985. [CrossRef]
15. Afshinnia, F.; Zeng, L.; Byun, J.; Wernisch, S.; Deo, R.; Chen, J.; Hamm, L.; Miller, E.R.; Rhee, E.P.; Fischer, M.J.; et al. Elevated lipoxygenase and cytochrome P450 products predict progression of chronic kidney disease. *Nephrol. Dial. Transplant.* **2018**, *35*, 303–312. [CrossRef]
16. Barbour, S.J.; Er, L.; Djurdjev, O.; Karim, M.; Levin, A. Differences in progression of CKD and mortality amongst Caucasian, Oriental Asian and South Asian CKD patients. *Nephrol. Dial. Transpl.* **2010**, *25*, 3663–3672. [CrossRef] [PubMed]
17. Chaplin, M.; Kirkham, J.J.; Dwan, K.; Sloan, D.J.; Davies, G.; Jorgensen, A.L. STrengthening the reporting of pharmacogenetic studies: Development of the STROPS guideline. *PLoS Med.* **2020**, *17*, e1003344. [CrossRef] [PubMed]
18. KDIGO, W.G.C. KDIGO 2012 clinical practice guideline for the evaluation and management of chronic kidney disease. *Kidney Int. Suppl.* **2012**, *3*, 1–150.
19. Vrijens, B.; De Geest, S.; Hughes, D.A.; Przemyslaw, K.; Demonceau, J.; Ruppar, T.; Dobbels, F.; Fargher, E.; Morrison, V.; Lewek, P.; et al. A new taxonomy for describing and defining adherence to medications. *Br. J. Clin. Pharmacol.* **2012**, *73*, 691–705. [CrossRef]
20. Lee, F.Y.; Islahudin, F.; Makmor-Bakry, M.; Wong, H.-S.; Bavanandan, S. Factors associated with the frequency of antihypertensive drug adjustments in chronic kidney disease patients: A multicentre, 2-year retrospective study. *Int. J. Clin. Pharm.* **2021**. [CrossRef] [PubMed]
21. Jones, C.; Roderick, P.; Harris, S.; Rogerson, M. Decline in kidney function before and after nephrology referral and the effect on survival in moderate to advanced chronic kidney disease. *Nephrol. Dial. Transpl.* **2006**, *21*, 2133–2143. [CrossRef] [PubMed]
22. Lemeshow, S.; Hosmer, D.W.; Klar, J.; Lwanga, S.K. *World Health Organization. Adequacy of Sample size in Health Studies/Stanley Lemeshow*; Wiley: Chichester, UK, 1990.
23. Lucena-Aguilar, G.; Sánchez-López, A.M.; Barberán-Aceituno, C.; Carrillo-Ávila, J.A.; López-Guerrero, J.A.; Aguilar-Quesada, R. DNA source selection for downstream applications based on DNA quality indicators analysis. *Biopreserv. Biobank.* **2016**, *14*, 264–270. [CrossRef]
24. Tahir, N.A.M.; Saffian, S.M.; Islahudin, F.H.; Gafor, A.H.A.; Othman, H.; Manan, H.A.; Makmor-Bakry, M. Effects of CST3 Gene G73A Polymorphism on Cystatin C in a Prospective Multiethnic Cohort Study. *Nephron* **2020**, *144*, 204–212. [CrossRef]
25. Ariffin, N.M.; Islahudin, F.; Kumolosasi, E.; Makmor-Bakry, M. Effects of MAO-A and CYP450 on primaquine metabolism in healthy volunteers. *Parasitol. Res.* **2019**, *118*, 1011–1018. [CrossRef] [PubMed]
26. Hosmer, D.W.J.; Lemeshow, S. Assessing the fit of the model. In *Applied Logistic Regression*; Hosmer, D.W.J., Lemeshow, S., Eds.; Wiley: Hoboker, NJ, USA, 2000; pp. 156–164.
27. Shrestha, N. Detecting multicollinearity in regression analysis. *Am. J. Appl. Math. Stat.* **2020**, *8*, 39–42. [CrossRef]
28. Givens, R.C.; Lin, Y.S.; Dowling, A.L.; Thummel, K.E.; Lamba, J.K.; Schuetz, E.G.; Stewart, P.W.; Watkins, P.B. CYP3A5 genotype predicts renal CYP3A activity and blood pressure in healthy adults. *J. Appl. Physiol.* **2003**, *95*, 1297–1300. [CrossRef]
29. Schjoedt, K.J.; Andersen, S.; Rossing, P.; Tarnow, L.; Parving, H.H. Aldosterone escape during blockade of the renin-angiotensin-aldosterone system in diabetic nephropathy is associated with enhanced decline in glomerular filtration rate. *Diabetologia* **2004**, *47*, 1936–1939. [CrossRef]
30. Knights, K.M.; Rowland, A.; Miners, J.O. Renal drug metabolism in humans: The potential for drug-endobiotic interactions involving cytochrome P450 (CYP) and UDP-glucuronosyltransferase (UGT). *Br. J. Clin. Pharmacol.* **2013**, *76*, 587–602. [CrossRef]
31. Higuchi, S.; Kohsaka, S.; Shiraishi, Y.; Katsuki, T.; Nagatomo, Y.; Mizuno, A.; Sujino, Y.; Kohno, T.; Goda, A.; Yoshikawa, T.; et al. Association of renin-angiotensin system inhibitors with long-term outcomes in patients with systolic heart failure and moderate-to-severe kidney function impairment. *Eur. J. Int. Med.* **2019**, *62*, 58–66. [CrossRef] [PubMed]
32. Caravaca-Fontán, F.; Azevedo, L.; Luna, E.; Caravaca, F. Patterns of progression of chronic kidney disease at later stages. *Clin. Kidney J.* **2018**, *11*, 246–253. [CrossRef]
33. Ali, I.; Chinnadurai, R.; Ibrahim, S.T.; Green, D.; Kalra, P.A. Predictive factors of rapid linear renal progression and mortality in patients with chronic kidney disease. *BMC Nephrol.* **2020**, *21*, 345. [CrossRef] [PubMed]
34. O'Hare, A.M.; Choi, A.I.; Bertenthal, D.; Bacchetti, P.; Garg, A.X.; Kaufman, J.S.; Walter, L.C.; Mehta, K.M.; Steinman, M.A.; Allon, M.; et al. Age affects outcomes in chronic kidney disease. *J. Am. Soc. Nephrol.* **2007**, *18*, 2758–2765. [CrossRef]
35. Tsuruya, K.; Yoshida, H.; Nagata, M.; Kitazono, T.; Iseki, K.; Iseki, C.; Fujimoto, S.; Konta, T.; Moriyama, T.; Yamagata, K.; et al. Impact of the triglycerides to high-density lipoprotein cholesterol ratio on the incidence and progression of CKD: A longitudinal study in a large Japanese population. *Am. J. Kidney Dis.* **2015**, *66*, 972–983. [CrossRef] [PubMed]
36. Lee, S.; Kang, S.; Joo, Y.S.; Lee, C.; Nam, K.H.; Yun, H.-R.; Park, J.T.; Chang, T.I.; Yoo, T.-H.; Kim, S.W.; et al. Smoking, smoking cessation, and progression of chronic kidney disease: Results from KNOW-CKD study. *Nicotine Tob. Res.* **2020**, *23*, 92–98. [CrossRef] [PubMed]
37. Lhotta, K.; Rumpelt, H.J.; König, P.; Mayer, G.; Kronenberg, F. Cigarette smoking and vascular pathology in renal biopsies. *Kidney Int.* **2002**, *61*, 648–654. [CrossRef]
38. Tangkiatkumjai, M.; Boardman, H.; Praditpornsilpa, K.; Walker, D.M. Association of herbal and dietary supplements with progression and complications of chronic kidney disease: A prospective cohort study. *Nephrol. (Carlton)* **2015**, *20*, 679–687. [CrossRef] [PubMed]

39. Lin, M.-Y.; Chiu, Y.-W.; Chang, J.-S.; Lin, H.-L.; Lee, C.T.-C.; Chiu, G.-F.; Kuo, M.-C.; Wu, M.-T.; Chen, H.-C.; Hwang, S.-J. Association of prescribed Chinese herbal medicine use with risk of end-stage renal disease in patients with chronic kidney disease. *Kidney Int.* **2015**, *88*, 1365–1373. [CrossRef]
40. Saeed, S.; Islahudin, F.; Makmor-Bakry, M.; Redzuan, A.M. The practice of complementary and alternative medicine among chronic kidney disease patients. *J. Adv. Pharm. Edu. Res.* **2018**, *8*, 30–36.

Article

Pharmacogenomic Biomarkers in US FDA-Approved Drug Labels (2000–2020)

Jeeyun A. Kim [1], Rachel Ceccarelli [2] and Christine Y. Lu [2,*]

1. Department of Epidemiology, Harvard T.H. Chan School of Public Health, Boston, MA 02115, USA; jeeyunkim@mail.harvard.edu
2. Department of Population Medicine, Harvard Pilgrim Health Care Institute and Harvard Medical School, Landmark Center, 401 Park Drive, Suite 401 East, Boston, MA 02215, USA; rachel.ceccarelli@umassmemorial.org
* Correspondence: christine_lu@hphci.harvard.edu; Tel.: +1-617-867-4989

Abstract: Pharmacogenomics (PGx) is a key subset of precision medicine that relates genomic variation to individual response to pharmacotherapy. We assessed longitudinal trends in US FDA approval of new drugs labeled with PGx information. Drug labels containing PGx information were obtained from Drugs@FDA and guidelines from PharmGKB were used to compare the actionability of PGx information in drug labels across therapeutic areas. The annual proportion of new drug approvals with PGx labeling has increased by nearly threefold from 10.3% ($n = 3$) in 2000 to 28.2% ($n = 11$) in 2020. Inclusion of PGx information in drug labels has increased for all clinical areas over the last two decades but most prominently for cancer therapies, which comprise the largest proportion (75.5%) of biomarker–drug pairs for which PGx testing is required. Clinically actionable information was more frequently observed in biomarker–drug pairs associated with cancer drugs compared to those for other therapeutic areas ($n = 92$ (59.7%) vs. $n = 62$ (40.3%), $p < 0.0051$). These results suggest that further evidence is needed to support the clinical adoption of pharmacogenomics in non-cancer therapeutic areas.

Keywords: pharmacogenomics; precision medicine; US Food and Drug Administration; clinical actionability

1. Introduction

Approximately 80% of the variability in drug efficacy and adverse effects can be explained by genomic variation, which creates major challenges for the appropriate selection and dosing of medications [1]. Genomic composition is an important factor for individual response to therapy by affecting the expression of drug targets, drug metabolizing enzymes, and other proteins involved in pathophysiological mechanisms pertaining to the drug's pharmacodynamic and pharmacokinetic processes [2,3]. As an applicable component of precision medicine, pharmacogenomics (PGx) incorporates genomic profiling to identify biomarkers based on relevant genotype–phenotype interactions that can predict drug response and risk of adverse drug reactions for individual patients. Novel next-generation sequencing techniques have enabled rapid growth of PGx knowledge, with over 200 genome-wide association studies (GWAS) of pharmacotherapy responses reported to date [4].

In particular, key somatic variants, such as the overexpression of *ERBB2* in breast cancer, can serve as markers for the selection of patient groups for which drugs like ado-trastuzumab emtansine and talazoparib tosylate are indicated. Pharmacogenomic testing for germline variants, such as those in the *DPYD* gene, can also predict the risk of toxicity and differential response to cancer therapies such as 5-fluorouracil, enabling prescribers to better tailor therapies with greater efficacy and safety for patients [5,6]. In other areas, PGx biomarkers have been used to specify dosing alterations, as in the example of the *CYP2C9* and *VKORC1* variants in warfarin use for treatment and prevention of thromboembolic events, as well as to prevent the occurrence of severe hypersensitivity effects, as with an *HLA-B* variant in relation to abacavir use for treatment of HIV infection [3,7].

Recent advances in the development of targeted therapies against specific variants have increased the efficiency of clinical trials by enabling smaller trial sizes, higher success rates, and expedited time to market [8–11]. Over the last two decades, the US Food and Drug Administration (FDA), the agency responsible for reviewing and approving a drug for marketing if it provides benefits that outweigh its known potential risks, has actively encouraged the incorporation of genomic data into drug development, including the issuance of several guidelines for industry regarding submission of PGx information as part of the drug review process [12]. This study examined trends in FDA approvals of new drugs labeled with PGx information from 2000 to 2020. We anticipated that the proportion of new drug approvals with PGx labeling would increase over time. We also compared the level of clinical actionability of biomarker information in drug labels across various therapeutic areas.

2. Materials and Methods

2.1. Data Extraction and Evaluation

All data came from publicly available sources on the FDA and PharmGKB websites. Initial drug and biologic approval reports from 1 January 2000 to 31 July 2020 were gathered from the Drugs@FDA database [13]. We extracted the following information in a standardized format from Drugs@FDA: drug brand name, active ingredient, approval date, submission classification, and therapeutic area. Among drug approvals with duplicate active ingredients, we included only the drug with the earliest initial approval date to our study. A drug can have several approval dates: one for each application submitted for FDA review. Among all retrieved entries, new drug applications (NDAs) with "Type 1 New Molecular Entity" and "Type 1/4 New Molecular Entity and New Combination" with the corresponding approval dates were examined in order to capture drug labels at the time of first approval. Because this classification does not exist for biologics, the earliest approval date and drug label were used for biologics. For drugs indicated for multiple diseases, we considered only the therapeutic areas that were relevant to the biomarker information.

Drug labels were reviewed for PGx information based on the FDA Table of Pharmacogenomic Biomarkers in Drug Labeling (called FDA Table hereafter) and the PharmGKB website; we included a biomarker for a drug if it was listed by either source [14]. The FDA Table lists approved products with PGx information in the drug labeling and specifies sections of the labeling that contained biomarker information [14]. The PharmGKB is a publicly available knowledgebase for PGx that provides annotations of medication prescribing guidelines based on published evidence for gene–drug associations [15]. We compared and verified the names of the listed biomarkers from both sources with the information provided in the first-approved drug labels extracted from Drugs@FDA. Since a drug can have multiple biomarkers and a single biomarker can be labeled for more than one drug product, we counted the number of unique biomarker–drug pairs mentioned in the first-approved drug label only; we did not include biomarkers included in labeling updates.

2.2. Drug Label Annotations of PGx Levels

PharmGKB provides four types of annotations (PGx Levels) for PGx information associated with specific gene–drug combinations:

1. "Required genetic testing", where labels state or imply that gene, protein, or chromosomal testing, including genetic testing, functional protein assays, cytogenetic studies, should be conducted prior to using the drug. Testing may only be required for a subset of patients. A label that states that the variant is an indication for the drug or that a test "should be performed" is also interpreted as requiring testing;
2. "Recommended genetic testing", where labels state or imply that gene, protein, or chromosomal testing, including genetic testing, functional protein assays, cytogenetic

studies, is recommended prior to using the drug. The recommendation may only be for a subset of patients. A label that states that testing "should be considered" or "consider genotyping or phenotyping" is also considered to recommend testing;

3. "Actionable PGx"—marked for labels that describe the impact of gene/protein/chromosomal variants or phenotypes on changes in efficacy, dosage, metabolism, or toxicity, including mention of contraindication of the drug in a subset of patients defined by particular variants/genotypes/phenotypes. However, labels with this annotation do not require or recommend gene, protein, or chromosomal testing;

4. "Informative PGx"—assigned to labels that state particular gene/protein/chromosomal variants or metabolizer phenotypes do not affect a drug's efficacy, dosage, metabolism, or toxicity, or that variants or phenotypes affect a drug's efficacy, dosage, metabolism, or toxicity, but this effect is not clinically significant. This level is also assigned to all other labels that have been listed in the FDA Table but do not currently meet the criteria for all other PharmGKB PGx annotations listed above [15].

We considered PGx information to be clinically actionable if they were categorized as "required genetic testing," "recommended genetic testing," or "actionable PGx." Biomarker–drug pairs were considered to lack actionability if they were assigned an "informative PGx" level by PharmGKB; examples of "informative" biomarker–drug pairs include those with labels that only describe the role of a variant in the drug's metabolism or state that dose adjustment or other actions were not necessary for a particular variant.

2.3. Statistical Analysis

Descriptive statistics were used to characterize trends in approval rates of new pharmacogenomic drugs and compared the clinical actionability of PGx information in drug labels between cancer therapies and drugs used in non-cancer therapeutic areas. We performed Fisher's exact tests to determine if PGx testing requirements and overall clinically actionable information were more frequently associated with cancer biomarker–drug pairs compared to biomarkers for all other clinical areas.

3. Results

Of 694 total new drug approvals identified from 1 January 2000 to 31 July 2020, new molecular entities accounted for 75.9% ($n = 527$) and biologics represented 24.1% ($n = 167$). Biosimilars comprised 16.8% ($n = 28$) of newly approved biologics. On average, there were about 33 new approvals per year and they ranged from a minimum of 18 drug approvals in 2007 to a maximum of 66 approvals in 2018. Cancer therapies comprised 23.1% ($n = 160$) of total drug approvals.

About a quarter of total new drug approvals (25.6%; $n = 178$) contained PGx biomarker information in initial approved labels. An estimated 74.7% ($n = 133$) of approvals with PGx labeling were for new molecular entities while the remaining 25.3% ($n = 45$) were for biologics. Biosimilars accounted for 15.6% ($n = 7$) of biologics approved with PGx labeling and 3.9% of overall initial drug approvals with PGx labels.

Figure 1 shows the distribution of therapeutic areas for 178 drug approvals with PGx labeling. Oncology was the most common therapeutic area, comprising 49.4% ($n = 88$) of all new drugs approved with PGx labeling. Other therapeutic areas included neurology ($n = 16$; 9.0%), infectious diseases ($n = 14$; 7.9%), psychiatry ($n = 10$; 5.6%), inborn errors of metabolism ($n = 9$; 5.1%), cardiology ($n = 8$; 4.5%), hematology ($n = 7$; 3.9%), and pulmonology ($n = 7$; 3.9%). The remaining clinical areas that each comprised less than 3% of PGx labels were gastroenterology, gynecology, rheumatology, urology, anesthesiology, dentistry, and dermatology.

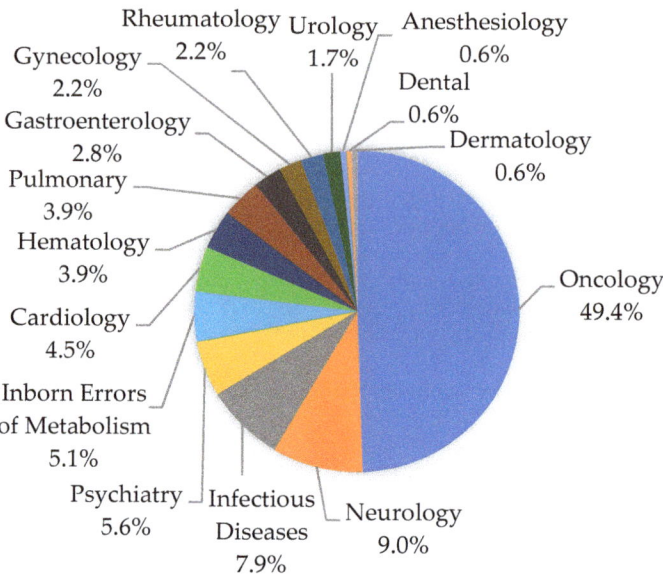

Figure 1. Therapeutic areas of new FDA drug approvals with pharmacogenomics (PGx) labeling from 2000 to 2020.

3.1. Yearly Trends in Drug Approvals with PGx Information

Overall, the average proportion of new drug approvals with PGx labeling was 23.8% per year from 2000 to 2020. The annual proportion of new drug approvals with PGx labeling increased by approximately threefold from 10.3% ($n = 3$) in 2000 to 33.9% ($n = 20$) in 2019 and 28.2% ($n = 11$) through July in 2020; with the lowest at 5.3% ($n = 1$) in 2005 and highest at 44.4% ($n = 12$) in 2013 (Table 1, Figure A1). This growth is emphasized in the latter half of the study period, during which there has also been a proliferation of regulatory guidance documents related to PGx (Figure 2).

Among cancer drugs, the average proportion of drug approvals with PGx labeling was 52.0% per year from 2000 to 2020. The annual proportion of new cancer drug approvals with PGx labeling increased from 33.3% ($n = 1$) in 2000 to 55.6% ($n = 10$) in 2019 and 47.1% ($n = 8$) through July in 2020 with the lowest at 0% in 2008 and highest at 100% ($n = 4$) in 2016 (Table 1).

Among non-cancer drugs, the average proportion of drug approvals with PGx labeling was 16.2% per year from 2000 to 2020. The annual proportion of new non-cancer drug approvals with PGx labeling increased from 7.7% ($n = 2$) in 2000 to 24.4% ($n = 10$) in 2019 and 13.6% ($n = 3$) through July in 2020 with the lowest at 0% in 2005 and highest at 38.9% ($n = 7$) in 2013 (Table 1).

Table 1. Annual proportion of drug approvals with PGx labeling for cancer vs. non-cancer indications.

Year	All			Cancer			Non-Cancer		
	Total Number of New Drugs Approved by FDA	Total No. of New Drugs with Biomarker Mentioned (%)		Number of New Drugs Approved by FDA	New Drugs with Biomarker Mentioned (%)		Number of New Drugs Approved by FDA	New Drugs with Biomarker Mentioned (%)	
2000	29	3 (10.3)		3	1 (33.3)		26	2 (7.7)	
2001	28	3 (10.7)		2	1 (50.0)		26	2 (7.7)	
2002	23	5 (21.7)		4	3 (75.0)		19	2 (10.5)	
2003	24	2 (8.3)		3	1 (33.3)		21	1 (4.8)	
2004	34	5 (14.7)		5	2 (40.0)		29	3 (10.3)	
2005	19	1 (5.3)		3	1 (33.3)		16	0	
2006	22	3 (13.6)		5	2 (40.0)		17	1 (5.9)	
2007	18	6 (33.3)		4	3 (75.0)		14	3 (21.4)	
2008	24	5 (20.8)		3	0		21	5 (23.8)	
2009	27	5 (18.5)		5	2 (40.0)		22	3 (13.6)	
2010	20	4 (20.0)		2	1 (50.0)		18	3 (16.7)	
2011	30	10 (33.3)		7	4 (57.1)		23	6 (26.1)	
2012	39	9 (23.1)		12	6 (50.0)		27	3 (11.1)	
2013	27	12 (44.4)		9	5 (55.6)		18	7 (38.9)	
2014	41	11 (26.8)		8	6 (75.0)		33	5 (15.2)	
2015	47	16 (34.0)		14	6 (42.9)		33	10 (30.3)	
2016	25	9 (36.0)		4	4 (100.0)		21	5 (23.8)	
2017	53	15 (28.3)		14	11 (78.6)		39	4 (10.3)	
2018	66	23 (34.8)		18	11 (61.1)		48	12 (25.0)	
2019	59	20 (33.9)		18	10 (55.6)		41	10 (24.4)	
2020[1]	39	11 (28.2)		17	8 (47.1)		22	3 (13.6)	

[1] Data through 31 July 2020.

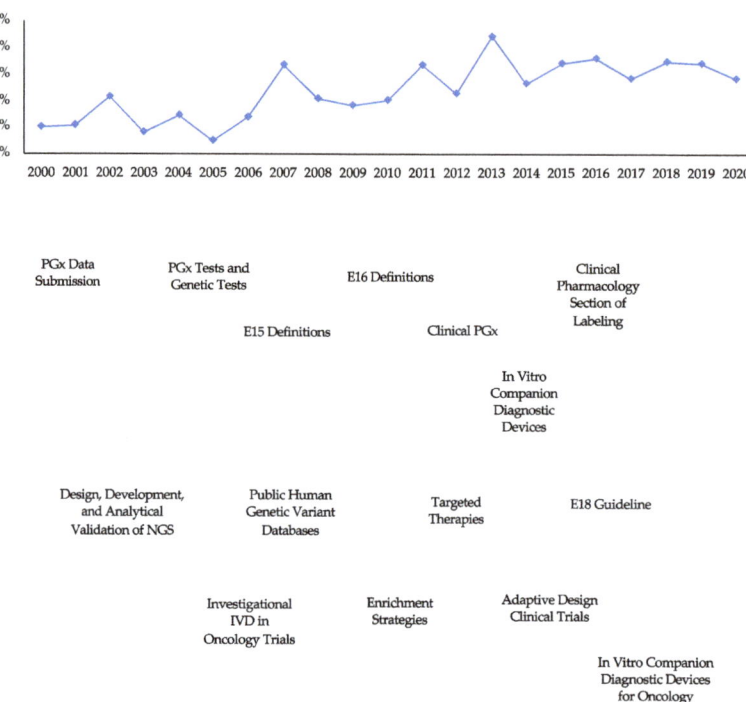

Figure 2. Trends in annual proportion of new drug approvals with PGx labeling and finalized regulatory guidance related to pharmacogenomics from 2000 to 2020, with data through 31 July 2020. E15, E16, and E18 Guidance were developed within the International Conference on Harmonisation of Technical Requirements for Registration of Pharmaceuticals for Human Use (ICH) and endorsed by the ICH Steering Committee at Step 4 of the ICH process [16].

3.2. Yearly Trends of Biomarker–Drug Pairs

Forty-three (24.2%) drugs of all drug approvals with PGx labeling contained multiple biomarkers at initial approval, with a maximum of 7 biomarkers in one drug label, resulting in a total of 258 unique biomarker–drug pairs identified from 2000 to 2020. Of these, 52.3% ($n = 135$) were for cancer indications. On average, there were 12.3 biomarker–drug pairs approved per year over the study period. The number of biomarker–drug pairs approved annually increased from 3 in 2000 to 35 in 2019 and 17 through July of 2020 with a minimum of 1 in 2005 and maximum of 43 in 2018.

The average annual proportion of biomarker–drug pairs indicated for cancer was 53%. Between 2000 and 2020, the annual proportion of biomarker–drug pairs with cancer indications increased from 33.3% ($n = 1$) in 2000 to 66% ($n = 23$) in 2019 and 65% ($n = 11$) in 2020 with the lowest at 0% in 2008 and highest at 100% ($n = 1$) in 2005 (Figure 3).

For the remaining 123 non-cancer biomarker–drug pairs, the average annual proportion of biomarker–drug pairs was 47%. The annual proportion of biomarker–drug pairs with indications for all other clinical areas decreased from 67% ($n = 2$) in 2000 to 34% ($n = 12$) in 2019 and 35% ($n = 6$) in 2020 with the lowest at 0% in 2005 and highest at 100% ($n = 6$) in 2008 (Figure 3).

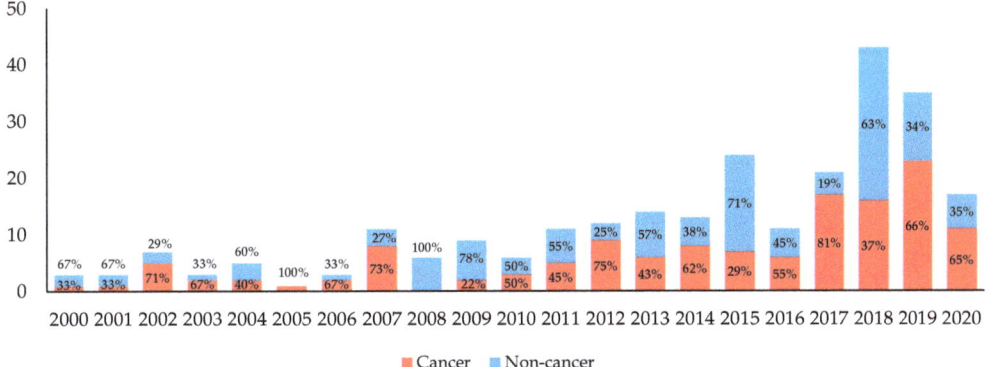

Figure 3. Trends in the number of new biomarker–drug pairs approved per year with annual proportions by cancer vs. non-cancer from 2000 to 2020. Data shown through July of 2020.

3.3. Clinical Actionability of PGx Information

Figure 4 depicts the distribution of biomarker–drug pairs across PGx levels of drug label information based on PharmGKB categories. Of 250 biomarker–drug pairs annotated with PGx levels, 61.6% ($n = 154$) are clinically actionable; of these, 59.7% ($n = 92$) were associated with cancer drugs while the remaining 40.3% ($n = 62$) were associated with drugs for non-cancer areas ($p < 0.0051$). Biomarker–drug pairs considered to be clinically actionable included 37.6% ($n = 94$) of total biomarker–drug pairs that require genetic testing (cancer accounted for 75.5% while non-cancer accounted for 24.5%; $p < 0.0001$), 0% recommend genetic testing, and 24.0% ($n = 60$) correspond to "actionable" information (cancer accounted for 35.0% while non-cancer accounted for 65.0%). The remaining 38.4% ($n = 96$) of biomarker–drug pairs were "informative" (cancer accounted for 42.7% and non-cancer 57.3%) but lacked clinical actionability.

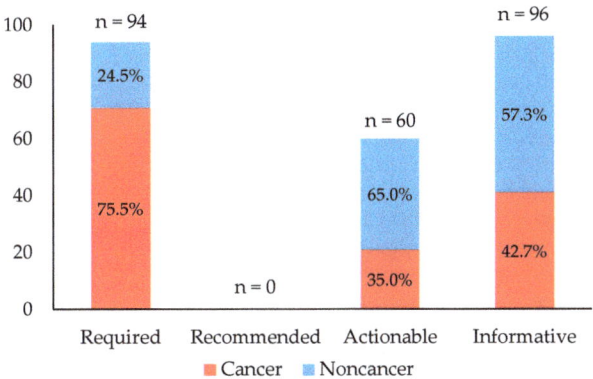

Figure 4. PharmGKB PGx Levels of biomarker–drug pairs for cancer and non-cancer therapies.

4. Discussion

With recent progress in genomic sciences and precision medicine along with regulatory guidance for pharmacogenomics, it is not surprising that we found PGx biomarkers have become increasingly prevalent in new drug labels for all therapeutic areas over the last two decades. Greater than half of all biomarker–drug pairs identified in our study were associated with clinically actionable measures of PGx information. Consistent with previous studies, this progress has continued to be most prominent in cancer therapies, which comprise the majority of new PGx drug approvals and account for the greatest proportion of biomarker–drug pairs with testing requirements [17–19].

In 2005, the FDA issued its first guidance for industry with information on how to submit PGx data during new drug application and review processes, including specific uses of PGx information in drug labeling [20]. Recommendations for co-development of new drugs and corresponding companion diagnostic devices (i.e., PGx tests), in the absence of available tests, were included in the initial document, with further guidance on in vitro diagnostics development published in 2014, 2019, and 2020 [21–23]. The majority of PGx-related guidance for industry, such as guidelines for including genetic information into appropriate sections of the labeling and the creation of the "Pharmacogenomics" subsection within the Clinical Pharmacology section, were issued in the latter half of the study period. There has been a corresponding substantial increase in the number of new drug approvals with PGx information in the labeling, with a total of 136 new drugs between 2011 and 2020 compared to 42 new drugs between 2000 and 2010 [24,25].

Cancer drugs have maintained a strong presence in PGx, as well as among targeted therapies in general. Greater knowledge of clinically significant gene–drug interactions (particularly in relation to somatic variants) has in part enabled the prediction of treatment efficacy in targeted patient subgroups and prompted industry investment in biomarker-based strategies for novel cancer drug development. A review of FDA-approved cancer therapies that required PGx testing demonstrated that two-thirds of drug approvals were based on an enrichment trial design [26]. Such trial designs have been associated with greater clinical trial success rates and lower costs associated with drug development, particularly for well-validated biomarkers such as *HER2* for the treatment of metastatic breast cancer [8–11]. Recent studies have further attributed improvements in cancer survival to the approval of several new PGx-based targeted treatments for metastatic cancer [27,28].

Targeted approaches to immunotherapy have recently changed the landscape of therapeutic strategies in cancer. For instance, immune-checkpoint inhibitors act against checkpoint protein (PD-1) or its partner protein (PD-L1), enabling the activation of an anti-tumor immune response. Identifying predictive biomarkers for checkpoint blockade response is critical for optimizing treatment efficacy and preventing drug-related toxic effects. These inhibitors have been associated with improved survival and fewer adverse events compared with chemotherapy for various tumor types, including metastatic melanoma, advanced non-small cell lung cancer (NSCLC), and head and neck squamous cell carcinoma [29,30]. Molecular diagnostics have been approved for the use of anti-PD-1/anti-PD-L1 therapies, particularly for pembrolizumab, nivolumab, and atezolizumab [31]. Several other biomarkers are also promising for predicting immunotherapy response. High tumor mutation burden identifies tumors with a greater number of variants that may be more easily recognized by the immune system, which has been correlated with benefit from anti-PD-1/anti-PD-L1 therapies for cancers such as melanoma and NSCLC [32]. Mismatch repair deficiency/microsatellite instability is a predictor of anti-PD-1/anti-PD-L1 treatment efficacy in solid tumors such as colorectal cancer [33,34]. Human leukocyte antigen (HLA) is another promising biomarker as it plays a major role in discerning foreign pathogens or tumor cells as part of the anti-tumor immune response [35]. Research suggests that a patient's HLA type might be indicative of response to immunotherapy and can be utilized in personalized cancer vaccine development and immunotherapy biomarker discovery [36].

The use of PGx is also important outside of cancer but their application may be limited by the following: the availability of other established biomarkers, such as blood pressure, hemoglobin A1C, and low-density lipoprotein used to assess patient prognostic risk in cardiovascular disease clinical trials, and the complexity of drug metabolism, particularly for conditions such as chronic kidney disease that can alter drug response phenotypes (e.g., phenoconversion) [7,37,38].

PGx-guided therapies in non-cancer areas (e.g., cardiovascular disease, mental illness) have primarily focused on the cytochrome P450 (CYP) family of pharmacogenes, which are involved in the metabolism of nearly 20% of commonly used drugs [39]. For example, variation in the *CYP2D6* gene influences drug metabolism activity such that individuals who carry deficient *CYP2D6* alleles have sub-optimal enzymatic activity and are at higher risk of developing adverse drug reactions. Among psychotropic medications, there are several drug substrates for *CYP2D6*, including atomoxetine (attention deficit hyperactivity disorder medication) and clozapine (antipsychotic for treatment of schizophrenia), for which drug labels recommend dose adjustments for patients who are *CYP2D6* poor metabolizers [40]. Studies provide accumulating evidence that PGx testing for CYP enzyme genes can inform drug dosing and selection and improve patient outcomes [41–44].

The vast majority of actionable drug labels with testing requirements provided genotype-based indication or contraindication. Although PGx labeling could help inform physicians determine an appropriate treatment plan for a patient, its impact on clinical practice may be hindered by the following considerations: the amount of evidence available to support the pharmacologic relevance of genomic associations is highly variable at the time of labeling [45,46]; and PGx information in some drug labels are informational only [46–48]. An example is the drug label for lenalidomide, which mentions a specific PGx variant as part of the indication but does not explicitly require testing prior to drug use. Other labels provide information on the impact of the variant on drug response without recommending a clinical action (e.g., the label for fesoterodine stated that a subset of individuals are poor metabolizers for *CYP2D6* and "Cmax and AUC of the active metabolite are increased 1.7- and 2-fold, respectively, in *CYP2D6* poor metabolizers, as compared to extensive metabolizers" [49]. The clinical significance of these increased concentrations was not stated, and it implies that prescribers need to order PGx testing for *CYP2D6* for some patients and modify the dosage according to individual genotype status).

In addition to PGx levels, PharmGKB provides clinical annotations of variant–drug associations that are assigned with "level of evidence" scores using several criteria to measure the confidence in the association based on literature findings such as replication of association, p value, and odds ratio [50]. The PharmGKB Clinical Annotation Levels of Evidence have been used to support other relevant guidelines, such as CPIC Levels for Genes/Drugs, which summarize literature-based evidence, strength of prescribing recommendation, and the corresponding clinical context for the use of PGx information in drug labels [51]. The degree of consistency between the levels of evidence and strength of prescribing recommendations is presently unclear and may be an area for further research. Notwithstanding, the application of actionable PGx information may depend on a range of other factors which may be context-dependent and subjective in nature. Hendricks-Sturrup et al. outlined several scenarios highlighting considerations such as therapeutic alternatives, timing of PGx testing with respect to diagnosis, and patient medical history and family history that influence decision-making for either incorporating or excluding certain PGx tests as part of patient management [52].

Our analysis suggests that we are likely to see continued growth in the prevalence of new drugs approved with PGx information, albeit with greater actionability for cancer treatment compared to all other clinical areas. We agree with the earlier commentary of Tutton that while actionable PGx information can help inform prescribing decisions, the increased approval of drugs containing PGx biomarkers serves only a partial role in facilitating large-scale adoption of PGx [18]. Additional challenges to the clinical adoption of PGx testing have been indicated in the literature, including the dearth of evidence supporting the clinical utility and cost-effectiveness of PGx testing [53–55]. Most salient of these is the underrepresentation of non-European ancestry in GWAS used to examine PGx traits and in clinical drug trials, which may result in ambiguity in the interpretation of PGx biomarkers for non-European patients and contribute to potential disparities in the utilization of PGx testing in cases where they are required [56,57]. A study conducted by Lynch et al. reported underutilization of guideline recommended PGx testing (e.g., *EGFR* testing in lung cancer) and substantial differences in the likelihood of getting tested based on the patient's race as well as other demographic factors, including socioeconomic status and zip code [58]. As the number of new drugs with actionable PGx information continues to expand, further research is needed to address the ethical and social implications of the current Eurocentric bias in pharmacogenomic research to ensure equitable benefit of PGx for all members of society.

There were several limitations related to the data analyzed. We studied only the approvals of new drug applications with a submission classification of Type 1 or Type 1,4 and initial submissions for biologics. Approvals of generic drug products and applications with other NDA classification codes for already marketed active ingredients were not assessed, such that new biomarkers added to labels in the post-market setting or included as part of approvals through other NDA classification codes were excluded from our study. Our rationale for focusing solely on these submission types was to assess the incorporation of PGx information in initial drug approvals. We also did not account for biomarkers associated with approved drugs that have been discontinued or labels that were changed due to reports of unexpected adverse effects or failure to verify clinical benefit.

We observed differences in drugs considered to have PGx labeling between PharmGKB and the FDA Table. At the time of our study, 11 drugs with PGx labeling corresponding to 16 unique biomarker–drug pairs were profiled in PharmGKB but were not listed in the FDA Table. Reasons for discrepancies in PGx biomarkers listed by these sources are unclear but may be attributed to different criteria for annotation of PGx biomarkers. Conversely, a total of five drugs corresponding to eight biomarker–drug pairs identified in our study lacked annotations for PharmGKB PGx levels: one of which (umeclidinium/vilanterol-*CYP2D6*) was annotated in a Swissmedic-approved drug label but not in an FDA-approved label, while the remaining seven biomarker–drug pairs (i.e., *TTR*-patisiran, *Deletion 17p*-venetoclax, *FGFR2*-pemigatinib, *ACADVL*-triheptanoin, *CPT2*-triheptanoin, *HADHA*-triheptanoin, *HADHB*-triheptanoin) were not annotated for reasons unknown [59–61].

Furthermore, none of the biomarkers identified in our study were assigned to the "recommended genetic testing" category. As of November 10, 2020, PharmGKB listed a total of five drug approvals with "recommended testing", of which two (i.e., azathioprine and thioguanine) were first approved prior to 2000 and to which biomarker information was added as part of subsequent labeling updates [62]. The remaining three approvals (i.e., dextromethorphan/quinidine, mercaptopurine, and oxcarbazepine) were approved with submission classifications such as Type 4 (new combination), Type 5 (new formulation/new manufacturer), and Type 3 (new dosage form), and were excluded from our analysis. Our findings suggest that there was sufficient evidence at initial approval to warrant testing requirements for relevant drugs, especially for therapies that were developed with indications based on specific genotypes; thus, those were assigned to the "required genetic testing" category instead.

5. Conclusions

Advances in genomics research have clearly affected how drugs are developed and approved. Our analysis demonstrates an upward trend in the inclusion of PGx labeling in new drug approvals in the US over the last two decades; the increased trend is more prominent in cancer drugs. Overall, we are likely to see continued growth in new drugs approvals with PGx information. More than half of PGx information in new drug approvals are clinically actionable, with the majority of testing requirements concentrated in cancer drugs. Further studies are warranted to examine the utilization of such tests in clinical practice as well as to generate evidence in support of utilizing PGx biomarkers for non-cancer therapeutic areas.

Author Contributions: Conceptualization, C.Y.L.; methodology, C.Y.L. and J.A.K.; validation, C.Y.L. and J.A.K.; formal analysis, J.A.K.; investigation, J.A.K.; resources, J.A.K. and R.C.; data curation, J.A.K. and R.C.; writing—original draft preparation, J.A.K.; writing—review and editing, C.Y.L., J.A.K. and R.C.; visualization, J.A.K.; supervision, C.Y.L.; project administration, C.Y.L. All authors have read and agreed to the published version of the manuscript.

Funding: This research received no external funding.

Institutional Review Board Statement: Not applicable for studies not involving humans or animals. All data used in this study are publicly available.

Informed Consent Statement: Not applicable.

Data Availability Statement: The data presented in this study are publicly available and can be downloaded from Drugs@FDA database (https://www.accessdata.fda.gov/scripts/cder/daf/ (accessed on 1 March 2021)) and PharmGKB (https://www.pharmgkb.org (accessed on 1 March 2021)).

Acknowledgments: Caitlin Lupton provided additional assistance in the preparation of the paper. C.Y.L. is supported in part by an Ebert Career Development Award at Harvard Pilgrim Health Care Institute & Harvard Medical School.

Conflicts of Interest: The authors declare no conflict of interest.

Appendix A

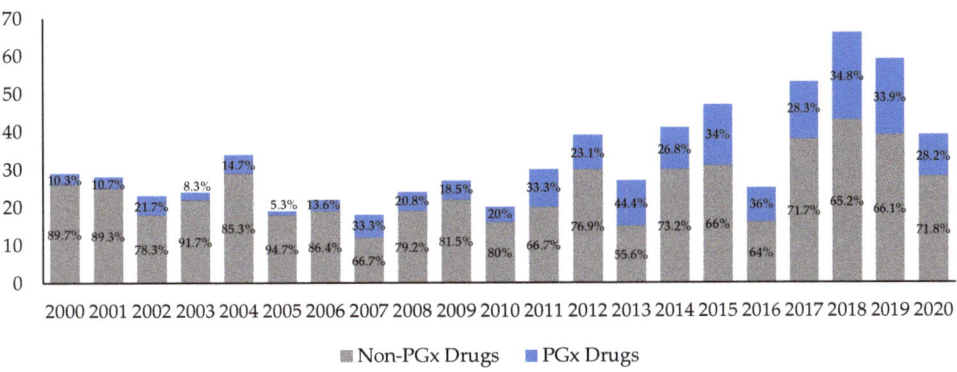

Figure A1. Trends in the number of new drug approvals with PGx labeling from 2000–2020. Data shown through July of 2020.

References

1. Cacabelos, R.; Cacabelos, N.; Carril, J.C. The role of pharmacogenomics in adverse drug reactions. *Expert Rev. Clin. Pharmacol.* **2019**, *12*, 407–442. [CrossRef]
2. Burt, T.; Dhillon, S. Pharmacogenomics in early-phase clinical development. *Pharmacogenomics* **2013**, *14*, 1085–1097. [CrossRef]
3. Lauschke, V.M.; Milani, L.; Ingelman-Sundberg, M. Pharmacogenomic Biomarkers for Improved Drug Therapy—Recent Progress and Future Developments. *AAPS J.* **2018**, *20*, 4. [CrossRef]
4. Giacomini, K.M.; Yee, K.M.G.S.W.; Mushiroda, T.; Weinshilboum, R.M.; Ratain, M.J.; Kubo, T.M.M. Genome-wide association studies of drug response and toxicity: An opportunity for genome medicine. *Nat. Rev. Drug Discov.* **2017**, *16*, 70. [CrossRef] [PubMed]
5. Kalia, M. Personalized oncology: Recent advances and future challenges. *Metabolism* **2013**, *62*, S11–S14. [CrossRef] [PubMed]
6. Lee, A.M.; Shi, Q.; Pavey, E.; Alberts, S.R.; Sargent, D.J.; Sinicrope, F.A.; Berenberg, J.L.; Goldberg, R.M.; Diasio, R.B. DPYD Variants as Predictors of 5-fluorouracil Toxicity in Adjuvant Colon Cancer Treatment (NCCTG N0147). *J. Natl. Cancer Inst.* **2014**, *106*, 106. [CrossRef]
7. Adams, S.M.; Crisamore, K.R.; Empey, P.E. Clinical Pharmacogenomics. *Clin. J. Am. Soc. Nephrol.* **2018**, *13*, 1561–1571. [CrossRef] [PubMed]
8. Falconi, A.; Lopes, G.; Parker, J.L. Biomarkers and Receptor Targeted Therapies Reduce Clinical Trial Risk in Non–Small-Cell Lung Cancer. *J. Thorac. Oncol.* **2014**, *9*, 163–169. [CrossRef] [PubMed]
9. Jardim, D.L.F.; Schwaederle, M.; Wei, C.; Lee, J.J.; Hong, D.S.; Eggermont, A.M.; Schilsky, R.L.; Mendelsohn, J.; Lazar, V.; Kurzrock, R. Impact of a Biomarker-Based Strategy on Oncology Drug Development: A Meta-analysis of Clinical Trials Leading to FDA Approval. *J. Natl. Cancer Inst.* **2015**, *107*. [CrossRef]
10. Parker, J.L.; Lushina, N.; Bal, P.S.; Petrella, T.; Dent, R.; Lopes, G. Impact of biomarkers on clinical trial risk in breast cancer. *Breast Cancer Res. Treat.* **2012**, *136*, 179–185. [CrossRef]

11. Schwaederle, M.; Zhao, M.; Lee, J.J.; Eggermont, A.M.; Schilsky, R.L.; Mendelsohn, J.; Lazar, V.; Kurzrock, R. Impact of Precision Medicine in Diverse Cancers: A Meta-Analysis of Phase II Clinical Trials. *J. Clin. Oncol.* **2015**, *33*, 3817–3825. [CrossRef]
12. Schuck, R.N.; Grillo, J.A. Pharmacogenomic Biomarkers: An FDA Perspective on Utilization in Biological Product Labeling. *AAPS J.* **2016**, *18*, 573–577. [CrossRef]
13. Drugs@FDA: FDA-Approved Drugs. Available online: https://www.accessdata.fda.gov/scripts/cder/daf/ (accessed on 10 November 2020).
14. US Food and Drug Administration. Table of Pharmacogenomic Biomarkers in Drug Labeling. Available online: https://www.fda.gov/drugs/science-and-research-drugs/table-pharmacogenomic-biomarkers-drug-labeling (accessed on 10 November 2020).
15. PharmGKB. Drug Label Information and Legend. Available online: https://www.pharmgkb.org/page/drugLabelLegend (accessed on 10 November 2020).
16. US Food and Drug Administration. Other FDA Resources Related to Pharmacogenomics. Available online: https://www.fda.gov/drugs/science-and-research-drugs/other-fda-resources-related-pharmacogenomics (accessed on 10 November 2020).
17. Mehta, D.; Uber, R.; Ingle, T.; Li, C.; Liu, Z.; Thakkar, S.; Ning, B.; Wu, L.; Yang, J.; Harris, S.; et al. Study of pharmacogenomic information in FDA-approved drug labeling to facilitate application of precision medicine. *Drug Discov. Today* **2020**, *25*, 813–820. [CrossRef]
18. Tutton, R. Pharmacogenomic biomarkers in drug labels: What do they tell us? *Pharmacogenomics* **2014**, *15*, 297–304. [CrossRef]
19. Vivot, A.; Boutron, I.; Ravaud, P.; Porcher, R. Guidance for pharmacogenomic biomarker testing in labels of FDA-approved drugs. *Genet. Med.* **2014**, *17*, 733–738. [CrossRef]
20. US Food and Drug Administration. Guidance for Industry. Pharmacogenomic Data Submissions. Available online: https://www.fda.gov/media/72420/download (accessed on 10 November 2020).
21. US Food and Drug Administration. Guidance for Industry. In Vitro Companion Diagnostic Devices. Available online: https://www.fda.gov/media/81309/download (accessed on 10 November 2020).
22. US Food and Drug Administration. Guidance for Industry. Developing and Labeling In vitro Companion Diagnostic Devices for a Specific Group of Oncology Therapeutic Products. Available online: https://www.fda.gov/media/120340/download (accessed on 10 November 2020).
23. US Food and Drug Administration. Guidance for Industry. Investigational In Vitro Diagnostics in Oncology Trials: Streamlined Submission Process for Study Risk Determination. Available online: https://www.fda.gov/media/120340/download (accessed on 10 November 2020).
24. US Food and Drug Administration. Guidance for Industry. Clinical Pharmacogenomics: Premarket Evaluation in Early-Phase Clinical Studies and Recommendations for Labeling. Available online: https://www.fda.gov/media/84923/download (accessed on 10 November 2020).
25. US Food and Drug Administration. Guidance for Industry. Clinical Pharmacology Section of Labeling for Human Prescription Drug and Biological Products—Content and Format. Available online: https://www.fda.gov/media/74346/download (accessed on 10 November 2020).
26. Vivot, A.; Boutron, I.; Béraud-Chaulet, G.; Zeitoun, J.-D.; Ravaud, P.; Porcher, R. Evidence for Treatment-by-Biomarker interaction for FDA-approved Oncology Drugs with Required Pharmacogenomic Biomarker Testing. *Sci. Rep.* **2017**, *7*, 1–9. [CrossRef]
27. Howlader, N.; Forjaz, G.; Mooradian, M.J.; Meza, R.; Kong, C.Y.; Cronin, K.A.; Mariotto, A.B.; Lowy, D.R.; Feuer, E.J. The Effect of Advances in Lung-Cancer Treatment on Population Mortality. *N. Engl. J. Med.* **2020**, *383*, 640–649. [CrossRef] [PubMed]
28. Siegel, R.L.; Miller, K.D.; Jemal, A. Cancer statistics, 2020. *CA Cancer J. Clin.* **2020**, *70*, 7–30. [CrossRef] [PubMed]
29. Wakabayashi, G.; Lee, Y.-C.; Luh, F.; Kuo, C.-N.; Chang, W.-C.; Yen, Y. Development and clinical applications of cancer immunotherapy against PD-1 signaling pathway. *J. Biomed. Sci.* **2019**, *26*, 1–13. [CrossRef]
30. Xia, L.; Liu, Y.; Wang, Y. PD-1/PD-L1 Blockade Therapy in Advanced Non-Small-Cell Lung Cancer: Current Status and Future Directions. *Oncologist* **2019**, *24*, S31–S41. [CrossRef] [PubMed]
31. US Food and Drug Administration. List of Cleared or Approved Companion Diagnostic Devices (In Vitro and Imaging Tools). Available online: https://www.fda.gov/medical-devices/vitro-diagnostics/list-cleared-or-approved-companion-diagnostic-devices-vitro-and-imaging-tools (accessed on 20 February 2021).
32. Greillier, L.; Tomasini, P.; Barlesi, F. The clinical utility of tumor mutational burden in non-small cell lung cancer. *Transl. Lung Cancer Res.* **2018**, *7*, 639–646. [CrossRef]
33. Tan, E.; Sahin, I.H. Defining the current role of immune checkpoint inhibitors in the treatment of mismatch repair-deficient/microsatellite stability-high colorectal cancer and shedding light on future approaches. *Exp. Rev. Gastroenterol. Hepatol.* **2021**, 1–8. [CrossRef]
34. Viale, G.; Trapani, D.; Curigliano, G. Mismatch Repair Deficiency as a Predictive Biomarker for Immunotherapy Efficacy. *BioMed Res. Int.* **2017**, *2017*, 1–7. [CrossRef] [PubMed]
35. Sabbatino, F.; Liguori, L.; Polcaro, G.; Salvato, I.; Caramori, G.; Salzano, F.A.; Casolaro, V.; Stellato, C.; Col, J.D.; Pepe, S. Role of Human Leukocyte Antigen System as A Predictive Biomarker for Checkpoint-Based Immunotherapy in Cancer Patients. *Int. J. Mol. Sci.* **2020**, *21*, 7295. [CrossRef]
36. Chowell, D.; Morris, L.G.T.; Grigg, C.M.; Weber, J.K.; Samstein, R.M.; Makarov, V.; Kuo, F.; Kendall, S.M.; Requena, D.; Riaz, N.; et al. Patient HLA class I genotype influences cancer response to checkpoint blockade immunotherapy. *Science* **2017**, *359*, 582–587. [CrossRef] [PubMed]

37. Adeniyi, O.; Ramamoorthy, A.; Schuck, R.; Sun, J.; Wilson, J.; Zineh, I.; Pacanowski, M. An Overview of Genomic Biomarker Use in Cardiovascular Disease Clinical Trials. *Clin. Pharmacol. Ther.* **2019**, *106*, 841–846. [CrossRef] [PubMed]
38. Lunenburg, C.A.; Gasse, C. Pharmacogenetics in psychiatric care, a call for uptake of available applications. *Psychiatry Res.* **2020**, *292*, 113336. [CrossRef] [PubMed]
39. Taylor, C.; Crosby, I.; Yip, V.; Maguire, P.; Pirmohamed, M.; Turner, R.M. A Review of the Important Role of *CYP2D6* in Pharmacogenomics. *Genes* **2020**, *11*, 1295. [CrossRef] [PubMed]
40. Kam, H.; Jeong, H. Pharmacogenomic Biomarkers and Their Applications in Psychiatry. *Genes* **2020**, *11*, 1445. [CrossRef] [PubMed]
41. Bättig, V.A.D.; Roll, S.C.; Hahn, M. Pharmacogenetic Testing in Depressed Patients and Interdisciplinary Exchange between a Pharmacist and Psychiatrists Results in Reduced Hospitalization Times. *Pharmacopsychiatry* **2020**, *53*, 185–192. [CrossRef]
42. Bradley, P.; Shiekh, M.; Mehra, V.; Vrbicky, K.; Layle, S.; Olson, M.C.; Maciel, A.; Cullors, A.; Garces, J.A.; Lukowiak, A.A. Improved efficacy with targeted pharmacogenetic-guided treatment of patients with depression and anxiety: A randomized clinical trial demonstrating clinical utility. *J. Psychiatr. Res.* **2018**, *96*, 100–107. [CrossRef]
43. Greden, J.F.; Parikh, S.V.; Rothschild, A.J.; Thase, M.E.; Dunlop, B.W.; DeBattista, C.; Conway, C.R.; Forester, B.P.; Mondimore, F.M.; Shelton, R.C.; et al. Impact of pharmacogenomics on clinical outcomes in major depressive disorder in the GUIDED trial: A large, patient- and rater-blinded, randomized, controlled study. *J. Psychiatr. Res.* **2019**, *111*, 59–67. [CrossRef] [PubMed]
44. Marshe, V.S.; Islam, F.; Maciukiewicz, M.; Bousman, C.; Eyre, H.A.; Lavretsky, H.; Mulsant, B.H.; Reynolds, C.F.; Lenze, E.J.; Müller, D.J. Pharmacogenetic Implications for Antidepressant Pharmacotherapy in Late-Life Depression: A Systematic Review of the Literature for Response, Pharmacokinetics and Adverse Drug Reactions. *Am. J. Geriatr. Psychiatry* **2020**, *28*, 609–629. [CrossRef]
45. Relling, M.V.; Evans, W.E. Pharmacogenomics in the clinic. *Nat. Cell Biol.* **2015**, *526*, 343–350. [CrossRef] [PubMed]
46. Zineh, I.; Pebanco, G.D.; Aquilante, C.L.; Gerhard, T.; Beitelshees, A.L.; Beasley, B.N.; Hartzema, A.G. Discordance Between Availability of Pharmacogenetics Studies and Pharmacogenetics-Based Prescribing Information for the Top 200 Drugs. *Ann. Pharmacother.* **2006**, *40*, 639–644. [CrossRef] [PubMed]
47. Frueh, F.W.; Amur, S.; Mummaneni, P.; Epstein, R.S.; Aubert, R.E.; DeLuca, T.M.; Verbrugge, R.R.; Burckart, G.J.; Lesko, L.J. Pharmacogenomic Biomarker Information in Drug Labels Approved by the United States Food and Drug Administration: Prevalence of Related Drug Use. *Pharmacother. J. Hum. Pharmacol. Drug Ther.* **2008**, *28*, 992–998. [CrossRef]
48. Mills, R.; Haga, S.B.; Moaddeb, J. Pharmacogenetic information for patients on drug labels. *Pharm. Pers. Med.* **2014**, *7*, 297–305. [CrossRef] [PubMed]
49. TOVIAZ Drug Label (Revised 11/2017). Available online: https://www.accessdata.fda.gov/drugsatfda_docs/label/2017/022030s014lbl.pdf (accessed on 10 November 2020).
50. Whirl-Carrillo, M.; McDonagh, E.M.; Hebert, J.M.; Gong, L.; Sangkuhl, K.; Thorn, C.F.; Altman, R.B.; Klein, T.E. Pharmacogenomics Knowledge for Personalized Medicine. *Clin. Pharmacol. Ther.* **2012**, *92*, 414–417. [CrossRef]
51. Caudle, K.E.; Gammal, R.S.; Whirl-Carrillo, M.; Hoffman, J.M.; Relling, M.V.; Klein, T.E. Evidence and resources to implement pharmacogenetic knowledge for precision medicine. *Am. J. Health Pharm.* **2016**, *73*, 1977–1985. [CrossRef]
52. Hendricks-Sturrup, R.M.; Linsky, A.; Lu, C.Y.; Vassy, J.L. Genomic testing is best integrated into clinical practice when it is actionable. *Pers. Med.* **2020**, *17*, 5–8. [CrossRef]
53. Hippman, C.; Nislow, C. Pharmacogenomic Testing: Clinical Evidence and Implementation Challenges. *J. Pers. Med.* **2019**, *9*, 40. [CrossRef] [PubMed]
54. Wang, B.; Canestaro, W.J.; Choudhry, N.K. Clinical Evidence Supporting Pharmacogenomic Biomarker Testing Provided in US Food and Drug Administration Drug Labels. *JAMA Intern. Med.* **2014**, *174*, 1938. [CrossRef]
55. Wong, W.B.; Carlson, J.J.; Thariani, R.; Veenstra, D.L.; Veenstra, D.L. Cost Effectiveness of Pharmacogenomics. *PharmacoEconomics* **2010**, *28*, 1001–1013. [CrossRef] [PubMed]
56. Zhang, H.; De, T.; Zhong, Y.; Perera, M.A. The Advantages and Challenges of Diversity in Pharmacogenomics: Can Minority Populations Bring Us Closer to Implementation? *Clin. Pharmacol. Ther.* **2019**, *106*, 338–349. [CrossRef] [PubMed]
57. De, T.; Park, C.S.; Perera, M.A. Cardiovascular Pharmacogenomics: Does It Matter If You're Black or White? *Annu. Rev. Pharmacol. Toxicol.* **2019**, *59*, 577–603. [CrossRef]
58. Lynch, J.A.; Berse, B.; Rabb, M.; Mosquin, P.; Chew, R.; West, S.L.; Coomer, N.; Becker, D.; Kautter, J. Underutilization and disparities in access to EGFR testing among Medicare patients with lung cancer from 2010–2013. *BMC Cancer* **2018**, *18*, 1–13. [CrossRef]
59. PharmGKB. Annotation of Swissmedic Label for Umeclidinium/Vilanterol and CYP2D6. Available online: https://www.pharmgkb.org/chemical/PA166184235/labelAnnotation/PA166184236 (accessed on 10 November 2020).
60. PharmGKB. Patisiran Drug Label Annotations. Available online: https://www.pharmgkb.org/chemical/PA166182884/labelAnnotation (accessed on 10 November 2020).
61. PharmGKB. Annotation of FDA Label for Venetoclax and FLT3, IDH1, IDH2, NPM1, TP53. Available online: https://www.pharmgkb.org/chemical/PA166153473/labelAnnotation/PA166163420 (accessed on 10 November 2020).
62. Clinical Pharmacogenetics Implementation Consortium. Genes-Drugs. Available online: https://cpicpgx.org/genes-drugs/ (accessed on 10 November 2020).

Article

Common Treatment, Common Variant: Evolutionary Prediction of Functional Pharmacogenomic Variants

Laura B. Scheinfeldt [1,*], Andrew Brangan [1], Dara M. Kusic [1], Sudhir Kumar [2,3,4] and Neda Gharani [1,5]

1. Coriell Institute for Medical Research, Camden, NJ 08003, USA; andrew.brangan@gmail.com (A.B.); dkusic@coriell.org (D.M.K.); neda.gharani@coriell.org (N.G.)
2. Institute for Genomics and Evolutionary Medicine, Temple University, Philadelphia, PA 19122, USA; s.kumar@temple.edu
3. Department of Biology, Temple University, Philadelphia, PA 19122, USA
4. Center for Excellence in Genome Medicine and Research, King Abdulaziz University, Jeddah 21577, Saudi Arabia
5. Gharani Consulting, Surrey KT139PA, UK
* Correspondence: lscheinfeldt@coriell.org

Abstract: Pharmacogenomics holds the promise of personalized drug efficacy optimization and drug toxicity minimization. Much of the research conducted to date, however, suffers from an ascertainment bias towards European participants. Here, we leverage publicly available, whole genome sequencing data collected from global populations, evolutionary characteristics, and annotated protein features to construct a new in silico machine learning pharmacogenetic identification method called XGB-PGX. When applied to pharmacogenetic data, XGB-PGX outperformed all existing prediction methods and identified over 2000 new pharmacogenetic variants. While there are modest pharmacogenetic allele frequency distribution differences across global population samples, the most striking distinction is between the relatively rare putatively neutral pharmacogene variants and the relatively common established and newly predicted functional pharamacogenetic variants. Our findings therefore support a focus on individual patient pharmacogenetic testing rather than on clinical presumptions about patient race, ethnicity, or ancestral geographic residence. We further encourage more attention be given to the impact of common variation on drug response and propose a new 'common treatment, common variant' perspective for pharmacogenetic prediction that is distinct from the types of variation that underlie complex and Mendelian disease. XGB-PGX has identified many new pharmacovariants that are present across all global communities; however, communities that have been underrepresented in genomic research are likely to benefit the most from XGB-PGX's in silico predictions.

Keywords: pharmacogenomic; machine learning; adaptation; human evolution

1. Introduction

There is a well-established contribution of genetic variation to drug response that has resulted in the expectation of personalized optimization of drug efficacy and the minimization of drug toxicity [1–7]. Unfortunately, there is also a well-documented ascertainment bias in the populations that have been included in genetic and genomic research to date [8–11]. As a result of recent human evolutionary history, the out of Africa migration and resulting population bottleneck, Europeans carry only a subset of human variation [12–16]. Given the overrepresentation of peoples of European descent in pharmacogenomic (PGx) research, there are likely to be a non-trivial number of variants that impact drug response that have not yet been identified, functionally characterized, or incorporated into clinical guidelines. This bias, therefore, limits the generalizability of results from genomic and PGx studies to all human populations [9,11,17]. Efforts to mitigate this bias will help ensure that communities of European descent are not the sole beneficiaries of PGx research findings [8,11].

An illustrative example of the implications of PGx ascertainment bias is the case of warfarin dosing. A variant in the gene calumenin (the rs339097 G allele), rare in individuals with European ancestry, increases the required therapeutic dose of the commonly prescribed blood thinner warfarin by up to 15% [18]. This variant, as well as other key variants in established genes such as CYP2C9*5, *6, *8, and *11, have been left out of several common dosing algorithms and, as a result, these predictive models perform poorly for individuals that carry these variants [19–21].

Computational or in silico prediction methods for PGx variants have the potential to alleviate PGx ascertainment bias. Several methods have been developed to predict pathogenic variants, variants thought to negatively impact protein function [22–25]. Li et al. [26] extended this computational prediction effort to develop a method for functional missense PGx variants, but found that PGx variants looked less like disease variants (which are thought to have been subjected to purifying selection) and more like neutral variants. More recently, Zhou et al. [27] applied an ensemble computational approach to predict deleterious PGx variants and successfully applied it to the minority subset of PGx variants with existing experimental data. Consistent with Li et al. [26], Zhou et al. [27] found that relaxing the requirement of evolutionary signatures of purifying selection improved the computational prediction of PGx variants.

Previous work by us and others has demonstrated the impact that positive selection has had on global human contemporary variation involved in immune response and metabolism [11,28–31]. Given the overlap between these gene categories and the genes involved in drug response, we present here a novel approach to in silico PGx variant prediction that leverages signatures of adaptation. Our computational approach is designed to mitigate ascertainment biases in PGx research and identify important PGx diversity that is currently missing from existing PGx resources.

2. Materials and Methods

2.1. Samples and Data

Whole-genome sequencing data from the Phase 3 of the 1000 Genomes Project [13] were used to identify global missense variation in previously annotated pharmacogenes in PharmGKB [32]; more detailed information about the 1000 Genomes Project Phase 3 population samples can be found in Table 1. Clinical Pharmacogenetics Implementation Consortium (CPIC) gene annotation information was downloaded from CPIC (https://cpicpgx.org/genes-drugs/) and was last annotated on 25 March 2020. Pharmacogene variant annotation information was downloaded from PharmGKB (https://www.pharmgkb.org/downloads/) on 28 October 2019. These data were compiled manually by PharmGKB scientific curators [32]. All of the available human UniProt feature annotations (ftp://ftp.uniprot.org/pub/databases/uniprot/current_release/knowledgebase/genome_annotation_tracks/UP000005640_9606_beds/) were downloaded on 6 December 2019 in bed format. Evolutionary probabilities were calculated as previously described for the subset of missense variant positions present in PharmGKB annotated pharmacogenes and in the UCSD 46 species vertebrate alignment [33,34], and candidate adaptive polymorphisms (CAPs) were identified as previously described [25,29]. Evolutionary rate, evolutionary time span, SIFT (Sorting Intolerant From Tolerant), and PolyPhen2 values were extracted from the e-GRASP Resource [35]. Version 1.5 CADD (Combined Annotation Dependent Depletion) values were downloaded from http://cadd.gs.washington.edu/download [36]. In total, 38,686 1000 Genomes Project Phase 3 whole-genome sequencing missense variants located in 1076 PharmGKB pharmacogenes with evolutionary probabilities were retained for downstream analyses (Supplementary Materials Table S1).

Table 1. 1000 Genomes Project Phase 3 data population samples.

Description	Label	Sample Size
African Caribbean in Barbados	ACB	96
Esan in Nigeria	ESN	99
Gambian in Western Division, Mandinka	GWD	113
Luhya in Webuye, Kenya	LWK	99
Mende in Sierra Leone	MSL	85
People with African Ancestry in Southwest USA	ASW	61
Yoruba in Ibadan, Nigeria	YRI	108
Colombians in Medellin, Colombia	CLM	94
People with Mexican Ancestry in Los Angeles, CA, USA	MXL	64
Peruvians in Lima, Peru	PEL	85
Puerto Ricans in Puerto Rico	PUR	104
Chinese Dai in Xishuangbanna, China	CDX	93
Han Chinese in Beijing, China	CHB	103
Japanese in Tokyo, Japan	JPT	104
Kinh in Ho Chi Minh City, Vietnam	KHV	99
Southern Han Chinese	CHS	105
British in England and Scotland	GBR	91
Finnish in Finland	FIN	99
Iberian Populations in Spain	IBS	107
Toscani in Italia	TSI	107
Utah residents (CEPH) with Northern and Western European ancestry	CEU	99
Bengali in Bangladesh	BEB	86
Gujarati Indians in Houston, TX, USA	GIH	103
Indian Telugu in the UK	ITU	102
Punjabi in Lahore, Pakistan	PJL	96
Sri Lankan Tamil in the UK	STU	102

2.2. Enrichment Testing

We used a publicly available human dataset of adaptive signatures [28] and tested for enrichment of annotated PharmGKB pharmacogenes using a permutation approach. More specifically, for each neutrality test statistic (iHS, XP-CLR, and D) we conducted 1000 permutations assuming 29,521 total genes (the number of genes within 100 kb of one of the Illumina 1M duo SNPs included in [28]). We used the R sample function without replacement (replace = FALSE) to randomly sample the respective number of adaptive signatures for each statistic (9593 iHS loci, 8636 XP-CLR loci, and 17,734 D loci, respectively, across all population samples). We retained the number of permuted adaptive signatures that were annotated in PharmGKB as pharmacogenes. We then counted the number of permutations that were equal to or more extreme than the actual number of PharmGKB pharmacogenes that overlapped adaptive signatures identified by each statistic. We additionally used the pnorm function in R to calculate an empirical P-value to measure whether the extent of overlap between the number of actual pharmacogenes and adaptive signatures is expected by chance given the permutation distribution.

2.3. Machine Learning Modeling

For each missense variant position, UniProt feature annotations were coded as present or absent, CAPs were coded as present or absent, global minor allele frequency ranging from 0 to 1 was included, evolutionary probabilities for reference and non-reference alleles ranging from 0 to 1 were included, evolutionary rate ranging from 0 to 57,405 was included, and evolutionary time span ranging from 0 to 2774 was included. The pharmacogenetic outcome was generated from existing PharmGKB annotation, such that each missense variant was annotated as a pharmacovariant or not.

The Caret package in R [37], including the associated randomForest [38] and xgboost [39] packages, were used for all machine learning PGx modeling. We partitioned the data into 70% for training and 30% for testing using the createDataPartition Caret function.

We used the DMwR package [40] smote method to balance the training data (using the Caret trainControl function with sampling = "smote"), and performed 5-fold cross validation and 10 repeats for the following models using the Caret train function: random forest (method = 'rf'), Logit Boost (method = 'LogitBoost'), and XG Boost (method = 'xgbTree'), which each offering classification-based modeling. Given our relatively higher confidence in 'true positives', we weighted the model evaluation on sensitivity (metric = "Sens").

3. Results

3.1. Annotated PGx Variation Is Negatively Impacted by Ascertainment Bias

To better characterize the potential impact of ascertainment bias on pharmacogene annotation, we performed a descriptive analysis of pharmacogenes annotated in CPIC (see methods for more detail) using the 1000 Genomes Project Phase 3 whole-genome sequencing data collected from worldwide populations (Table 1) [13]. We found that 70% of the genetic variants present in pharmacogenes annotated in CPIC are carried by non-Europeans, as displayed in Figure 1. This result is consistent with our expectation from global patterns of human genetic variation [12–16]. This result is also consistent with expectations from previous analyses of pharmacogene variation in worldwide populations [41] that the pharmacogene variation carried by Europeans alone is an incomplete picture of pharmacogene variation worldwide.

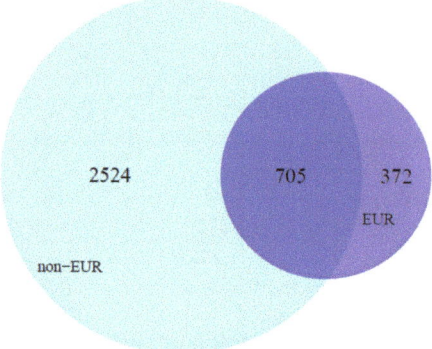

Figure 1. Venn diagram of 1000 Genomes Project Phase 3 pharmacogene variants.

Figure 1 displays a Venn diagram of all of the single nucleotide polymorphisms (SNPs) included in the 1000 Genomes Project Phase 3 whole-genome sequencing dataset for all of the pharmacogenes that have at least one CPIC annotation. The light blue shaded area represents all of the variants present only in non-European population samples, the dark blue represents all of the variants present only in European population samples, and the overlapping area represents all of the variants present in both European and non-European population samples.

3.2. Pharmacogenes Are Enriched for Adaptive Signatures

Previous work by us and others has demonstrated the impact that positive selection has had on contemporary worldwide human variation involved in immune response and metabolism [11,28–31]. Moreover, in a study of 62 global human population samples, Li et al. [42] demonstrate signatures of positive selection in many pharmacogenes. To further explore the extent to which genome-wide signatures of adaptation are enriched for pharmacogenes, we leveraged the publicly available dataset of adaptive signatures identified in Scheinfeldt et al. [28]. This set of adaptive signatures was generated using three complementary approaches for the identification of adaptive signatures that are sensitive to classic selective sweeps and selection on standing variation and includes many genes known to play a role in immune response and metabolism across diverse African communities [28]. In this case, we have chosen to focus on signatures of past adaptation in Africa because our human ancestors emerged in Africa over two hundred thousand years ago and lived in Africa for tens of thousands of years before a subset migrated out of Africa over the past eighty thousand years; because of this bottleneck, non-Africans carry only a subset of human variation [12–16,28]. Consistent with Li et al.'s [42] results, our permutation enrichment test was significant for all three test statistics: iHS ($p < 0.001$), XP-CLR ($p < 0.001$), and D ($p < 0.001$). We found comparable results with our empirical P-value approach: iHS (empirical $p < 0.001$), XP-CLR (empirical $p < 0.001$), and D (empirical $p < 0.001$).

3.3. In Silico Model Development

Given the extensive pharmacogene variation in non-Europeans (Figure 1), the limited representation of non-Europeans in genomic and pharmacogenomic research to date, and the significant enrichment of pharmacogenes in adaptive signatures across the human genome, we next used a range of evolutionary statistics for each variable missense position in each pharmacogene (evolutionary rate, evolutionary time, evolutionary probability of the reference and non-reference allele, and whether the position contains a candidate adaptive polymorphism (CAP) according to Patel et al. [29]) together with global minor allele frequency and all available functional annotations included in the human subset of UniProt feature annotations to develop an in silico prediction method for functionally important pharmacogene variants (Table S1 includes more detail on the included pharmacogenes, and Table S2 includes more detail on the included pharmacogene variants).

We compared three machine learning model approaches and assessed which had the highest sensitivity to detect true positive pharmacogenes in a cross validation of both the training data and the testing data. Overall, the XG Boost model (XGB) performed the best on the training data (Table 2) as measured by ROC. While RF performed marginally better in terms of sensitivity (median 0.97 vs. 0.95, respectively), XGB performed significantly better in terms of specificity (median 0.70 vs. 0.45, respectively). The XGB model also performed better than the RF and LB models on the testing data with respect to sensitivity. As displayed in Table 3, XGB correctly identified more 'true positive' pharmacovariants annotated in PharmGKB (140 vs. 98 and 125, respectively, for RF and LB).

Table 2. Machine learning model comparison using training data.

Statistic	Model	Minimum	1st Quartile	Median	Mean	3rd Quartile	Maximum
ROC	Random Forest	0.80	0.84	0.85	0.85	0.87	0.90
	LogitBoost	0.83	0.86	0.87	0.87	0.89	0.92
	XGBoost	0.88	0.90	0.91	0.91	0.92	0.94
Sensitivity	Random Forest	0.96	0.97	0.97	0.97	0.98	0.98
	LogitBoost	0.90	0.92	0.93	0.93	0.94	0.96
	XGBoost	0.93	0.94	0.95	0.95	0.95	0.96
Specificity	Random Forest	0.31	0.40	0.45	0.45	0.50	0.57
	LogitBoost	0.53	0.62	0.69	0.68	0.72	0.82
	XGBoost	0.61	0.67	0.70	0.69	0.72	0.78

We additionally reviewed the variables that contributed to the XGB model. Table 4 includes the list of variables in order of importance. As shown, minor allele frequency (MAF) was the most impactful variable, followed by three evolutionary summary statistics: whether the position contains a CAP [25,29], evolutionary time [35], and the evolutionary probability of the non-reference allele [25]. The UniProtKB topological (Topo) domain feature (the location of non-membrane regions of membrane-spanning proteins) was the next most impactful variable, followed by evolutionary rate [35], the UniProtKB topological chain feature (the extent of a polypeptide chain in the mature protein), and the evolutionary probability of the reference allele [25]. Six additional UniProtKB features provide lower levels of impact on the XGB model.

Table 3. Machine learning model comparison using test data.

Model	Prediction	Not Annotated in PharmGKB	PharmGKB PGx
Random Forest	neutral	11,076	105
	PGx	326	98
LogitBoost	neutral	10,877	539
	PGx	525	125
XGBoost	neutral	10,716	63
	PGx	686	140

Table 4. Overall variable importance for XGB-PGx.

Variable	Overall Variable Importance (XGBoost)
Global minor allele frequency	100.00
Candidate adaptive polymorphism (CAP)	10.00
Evolutionary time	4.66
Non-reference evolutionary probability	1.81
Uniprot Topo domain	1.62
Evolutionary rate	1.21
Uniprot chain	1.16
Reference evolutionary probability	0.77
Uniprot domain	0.50
Uniprot helix	0.21
Uniprot repeat	0.18
Uniprot proteome	0.10
Uniprot disulfide	0.07
Uniprot variants	0.07

3.4. Comparison with Existing Methods

Existing computational prediction methods have already been shown to perform poorly when applied to PGx data [43]. Our new XGB-PGX model outperforms SIFT, PolyPhen, and EVOD with respect to sensitivity, specificity, accuracy, and AUC (area under the receiver operating characteristic (ROC) curve) (Table 5). CADD performs marginally better with respect to specificity; however, XGB-PGX outperforms CADD with respect to sensitivity, accuracy, and AUC (Table 5). Given our lower confidence in our ability to identify 'true negatives', we consider the specificity results with additional caution.

3.5. Annotation Trends in PGx Variant Prediction

We were interested in determining whether there were any trends involving the new XGB-PGX 'predicted' PGx variants. In particular, we asked if clinically well-studied pharmacogenes annotated in CPIC and PharmGKB have fewer 'newly predicted' PGx variants relative to pharmacogenes annotated in PharmGKB with less or no clinical annotation in CPIC. We reasoned that PGx variants in pharmacogenes that have been studied more extensively for clinical applications may be better understood than PGx variants in pharmacogenes that have been included in fewer clinical studies. We evaluated whether the PharmGKB pharmacogenes implicated in more CPIC drug-gene pairs have fewer 'newly predicted' PGx variants relative to pharmacogenes implicated in fewer CPIC drug–gene pairs, and used this comparison as a proxy to capture PGx variants in pharmacogenes that have been studied more or less extensively for clinical applications. Figure 2 displays the boxplot distributions of newly 'predicted' XGB-PGX pharmacogenetic variants for each category of drug–gene pair. While there is no exact linear relationship between the number of annotated CPIC drug/gene pairs and the number of newly 'predicted' PGx variants, pharmacogenes associated with more than 10 medications display a noticeable reduction in newly 'predicted' PGx variants: CYP2D6 (2 new), CYP2C9 (0), CYP2C19 (0), G6PD (0), ABCB1 (0). The full list of included genes, number of PharmGKB-annotated missense variants, number of newly predicted variants, number of putatively neutral missense variants, total number of variants included in the analysis, and total number of annotated CPIC drugs associated with each gene is included in Table S1. Table S2 includes variant-level information, including all of the variables included in the machine learning analyses, whether a given variant is annotated in PharmGKB, whether a given variant is a newly predicted pharmacogenetic variant according to XGB-PGX, and global minor allele frequency.

Table 5. PGx prediction performance comparison of in silico approaches.

Method	Sensitivity	Specificity	Accuracy	AUC
SIFT	0.59	0.42	0.50	0.51
PolyPhen2	0.60	0.44	0.52	0.53
CADD	0.73	0.78	0.75	0.56
EVOD	0.64	0.50	0.57	0.57
XGB-PGX	0.95	0.68	0.82	0.84

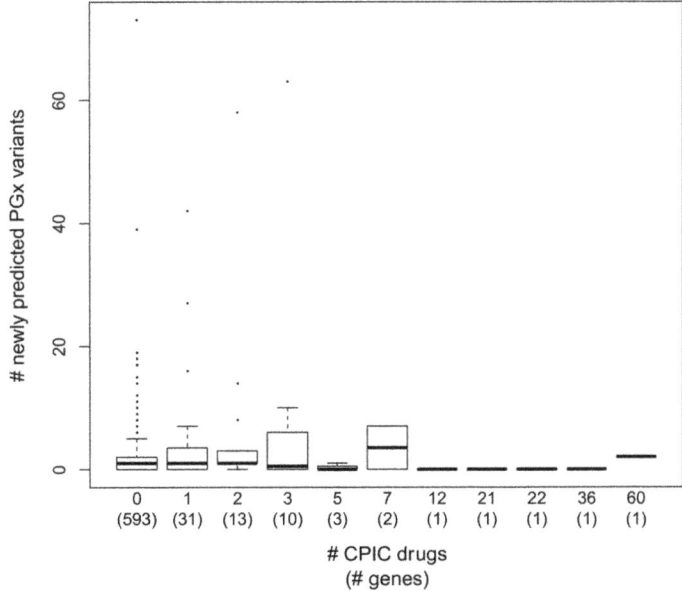

Figure 2. Boxplots of newly predicted pharmacogenetic variants across CPIC drug annotation categories.

Figure 2 displays boxplot distributions of the number of newly predicted pharmacogenetic variants (along the Y-axis) for each category of pharmacogene (along the X-axis), each defined by the number of annotated CPIC drugs associated with a given gene. The X-axis labels denote the number of annotated CPIC drugs associated with a given gene category, and below in parentheses, the number of genes included in each category is included.

3.6. Allele Frequency Trends in PGx Variant Prediction

We were also interested in comparing allele frequency distributions between already known (PharmGKB annotated) and newly predicted pharmacogenetic variants, particularly given the impact that minor allele frequency had on the XGB-PGX model. If only a fraction of pharmacogenetic variation is known due to ascertainment bias, we would expect known pharmacogenetic variants to have relatively high allele frequencies in European population samples. To test this prediction, we calculated non-reference allele frequencies in each of the 1000 Genomes Project population samples.

Figure 3 displays the distributions of PharmGKB annotated PGx variant allele frequencies, newly predicted PGx variant allele frequencies, and putatively neutral PGx variant allele frequencies across all 261,000 Genomes Project population samples. There do not appear to be meaningful differences in allele frequency distribution across population samples for already annotated pharmacovariants (Figure 3); however, XGB-PGX predicted variants are more common in African Caribbeans living in Barbados (ACB), people with African Ancestry living in Southwest USA (ASW), Esan living in Nigeria (ESN), Luhya living in Webuye, Kenya (LWK), Gambians living in Western Division, Mandinka (GWD), Mende living in Sierra Leone (MSL), and in Yoruba living in Ibadan, Nigeria (YRI). More notable is the dramatic increase in allele frequency in the annotated and predicted PGx variants relative to the putatively neutral variants.

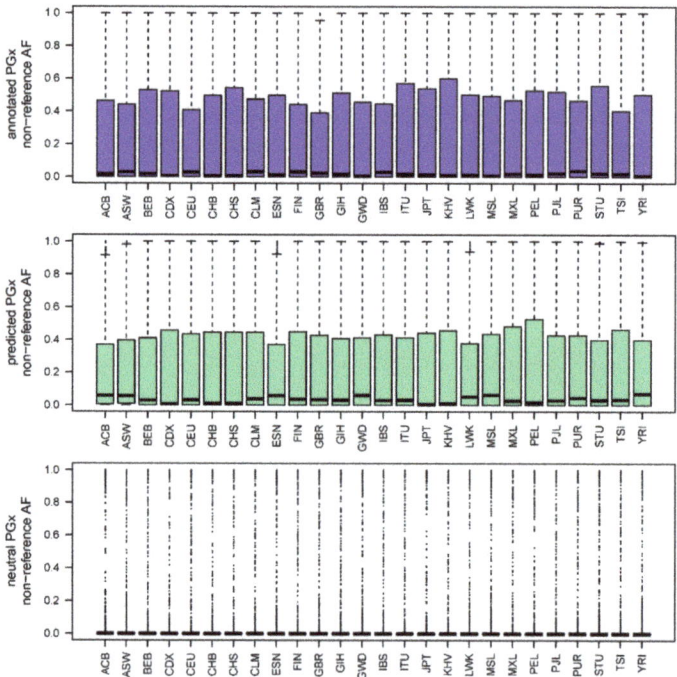

Figure 3. Allele frequency distributions across functional variant categories and population samples.

The top panel of Figure 3 displays boxplot distributions of the non-reference allele frequency (along the *Y*-axis) of each PharmGKB annotated pharmacogenetic variant in each 1000 Genomes Project Phase 3 population sample (along the *X*-axis) in purple. The middle panel of Figure 3 displays boxplot distributions of the non-reference allele frequency (along the *Y*-axis) of each XGB-PGX predicted pharmacogenetic variant in each 1000 Genomes Project Phase 3 population sample (along the *X*-axis) in green. The bottom panel of Figure 3 displays boxplot distributions of the non-reference allele frequency (along the *Y*-axis) of each putatively neutral variant in each 1000 Genomes Project Phase 3 population sample (along the X-axis) in grey.

4. Discussion

The new in silico PGx variant prediction method, XGB-PGX, described here leverages identifiable adaptive signatures that have impacted missense variants across the human genome together with functional protein annotation information. Our approach is designed to mitigate ascertainment biases in PGx research and identify important global PGx diversity that is currently underrepresented or missing in existing PGx resources. This approach complements existing, annotated PGx resources and contributes to ongoing efforts to maximize drug efficacy and minimize drug toxicity in clinical care by identifying a more comprehensive set of PGx variants for functional characterization and clinical application.

XGB-PGX outperforms existing in silico functional variant prediction methods when applied specifically to PGx missense variation data. This performance improvement is likely due to the common assumption by existing methods that functional variants are deleterious and therefore rare in the general population. This assumption does not hold for PGx variation—presumably, at least in part, because of the documented impact of positive selection—and therefore needed to be adjusted in XGB-PGX for better performing PGx variant prediction.

We explored whether the number of newly predicted PGx variants followed any pattern related to clinical annotation. We found that CPIC annotated genes associated with seven or fewer medications had noticeably higher numbers of newly predicted PGx variants relative to CPIC annotation genes with more than ten associated medications. In particular, XGB-PGX identified no newly predicted PGx variants in ABCB1 (associated with 12 medications), CYP2C19 (associated with 21 medications), CYP2C9 (associated with 22 medications), and G6PD (associated with 36 medications), while XGB-PGX identified only two newly predicted PGx variants in CYP2D6 (associated with 60 medications). We interpret these results to suggest that the majority of the functional variation present in the most clinically studied pharmacogenes may already be known despite the ascertainment bias described above.

Interestingly, genes known to play important roles in immune response, such as the pharmacogenes that belong to the major histocompatibility complex (HLA-A, HLA-C, HLA-DQA1, and HLA-DRB1) have over 25 newly predicted missense PGx variants. Alternately, only one of the pharmacogenes (CYP4F2) belonging to the cytochrome p450 gene family (CYP2D6, CYP2B6, CYP2C9, CYP2C8, CYP2C19, CYP4F2), which is known to play a role in toxin metabolism, has more than two newly predicted missense PGx variants. These results suggest that further investigation of functionally predicted immune response variation is an intriguing new area for pharmacogenomic investigation.

We expected that our XGB-PGX prediction method would identify new PGx variants that would be more common in communities that have been underrepresented in PGx research. We found that the allele frequency distributions of already annotated and newly predicted PGx variants across 1000 Genomes Project global population samples include a range of allele frequencies, including both common and rare variation. We identified a modest increase in the newly predicted PGx variant allele frequencies in African Caribbeans living in Barbados (ACB); people with African Ancestry living in Southwest USA (ASW); Esan living in Nigeria (ESN); Luhya living in Webuye, Kenya (LWK); Gambians living in Western Division, Mandinka (GWD); Mende living in Sierra Leone (MSL); and in Yoruba living in Ibadan, Nigeria (YRI), as displayed in Figure 3. This trend is consistent with our initial assumption that existing PGx annotations are likely missing important variation, particularly in underrepresented communities (Figure 3).

The most striking difference among allele frequency distributions is between the relatively rare putatively neutral variants and the more common annotated and predicted functional PGx variants, regardless of population affiliation. The presence of a CAP at a given pharmacogene position is the second most important variable in XGB-PGX (Table 4), and this allele frequency pattern is consistent with our previous analyses of CAPs that demonstrated the majority of these adaptive variants to be common and shared across worldwide populations [29]. This pattern is also consistent with an older signature of adaptation that predates the out of Africa migration of modern humans [29]. More generally, these findings lend further support to a focus on individual pharmacogenetic testing rather than on presumptions about patient race, ethnicity, or ancestral migration history.

To date, a disproportionate amount of in silico modeling of functional variation implicated in disease and drug response has focused on rare, deleterious mutations [27,36,44,45]; however, we and others have demonstrated the important impact that positive selection has had in shaping variation at pharmacogenetic loci [28,29,42]. While negative or purifying selective pressure tends to suppress deleterious variation, positive or adaptive selective pressure tends to increase allele frequencies over time [46]. We therefore encourage more attention to be given to the important role that common genetic variation plays in pharmacogenomics and suggest a 'common treatment, common variant' perspective for pharmacogenetics that leverages the characteristics of pharmacovariants that are distinct relative to the deleterious genetic variants involved in disease.

While complementary to existing computational functional variant prediction methods that perform well in identifying rare, deleterious mutations involved in disease and drug response [27,36,44,45], there are several limitations to XGB-PGX. First, XGB-PGX is a predictive, in silico approach that requires functional validation and exploration of clinical relevance prior to any application to clinical interpretation. Second, XGB-PGX was developed using known pharmacogenes and the subset of missense variants that are in genomic regions that align to the vertebrate phylogeny; thus, variants located in alignment gaps will not be identified by our method. For example, none of the CYP2C9 and CYP2C19 variants that were functionally assessed by Devarajan et al. [47] were present in the aligned vertebrate phylogeny and the 1000 Genomes Project Phase 3 whole genome sequencing datasets used for XGB-PGX. In addition, XGB-PGX was trained on known PGx variants, and this subset is likely to be impacted by the same ascertainment bias we note above. We therefore have more confidence in true positives and less confidence in non-annotated 'negatives'.

5. Conclusions

XGB-PGX has identified over 2000 new putative pharmacovariants that are equally relevant to worldwide communities regardless of geographic affiliation; however, communities that have been left out of past research may benefit the most from in silico prediction methods such as XGB-PGX until ascertainment bias in genomics and pharmacogenomics is solved.

Supplementary Materials: The following are available online at https://www.mdpi.com/2075-4426/11/2/131/s1: Table S1 includes the full list of genes included in the machine learning analyses, the number of PharmGKB-annotated missense variants, the number of newly predicted variants, the number of putatively neutral missense variants, the total number of variants included in the analysis, and the total number of annotated CPIC drugs associated with each gene. Table S2 includes all of the variables included in the machine learning analyses, whether a given variant is annotated in PharmGKB, whether a given variant is newly predicted pharmacogenetic variant according to XGB-PGX, and the global minor allele frequencies for all variants included in the machine learning analyses.

Author Contributions: L.B.S. designed XGB-PGX with input from S.K. and N.G. L.B.S. performed data analysis with assistance from D.M.K., A.B. and N.G. L.B.S., D.M.K., A.B., S.K. and N.G., all contributed to the manuscript writing. All authors have read and agreed to the published version of the manuscript.

Funding: Support was provided by the National Institutes of Health to S.K. (R01LM013385-02 and R35GM139540-01) and to L.B.S. (U41HG008736-05).

Institutional Review Board Statement: Not applicable.

Informed Consent Statement: Not applicable.

Data Availability Statement: Original/source data used in the analyses described in the paper are available as follows: 1000 Genomes Project Phase 3 whole-genome sequencing data are available at the following website: ftp://ftp.1000genomes.ebi.ac.uk/vol1/ftp/phase3/; Uniprot functional annotations can be accessed at the following website: ftp://ftp.uniprot.org/pub/databases/uniprot/current_release/knowledgebase/genome_annotation_tracks/UP000005640_9606_beds/; mypeg annotations can be accessed at the following website: http://www.mypeg.info/evod; PharmGKB annotations can be accessed at the following website: https://www.pharmgkb.org/downloads/; CPIC annotations can be accessed at the following website: https://cpicpgx.org/genes-drugs/; CADD values can be accessed at the following website: http://cadd.gs.washington.edu/download.

Acknowledgments: We would like to thank Jean-Pierre Issa's laboratory, and, in particular, Jozef Madzo and Kelsey Keith for their helpful discussions. We would also like to thank Coriell's bioinformatic team for their support and generous bioinformatics server availability. This work was supported by the Coriell Institute for Medical Research and by R01LM013385-02 and R35GM139540-01 to SK and by U41HG008736-05 to LBS.

Conflicts of Interest: The authors declare no conflict of interest.

References

1. Crews, K.R.; Hicks, J.K.; Pui, C.H.; Relling, M.V.; Evans, W.E. Pharmacogenomics and individualized medicine: Translating science into practice. *Clin. Pharmacol. Ther.* **2012**, *92*, 467–475. [CrossRef]
2. Relling, M.V.; Evans, W.E. Pharmacogenomics in the clinic. *Nature* **2015**, *526*, 343–350. [CrossRef] [PubMed]
3. Relling, M.V.; Krauss, R.M.; Roden, D.M.; Klein, T.E.; Fowler, D.M.; Terada, N.; Lin, L.; Riel-Mehan, M.; Do, T.P.; Kubo, M.; et al. New Pharmacogenomics Research Network: An Open Community Catalyzing Research and Translation in Precision Medicine. *Clin. Pharmacol. Ther.* **2017**, *102*, 897–902. [CrossRef] [PubMed]
4. Rasmussen-Torvik, L.J.; Stallings, S.C.; Gordon, A.S.; Almoguera, B.; Basford, M.A.; Bielinski, S.J.; Brautbar, A.; Brilliant, M.H.; Carrell, D.S.; Connolly, J.J.; et al. Design and anticipated outcomes of the eMERGE-PGx project: A multicenter pilot for preemptive pharmacogenomics in electronic health record systems. *Clin. Pharmacol. Ther.* **2014**, *96*, 482–489. [CrossRef] [PubMed]
5. Gharani, N.; Keller, M.A.; Stack, C.B.; Hodges, L.M.; Schmidlen, T.J.; Lynch, D.E.; Gordon, E.S.; Christman, M.F. The Coriell personalized medicine collaborative pharmacogenomics appraisal, evidence scoring and interpretation system. *Genome Med.* **2013**, *5*, 93. [CrossRef] [PubMed]
6. Dunnenberger, H.M.; Crews, K.R.; Hoffman, J.M.; Caudle, K.E.; Broeckel, U.; Howard, S.C.; Hunkler, R.J.; Klein, T.E.; Evans, W.E.; Relling, M.V. Preemptive clinical pharmacogenetics implementation: Current programs in five US medical centers. *Annu. Rev. Pharmacol. Toxicol.* **2015**, *55*, 89–106. [CrossRef]
7. Bank, P.C.D.; Swen, J.J.; Guchelaar, H.J. Implementation of Pharmacogenomics in Everyday Clinical Settings. *Adv. Pharmacol.* **2018**, *83*, 219–246. [CrossRef] [PubMed]
8. Bentley, A.R.; Callier, S.; Rotimi, C.N. Diversity and inclusion in genomic research: Why the uneven progress? *J. Community Genet.* **2017**, *8*, 255–266. [CrossRef]
9. Martin, A.R.; Gignoux, C.R.; Walters, R.K.; Wojcik, G.L.; Neale, B.M.; Gravel, S.; Daly, M.J.; Bustamante, C.D.; Kenny, E.E. Human Demographic History Impacts Genetic Risk Prediction across Diverse Populations. *Am. J. Hum. Genet.* **2017**, *100*, 635–649. [CrossRef]
10. Popejoy, A.B.; Fullerton, S.M. Genomics is failing on diversity. *Nature* **2016**, *538*, 161–164. [CrossRef]
11. Scheinfeldt, L.B.; Tishkoff, S.A. Recent human adaptation: Genomic approaches, interpretation and insights. *Nat. Rev. Genet.* **2013**, *14*, 692–702. [CrossRef]
12. Scheinfeldt, L.B.; Soi, S.; Tishkoff, S.A. Colloquium paper: Working toward a synthesis of archaeological, linguistic, and genetic data for inferring African population history. *Proc. Natl. Acad. Sci. USA* **2010**, *107* (Suppl. 2), 8931–8938. [CrossRef]
13. Genomes Project, C.; Auton, A.; Brooks, L.D.; Durbin, R.M.; Garrison, E.P.; Kang, H.M.; Korbel, J.O.; Marchini, J.L.; McCarthy, S.; McVean, G.A.; et al. A global reference for human genetic variation. *Nature* **2015**, *526*, 68–74. [CrossRef]
14. Biswas, S.; Scheinfeldt, L.B.; Akey, J.M. Genome-wide insights into the patterns and determinants of fine-scale population structure in humans. *Am. J. Hum. Genet.* **2009**, *84*, 641–650. [CrossRef] [PubMed]
15. Scheinfeldt, L.B.; Biswas, S.; Madeoy, J.; Connelly, C.F.; Schadt, E.E.; Akey, J.M. Population genomic analysis of ALMS1 in humans reveals a surprisingly complex evolutionary history. *Mol. Biol. Evol.* **2009**, *26*, 1357–1367. [CrossRef]
16. Choudhury, A.; Aron, S.; Botigue, L.R.; Sengupta, D.; Botha, G.; Bensellak, T.; Wells, G.; Kumuthini, J.; Shriner, D.; Fakim, Y.J.; et al. High-depth African genomes inform human migration and health. *Nature* **2020**, *586*, 741–748. [CrossRef] [PubMed]
17. Baker, J.L.; Shriner, D.; Bentley, A.R.; Rotimi, C.N. Pharmacogenomic implications of the evolutionary history of infectious diseases in Africa. *Pharmacogenom. J.* **2017**, *17*, 112–120. [CrossRef] [PubMed]

18. Voora, D.; Koboldt, D.C.; King, C.R.; Lenzini, P.A.; Eby, C.S.; Porche-Sorbet, R.; Deych, E.; Crankshaw, M.; Milligan, P.E.; McLeod, H.L.; et al. A polymorphism in the VKORC1 regulator calumenin predicts higher warfarin dose requirements in African Americans. *Clin. Pharmacol. Ther.* **2010**, *87*, 445–451. [CrossRef]
19. Shahabi, P.; Scheinfeldt, L.B.; Lynch, D.E.; Schmidlen, T.J.; Perreault, S.; Keller, M.A.; Kasper, R.; Wawak, L.; Jarvis, J.P.; Gerry, N.P.; et al. An expanded pharmacogenomics warfarin dosing table with utility in generalised dosing guidance. *Thromb. Haemost.* **2016**, *116*, 337–348. [CrossRef]
20. Kaye, J.B.; Schultz, L.E.; Steiner, H.E.; Kittles, R.A.; Cavallari, L.H.; Karnes, J.H. Warfarin Pharmacogenomics in Diverse Populations. *Pharmacotherapy* **2017**, *37*, 1150–1163. [CrossRef]
21. Kimmel, S.E.; French, B.; Kasner, S.E.; Johnson, J.A.; Anderson, J.L.; Gage, B.F.; Rosenberg, Y.D.; Eby, C.S.; Madigan, R.A.; McBane, R.B.; et al. A pharmacogenetic versus a clinical algorithm for warfarin dosing. *N. Engl. J. Med.* **2013**, *369*, 2283–2293. [CrossRef]
22. Ng, P.C.; Henikoff, S. Predicting deleterious amino acid substitutions. *Genome Res.* **2001**, *11*, 863–874. [CrossRef] [PubMed]
23. Adzhubei, I.A.; Schmidt, S.; Peshkin, L.; Ramensky, V.E.; Gerasimova, A.; Bork, P.; Kondrashov, A.S.; Sunyaev, S.R. A method and server for predicting damaging missense mutations. *Nat. Methods* **2010**, *7*, 248–249. [CrossRef]
24. Rentzsch, P.; Witten, D.; Cooper, G.M.; Shendure, J.; Kircher, M. CADD: Predicting the deleteriousness of variants throughout the human genome. *Nucleic Acids Res.* **2019**, *47*, D886–D894. [CrossRef] [PubMed]
25. Liu, L.; Tamura, K.; Sanderford, M.; Gray, V.E.; Kumar, S. A Molecular Evolutionary Reference for the Human Variome. *Mol. Biol. Evol.* **2016**, *33*, 245–254. [CrossRef]
26. Li, B.; Seligman, C.; Thusberg, J.; Miller, J.L.; Auer, J.; Whirl-Carrillo, M.; Capriotti, E.; Klein, T.E.; Mooney, S.D. In silico comparative characterization of pharmacogenomic missense variants. *BMC Genom.* **2014**, *15* (Suppl. 4), S4. [CrossRef]
27. Zhou, Y.; Mkrtchian, S.; Kumondai, M.; Hiratsuka, M.; Lauschke, V.M. An optimized prediction framework to assess the functional impact of pharmacogenetic variants. *Pharmacogenom. J.* **2019**, *19*, 115–126. [CrossRef]
28. Scheinfeldt, L.B.; Soi, S.; Lambert, C.; Ko, W.Y.; Coulibaly, A.; Ranciaro, A.; Thompson, S.; Hirbo, J.; Beggs, W.; Ibrahim, M.; et al. Genomic evidence for shared common ancestry of East African hunting-gathering populations and insights into local adaptation. *Proc. Natl. Acad. Sci. USA* **2019**, *116*, 4166–4175. [CrossRef]
29. Patel, R.; Scheinfeldt, L.B.; Sanderford, M.D.; Lanham, T.R.; Tamura, K.; Platt, A.; Glicksberg, B.S.; Xu, K.; Dudley, J.T.; Kumar, S. Adaptive Landscape of Protein Variation in Human Exomes. *Mol. Biol. Evol.* **2018**, *35*, 2015–2025. [CrossRef]
30. Fumagalli, M.; Sironi, M.; Pozzoli, U.; Ferrer-Admetlla, A.; Pattini, L.; Nielsen, R. Signatures of environmental genetic adaptation pinpoint pathogens as the main selective pressure through human evolution. *PLoS Genet.* **2011**, *7*, e1002355. [CrossRef]
31. Grossman, S.R.; Andersen, K.G.; Shlyakhter, I.; Tabrizi, S.; Winnicki, S.; Yen, A.; Park, D.J.; Griesemer, D.; Karlsson, E.K.; Wong, S.H.; et al. Identifying recent adaptations in large-scale genomic data. *Cell* **2013**, *152*, 703–713. [CrossRef]
32. McDonagh, E.M.; Whirl-Carrillo, M.; Garten, Y.; Altman, R.B.; Klein, T.E. From pharmacogenomic knowledge acquisition to clinical applications: The PharmGKB as a clinical pharmacogenomic biomarker resource. *Biomark. Med.* **2011**, *5*, 795–806. [CrossRef] [PubMed]
33. Kent, W.J.; Sugnet, C.W.; Furey, T.S.; Roskin, K.M.; Pringle, T.H.; Zahler, A.M.; Haussler, D. The human genome browser at UCSC. *Genome Res.* **2002**, *12*, 996–1006. [CrossRef] [PubMed]
34. Murphy, W.J.; Eizirik, E.; O'Brien, S.J.; Madsen, O.; Scally, M.; Douady, C.J.; Teeling, E.; Ryder, O.A.; Stanhope, M.J.; de Jong, W.W.; et al. Resolution of the early placental mammal radiation using Bayesian phylogenetics. *Science* **2001**, *294*, 2348–2351. [CrossRef]
35. Karim, S.; NourEldin, H.F.; Abusamra, H.; Salem, N.; Alhathli, E.; Dudley, J.; Sanderford, M.; Scheinfeldt, L.B.; Chaudhary, A.G.; Al-Qahtani, M.H.; et al. e-GRASP: An integrated evolutionary and GRASP resource for exploring disease associations. *BMC Genom.* **2016**, *17*, 770. [CrossRef]
36. Kircher, M.; Witten, D.M.; Jain, P.; O'Roak, B.J.; Cooper, G.M.; Shendure, J. A general framework for estimating the relative pathogenicity of human genetic variants. *Nat. Genet.* **2014**, *46*, 310–315. [CrossRef]
37. Kuhn, M. Building Predictive Models in R Using the caret Package. *J. Stat. Softw.* **2008**, *28*, 1–26. [CrossRef]
38. Liaw, A.; Wiener, M. Classification and Regression by randomForest. *R News* **2002**, *2*, 18–22.
39. Chen, T.; Guestrin, C. XGBoost: A Scalable Tree Boosting System. In Proceedings of the 22nd ACM SIGKDD International Conference on Knowledge Discovery and Data Mining, New York, NY, USA, 13 August 2016; Association for Computing Machinery: New York, NY, USA, 2016; pp. 785–794. [CrossRef]
40. Torgo, L. *Data Mining with R, Learning with Case Studies*; Chapman and Hall/CRC: Boca Raton, FL, USA, 2010.
41. Wright, G.E.B.; Carleton, B.; Hayden, M.R.; Ross, C.J.D. The global spectrum of protein-coding pharmacogenomic diversity. *Pharmacogenom. J.* **2018**, *18*, 187–195. [CrossRef] [PubMed]
42. Li, J.; Zhang, L.; Zhou, H.; Stoneking, M.; Tang, K. Global patterns of genetic diversity and signals of natural selection for human ADME genes. *Hum. Mol. Genet.* **2011**, *20*, 528–540. [CrossRef]
43. Gerek, N.Z.; Liu, L.; Gerold, K.; Biparva, P.; Thomas, E.D.; Kumar, S. Evolutionary Diagnosis of non-synonymous variants involved in differential drug response. *BMC Med. Genomics* **2015**, *8* (Suppl. 1), S6. [CrossRef]
44. Ng, P.C.; Henikoff, S. SIFT: Predicting amino acid changes that affect protein function. *Nucleic Acids Res.* **2003**, *31*, 3812–3814. [CrossRef] [PubMed]
45. Nickerson, D.A.; Tobe, V.O.; Taylor, S.L. PolyPhred: Automating the detection and genotyping of single nucleotide substitutions using fluorescence-based resequencing. *Nucleic Acids Res.* **1997**, *25*, 2745–2751. [CrossRef] [PubMed]

46. Biswas, S.; Akey, J.M. Genomic insights into positive selection. *Trends Genet.* **2006**, *22*, 437–446. [CrossRef] [PubMed]
47. Devarajan, S.; Moon, I.; Ho, M.F.; Larson, N.B.; Neavin, D.R.; Moyer, A.M.; Black, J.L.; Bielinski, S.J.; Scherer, S.E.; Wang, L.; et al. Pharmacogenomic Next-Generation DNA Sequencing: Lessons from the Identification and Functional Characterization of Variants of Unknown Significance in CYP2C9 and CYP2C19. *Drug Metab. Dispos.* **2019**, *47*, 425–435. [CrossRef]

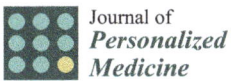

Article

Combination of Genome-Wide Polymorphisms and Copy Number Variations of Pharmacogenes in Koreans

Nayoung Han, Jung Mi Oh and In-Wha Kim *

College of Pharmacy and Research Institute of Pharmaceutical Sciences,
Seoul National University, Seoul 08826, Korea; hans1217@gmail.com (N.H.); jmoh@snu.ac.kr (J.M.O.)
* Correspondence: iwkim2@hanmail.net; Tel.: +82-2-880-7736

Abstract: For predicting phenotypes and executing precision medicine, combination analysis of single nucleotide variants (SNVs) genotyping with copy number variations (CNVs) is required. The aim of this study was to discover SNVs or common copy CNVs and examine the combined frequencies of SNVs and CNVs in pharmacogenes using the Korean genome and epidemiology study (KoGES), a consortium project. The genotypes (N = 72,299) and CNV data (N = 1000) were provided by the Korean National Institute of Health, Korea Centers for Disease Control and Prevention. The allele frequencies of SNVs, CNVs, and combined SNVs with CNVs were calculated and haplotype analysis was performed. *CYP2D6* rs1065852 (c.100C>T, p.P34S) was the most common variant allele (48.23%). A total of 8454 haplotype blocks in 18 pharmacogenes were estimated. *DMD* ranked the highest in frequency for gene gain (64.52%), while *TPMT* ranked the highest in frequency for gene loss (51.80%). Copy number gain of *CYP4F2* was observed in 22 subjects; 13 of those subjects were carriers with *CYP4F2**3 gain. In the case of *TPMT*, approximately one-half of the participants (N = 308) had loss of the *TPMT**1*1 diplotype. The frequencies of SNVs and CNVs in pharmacogenes were determined using the Korean cohort-based genome-wide association study.

Keywords: polymorphisms; pharmacogenes

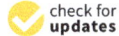

Citation: Han, N.; Oh, J.M.; Kim, I.-W. Combination of Genome-Wide Polymorphisms and Copy Number Variations of Pharmacogenes in Koreans. *J. Pers. Med.* **2021**, *11*, 33. https://doi.org/10.3390/jpm11010033

Received: 13 November 2020
Accepted: 4 January 2021
Published: 7 January 2021

Publisher's Note: MDPI stays neutral with regard to jurisdictional claims in published maps and institutional affiliations.

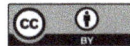

Copyright: © 2021 by the authors. Licensee MDPI, Basel, Switzerland. This article is an open access article distributed under the terms and conditions of the Creative Commons Attribution (CC BY) license (https://creativecommons.org/licenses/by/4.0/).

1. Introduction

It is well established that human genetic diversity is important for our understanding population histology [1], variability in disease susceptibility, and treatment response or adverse reactions to medications [2]. Single nucleotide variants (SNVs) are the most widely studied form of genetic variations and several SNVs have been linked to disease susceptibility and drug responses. Therefore, genome-wide association (GWA) studies have led to the identification of multiple genetic variants correlated with traits, such as body mass index, skin color [3], fat distribution [4], and glomerular filtration rate [5], and with diseases, such as autoimmune disease [6] and non-alcoholic fatty liver disease [7].

Additionally, these SNV markers from GWA studies can be used in pharmacogenomic research as a means of directly predicting interindividual responses to medicines [8]. Research has identified successfully the loci of genetic variants associated with responses to tumor necrosis factor inhibitors [9], antidepressants [10], and antipsychotics [11], and with adverse reactions induced by medicines, such as thiopurine-induced myelosuppression [12], statin-induced myopathy [13], and carbamazepine-induced hypersensitivity [14]. These genetic variations alter the structure and function of proteins such as drug-metabolizing enzymes, drug transporters, receptors, and response targets, collectively referred to as pharmacogenes [15].

Common copy number variations (CNVs) were estimated to occur in approximately 9.5% of the human reference genome and have non-random distribution [16]. CNVs account for at least five times more variable base pairs compared to that of SNVs when two human genomes are compared to each other [17,18]. As with SNVs, CNVs were found to influence susceptibility to cancer [19] as well as neurodegenerative disease [20] and psychiatric disease [21]. Despite their clinical significance, CNVs remain understudied compared to SNVs. The reasons may be that the detection of CNVs is more difficult and CNVs only occur with low-to-intermediate frequency [22]. However, for predicting phenotypes and executing precision medicine, combination analysis of SNVs genotyping with CNVs is required. There have been several studies to detect both CNVs and SNVs in *CYP2D6* [23,24]. However, CNV information integrated with polymorphisms on pharmacogenes is still not fully characterized [25]. Traditional methods are time-consuming and labor-intensive and a large number of participants are required.

The Korean genome and epidemiology study (KoGES) is a consortium project that was established as a genome epidemiological study for the research community with a health database and biobank to help investigate Korean population-based and gene–environment model studies [26–28]. Because this dataset contains a significant collection of SNVs and CNVs data from normal tissue and blood samples, KoGES is appropriate for combined pharmacogenomic studies. Thus, this study aimed to discover SNVs and CNVs and to examine the combined frequencies of SNVs and CNVs in pharmacogenes in the Korean population using this large public dataset.

2. Materials and Methods

2.1. Study Subjects

The study subjects were selected from the Ansan and Ansung study (N = 5836), the Health Examinee cohort (HEXA, N = 58,701), and the cardiovascular disease association study (CAVAS, N = 8105) that constitute the KoGES [29]. Epidemiologic data were provided by the Korean National Institute of Health, Korea Centers for Disease Control and Prevention (KCDC). Socio-demographic, medical history, health conditions, and family history of disease information were collected by trained interviewers using structured questionnaires. All physical examinations were administered by health professionals trained to follow standardized protocols. The participants who had cancer were excluded from the analysis. All subjects were middle-aged adults between 40 and 69 years of age. All study participants provided written informed consent.

2.2. Pharmacogenes

The pharmacogenomics-related genes were selected by the Very Important Pharmacogene summaries in the Pharmacogenomics Knowledge Base (as of March 2020) [30] and the Clinical Pharmacogenetics Implementation Consortium (CPIC) guideline (as of March 2020) [31]. The genes from the U.S. Food and Drug Administration (FDA) Table of Pharmacogenomic Biomarkers in Drug Labels (as of March 2020) were included [32]. A total of 191 genes were analyzed and are listed in Supplementary Table S1.

2.3. Data Collection and Preprocessing

The genotypes (N = 72,299) and CNV data (N = 1000) were provided by the KCDC. These imputated genotypes were produced by the Korea BioBank Array (referred to as KoreanChip, KCHIP, Seoul, The Republic of Korea) project, optimized for the Korean population [33]. A KCHIP array includes a total of 833,535 SNVs for autosomal chromosomes. Quality-controlled data were used for imputation analysis with 1000 Genomes Phase 3 data as a reference panel using ShapeIT v2 [34] and IMPUTE v2 [35]. An SNV missing rate greater than 0.05, SNVs with a minor allele frequency less than 0.01, or a Hardy–Weinberg equilibrium (HWE) of P less than 10^{-6} were excluded according to standard quality control procedures. The SNV position aligned to human reference genomes hg19 using the Bioconductor BiomaRt R package [36]. For each gene, 10 kb bases of region were added both upstream and downstream of the defined gene location. The CNV data of 1000 subjects were produced from the Ansan and Ansung study [37]. The CNV data were genotyped with the NimbleGen HD2 3 × 720 K comparative genomic hybridization array (aCGH) (Roche NimblGen, Madison, WI, USA) [37]. For the combination analysis of genotypes and CNVs, the variants from gene–drug pairs from CPIC were searched for their clinical effects. The functional effects of variants were predicted by SIFT (Sorting Intolerance From Tolerant) [38] and POLYPHEN-2 (Polymorphism Phenotyping v2) [39].

2.4. CNV Calling

R package that implements the Genome Alteration Detection Analysis algorithm (GADA) was used for CNV discovery [40]. To overcome the limitation of single algorithm detection, we tested different thresholds, T, from 3 to 8. CNV discovery with several parameters was tested to find the best parameters using known CNV regions [41]. Consequently, we selected the best parameter with high concordance with known CNV regions with T = 4.5, alpha = 0.2, and MinSegLen = 6. CNV regions longer than 50 bp in length were included for further analysis. A log 2 ratio cut-off of ±0.25 was used to define copy number gain and loss and cut-offs of ±0.8 were used to define amplification and deletion, respectively [42,43].

2.5. Data Analysis

Categorical variables such as gender and variant occurrences are presented in percentages and frequencies. Continuous variables such as age are presented with average and standard variations. The chi-squared test with one degree of freedom was used to test the departure from HWE for each variant. Data were analyzed with PLINK 1.9 or 2.0 [44] and R (version 3.6.3). Linkage disequilibrium analysis among pairs of SNVs was performed to identify the haplotype. Estimation of haplotype blocks and their frequencies were performed with PLINK and Haploview [45].

3. Results

3.1. Characteristics of the Study Population

For the KCHIP study, among the Ansan and Ansung study (N = 5493), HEXA (N = 58,701), and CAVAS (N = 8105), after excluding patients with cancer, 5182 of the Ansan and Ansung study subjects, 55,955 of HEXA, and 7890 of CAVAS remained. For the CNV data, 945 subjects remained after excluding patients with cancer. Among them, 614 subjects had SNV and CNV data. The characteristics of the subjects from the SNV and CNV data are presented in Table 1. The average ages of the subjects with SNV and CNV data were 54.08 and 54.05 years, respectively. The frequencies of female subjects (63.78%) was higher than that of male subjects (36.22%) in the SNV data, while that of female subjects (49.95%) was similar to that of male subjects (50.05%) in the CNV data.

Table 1. Demographic characteristics of study subjects.

Characteristics	SNV	CNV	Combination of SNV with CNV
Number of patients, n	69,027	947	614
Age, years	54.08 ± 8.31	54.05 ± 9.08	52.82 ± 8.80
Gender			
male	25,004 (36.22)	474 (50.05)	311 (50.65)
female	44,023 (63.78)	473 (49.95)	303 (49.35)

Values are reported as n (%) or mean ± standard deviation; SNV, single nucleotide variation; CNV, copy number variation.

3.2. Genotype Variants

A total of 36,853 SNVs in pharmacogenes were included for the further analysis. The allele frequencies of SNVs of more than 10% are listed in Supplementary Table S2. *VKORC1* rs9923231 (−1639G>A or G3673A) was found to be the most common alternative allele (92.42%). *CYP2D6* rs1065852 (c.100C>T, p.P34S) was the next common allele (48.23%). The allelic frequencies of *CYP2C19*2* (rs4244285, c.681G>A, p.P227P) and *CYP2C19*3* (rs4986893, c.636G>A, p.W212X) were 28.29% and 10.04%, respectively. The allelic frequency of *CYP3A5*3* (rs776746, c.6986A>G) was 23.47%. *CYP4F2*3* (rs2108622, c.1297C>T, p.V433M) and *CYP4F2*2* rs3093105 (c.34T>G, p.W12G) were 32.41% and 13.40%, respectively. Among SNVs in pharmacogenes, those that were assigned as having level A evidence of gene–drug pairs by CPIC are shown in Figure 1. The median alternative allele frequency of *CYP2D6* variants was ranked the highest (46.17%, ranged from 1.02% to 87.34%), followed by *SLCO1B1* variants (39.32%, ranged from 1.07% to 86.62%). SNVs with frequencies less than 10% that were also assigned as having level A evidence of gene–drug pairs by CPIC or predicted to be deleterious by SIFT and POLYPHEN-2 are listed in Supplementary Table S3. *CACNA1S* rs3850625 (c.4615G>A (p.R1539C), *CFTR* rs121909046 (c.650A>G, p.E217G) and rs113857788 (c.4056G>C p.Q1352H), and *CYP2B6* rs8192709 (c.64C>T, p.R22C) were predicted to be deleterious by SIFT.

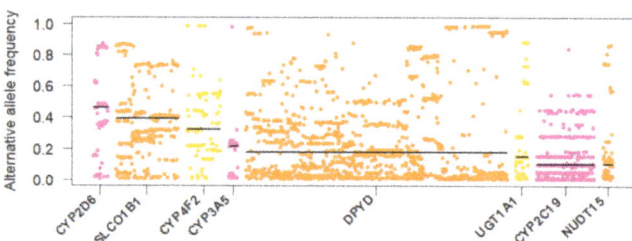

Figure 1. Single-nucleotide variants of pharmacogenes with alternative allele frequencies of more than 10% in a Korean population. Horizontal lines indicate median values.

3.3. Haplotype Analysis

The frequency distributions of the variants or haplotypes were found to be significantly different among ethnic populations. Therefore, haplotype analysis was performed on about 18 pharmacogenomic genes from 73 gene–drug pairs with level A evidence by CPIC. A total of 8454 haplotype blocks in 18 genes were estimated, and the number varied from 2 to 3924 blocks per each gene, with an average of 4378. *CYP2B6* rs8192709 (c.64C>T, p.R22C) constructed a haplotype block with rs8192711 (G>A), rs34801721 (A>T), rs2279341 (G>C), rs12985017 (T>C), and rs12985269 (T>C) (Figure 2). The haplotype block of *CYP2B6* in Caucasians was constructed with rs2279341, rs12985017, and rs12985269. Carriers with the alternative haplotype T-A-T-C-C-C were found in 3.98% of this study population.

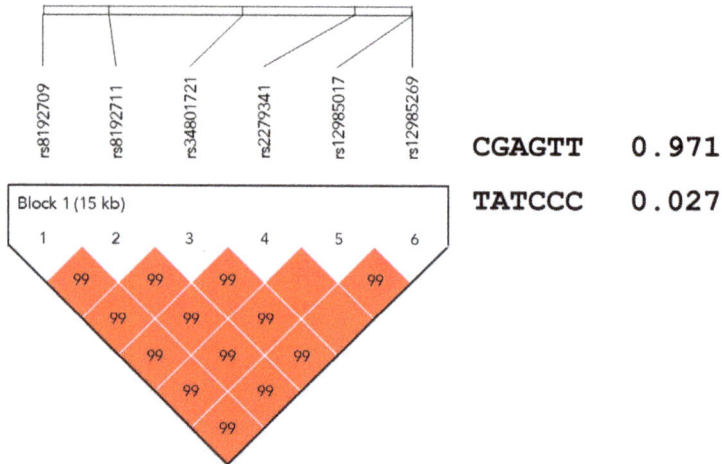

Figure 2. Haplotype block map constructed by candidate single-nucleotide variations in *CYP2B6*. Notes: Block 1 includes rs8192709, rs8192711, rs34801721, rs2279341, rs12985017, and rs12985269; the linkage disequilibrium between two SNPs is indicated by the standardized r^2 (red boxes).

3.4. Copy Number Variation Profiling

In the 947 subjects, segments with more than 1 CNV were determined in 937 subjects using GADA. In total, 448 segments were detected in 937 individuals with an average of 22.58 copy number segments in each individual. CNV regions of more than 50 bp were included for the further analysis. The mean and median lengths of these CNV regions were 4.29 and 2.21 kb, respectively. Figure 3 shows the distribution of the 333 CNV regions by frequency rate. Of the 333 CNV regions, 92 had frequency rates of >1%. The frequencies of CNVs were calculated and genes with a frequency of more than 1% are summarized in Table 2. *DMD* ranked the highest in frequency for gene gain (64.52%), while *TPMT* ranked the highest in frequency for gene loss (51.80%), and the frequency of *TPMT* deletion was 3.58%. There were gene gains in *G6PD* (17.21%), *KIT* (21.12%), and *OTC* (57.76%), while there was gene loss in *ABCB1* (15.31%), *BCR* (19.01%), *DMD* (20.27%), *EGFR* (41.39%), *HLA-B* (36.54%), *HLA-DRB1* (40.65%), *PDGFRA* (21.44%), and *SULT1A1* (19.75%) with a frequency of more than 10%. The genes with a CNV frequency of less than 1% are listed in Supplementary Table S4. Gene losses of *ABCG2* and *CYP2E1* were found in 0.63% of subjects, while the gene gain of *CYP2B6* was found in 0.21% of subjects.

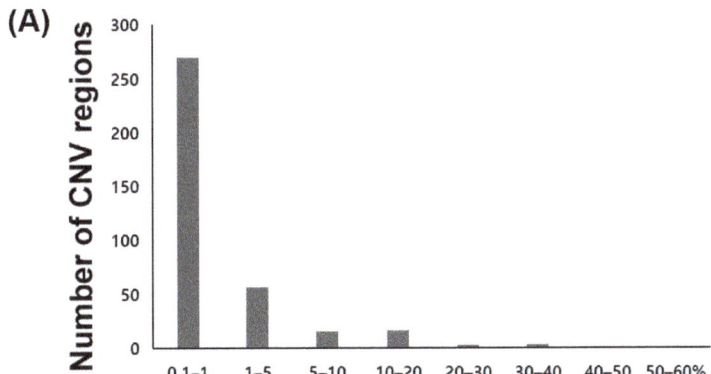

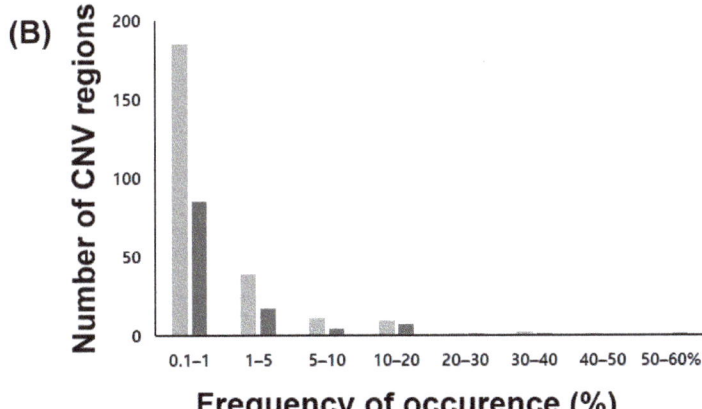

Figure 3. Distribution of copy number variation frequencies for the copy number variation regions in a Korean population. (**A**) Frequencies of copy number variation regions. (**B**) Copy number variation frequencies of the detected copy number variation regions, divided into gains and losses.

Table 2. Copy number variations for pharmacogenes with a frequency of more than 1% in Koreans.

Gene	Position	Gain Frequency (%)	Loss Frequency (%)
ABCB1	7: 87133179–87342639	0.11	15.31
ALK	2: 29415640–30144477	6.12	1.06
ALOX5	10: 45869624–45941567	6.65	1.58
BCR	11: 23522552–23660224	0.11	19.01
BRCA	17: 41196312–41277500	2.22	2.64
COMT	19: 19929263–19957498	7.07	0.32
CYP2A6	19: 41349443–41356352	1.27	1.48
CYP4F2	19: 15988834–16008884	3.80	0.42
DMD	X: 31137345–33229673	64.52	20.27
EGFR	7: 55086725–55275031	2.32	41.39
ESR1	6: 152128814–152424408	0	1.48
G6PD	X: 153759606–153775233	17.21	0.42
HLA-B	6: 31237743–31324989	0.42	36.54
HLA-DRB1	6: 32489683–32557613	0.32	40.65
KIT	4: 55524095–55606881	21.12	2.22
OTC	X: 38211736–38280703	57.76	0.42
PDGFRA	4: 55095264–55164412	0.11	21.44
RYR1	19: 38924340–39078204	5.07	2.11
SMN2	5: 70220768–70248842	2.11	0.11
SULT1A1	16: 28616908–28620649	7.71	19.75
TPMT	6: 18128545–18155374	0	51.80

3.5. Combination of Genotype Variants and CNVs

A total of 22 pharmacogenomic genes from 73 gene–drug pairs with level A evidence by CPIC were selected for the combination analysis of SNVs and CNVs in 614 subjects. CYP4F2*1*3 (24.43%) was most common CYP4F2 diplotype followed by CYP4F2*2*3 (18.57%) (Table 3). Among the CYP4F2 gains observed in 22 subjects, 13 subjects were carriers with a CYP4F2*3 gain. The frequency of CYP4F2 loss was 0.49%. In the TPMT case, approximately half of the participants ($N = 308$) showed a loss of the TPMT*1*1 diplotype.

Table 3. Copy number variation combined with single nucleotide variations in Koreans ($N = 614$).

Gene Allele	Subjects (N)	Frequency (%)
CYP4F2*1*1	258	42.02
CYP4F2*1*2	1	0.16
CYP4F2*1*3	150	24.43
CYP4F2*3*3	22	3.58
CYP4F2*2*3	114	18.57
CYP4F2*1*2-*3*3	31	5.05
CYP4F2*2*2-*3*3	13	2.12
CYP4F2*1*1 gain	9	1.47
CYP4F2*1*3 gain	6	0.98
CYP4F2*2*3 gain	6	0.98
CYP4F2*3*3 gain	1	0.16
CYP4F2*1*1 loss	2	0.33
CYP4F2*2*3 loss	1	0.16
TPMT*1*1	287	46.74
TPMT*1*3C	8	1.30
TPMT*1*1 loss	308	50.16
TPMT*1*3C loss	11	1.79

4. Discussion

Pharmacogenomic studies represent a critical component of precision medicine. Compared to SNVs, CNVs or the combined study of SNVs and CNVs all both relatively less studied. With regard to SNV or CNV data from genome epidemiological research,

KoGES in Korea can be used for pharmacogenomic studies. The purpose of this study was to discover SNVs and CNVs and to examine the combined frequencies of SNVs and CNVs in pharmacogenes in Korea using KoGES.

For 191 pharmacogenes, a total of 36,853 SNVs from 69,027 subjects, 333 CNVs from 947 subjects, and combined data of SNVs and CNVs from 614 subjects were available in this study. The SNV rs9923231 (−1639G>A or G3673A) is known to alter a transcription factor binding site in the *VKORC1* promoter region, and this allele frequency in Asians was found to be approximately 0.92 [46], similar with our result. This variant was associated with decreased gene expression, resulting in decreased warfarin dose requirements. *CYP2D6* rs1065852 (c.100C>T, p.P34S) was the next most common allele (48.23%), and it appeared in *4, *10, *14A, and *36 alleles, with lower enzyme activities compared to the wild type [47]. This enzyme is involved in the metabolism of approximately 25% of commonly prescribed drugs, including antidepressants, antipsychotics, antiarrhythmics, β-blockers, and opioids [24]. The allelic frequencies of *CYP2C19*2 and *CYP2C19*3 were 28.29% and 10.04%, respectively, in our study, similar to earlier findings [48], and indicate that genomic data from the KoGES study are appropriate for pharmacogenomics studies in Korea. These losses of functional alleles of *CYP2C19* can increase the risks for serious cardiovascular events among patients treated with clopidogrel [49].

In our study, *CACNA1S* rs3850625 and *CFTR* rs121909046 and rs113857788 were predicted to be deleterious by SIFT. *CACNA1S* rs3850625 was associated with malignant hyperthermia accelerated by inhalational anesthetics and muscle relaxants [50]. Those two variants in the *CFTR* gene were found to have the strongest association with bronchiectasis and chronic pancreatitis in the Korean population [51].

According to a haplotype analysis, the haplotype block *CYP2B6*2 (rs8192709) was constructed and the corresponding frequency was found to be 3.98 in this study. Approximately 3.4% of *CYP2B6*2 variants were found in Han and Uygur Chinese [52]. Although the level of evidence for clinical annotations of *CYP2B6*2 was lower than that for the *CYP2B6*6 allele according to CPIC, this minor allele is known to decrease the clearance of methadone [53] or efavirenz [54].

The activities of several important drug-metabolizing genes, such as *CYP2B6*, *CYP2E1*, *CYP2D6*, *GSTM1*, and *SULT1A1*, are known to be related to variable copy numbers. In our study, CNVs of *CYP2B6*, *CYP2E1*, and *SULT1A1* were detected, whereas CNV data from KoGES did not cover *CYP2D6* and *GSTM1* genes. Accordingly, alternative methods during a CNV analysis are needed to detect those genes.

The *DMD* gene found to be the most frequent in terms of the copy number gain in our study is the largest gene in the human genome, encompassing 2.2 Mb and encoding for a muscular protein, dystrophin, which is related to the X-linked recessive disorders Duchenne muscular dystrophy and Becker muscular dystrophy [55]. Deletions or complex rearrangements usually occur between exons 43 and 55 or exons 2 and 23 [55]. Most carriers with mutations or deletions of the *DMD* gene are asymptomatic [56]. One hundred and seventeen different deletions and 48 duplications in the *DMD* gene were found in 507 Korean patients with Duchenne muscular dystrophy or Becker muscular dystrophy [57].

TPMT ranked highest here in terms of the frequency of gene loss at 3.58% in our results. This is most likely due to a variable number of tandem repeats (VNTR) within a G/C-rich region in the promotor of *TPMT* [58]. The frequency of the VNTR allele, consisting of two repeat sequence motifs A, one motif B, and one motif C, was reported to be 48.2% in an Asian British cohort [59]. The patterns and total number of VNTR alleles were associated with the level of TPMT activity [59]. The *TPMT* gene encoding thiopurine S-methyltransferase is a crucial enzyme during the metabolism of thiopurine drugs such as azathioprine and 6-mercaptopurine [60].

In the next step, the CNV data were combined with SNVs for pharmacogenes. The loss frequency of *TPMT*3C (rs1142345, c.A719G, p.Y240C) was 1.79%. The *TPMT*3C variant, with moderate activity, was found to be the most frequent alternative allele in Koreans, and TPMT deficiency can increase certain fatal adverse reaction risks, such as bone marrow toxicity and myelosuppression induced by 6-mercaptopurine [61]. Thiopurine-associated leukopenia (more than 30%) was found to be considerably higher than expected according to the frequency of the *TPMT* variant (~1%) in Koreans with Crohn's disease [62]. This result may be related to the copy number variation in the *TPMT* gene. Despite the fact that less than 5% of the samples showed gene gains or losses in these genes, the corresponding clinical impacts should be considered when medicines associated with these genes are administered.

A limitation of this study was that the CNV frequencies of some genes differed from those in previous studies [63]. This difference may have been caused by the different assay methods. There are many different methods for determining the CNVs of genes, and each method has advantages and pitfalls. The array CGH methods and SNP arrays and CNV arrays are excellent for initial scans along the lines of the SNP GWA study, and other PCR-based methods such as multiplex ligation-dependent probe amplification (MLPA) are used for conformation to genotype copy numbers [64]. The KCHIP array did not contain SNVs for sex chromosomes, meaning that pharmacogenes such as *DMD* and *G6PD* could not be included in the analysis of the combinations of genotype variants and CNVs. Another limitation in our study was that hybrid pseudogene, conversion, or tandem alleles cannot be determined due to the assay method used in this study. Additionally, as subjects with common complex diseases such as diabetic mellitus, hypertension, and cardiovascular disease were not excluded, this could affect the results of this study. Further studies with regard to functional variation evaluations and associated determinations are needed to manage patients more efficiently.

The 1000 Genomes Project and the Encyclopedia of DNA Elements Project produced comprehensive maps outlining the regions of the human genome containing SNVs, multi-nucleotide variants, and CNVs [65]. However, combination analyses of SNVs with CNVs in pharmacogenetic studies are limited. Here, we conducted a combined analysis of SNVs with CNVs in pharmacogenes in Koreans.

In conclusion, the frequencies of SNVs and CNVs in pharmacogenes were determined by means of a Korean cohort-based GWA study. Though further assessments of correlations with phenotype changes are necessary, the results here may be useful for the identification of genetic causes of cases involving severe drug-induced toxicity or reduced therapeutic benefits from a drug.

Supplementary Materials: The following are available online at https://www.mdpi.com/2075-4426/11/1/33/s1, Table S1: List of 129 pharmacogenes in this study. Table S2: Single nucleotide variants of pharmacogenes with an allele frequency of more than 10% in Koreans. Table S3: Single nucleotide variants of pharmacogenes with an allele frequency of more than 10% in Koreans. Table S4. Copy number variations for pharmacogenes with a frequency of less than 1% in Koreans.

Author Contributions: Conceptualization, I.-W.K. and J.M.O.; methodology, N.H.; validation, I.-W.K.; formal analysis, N.H.; investigation, N.H.; data curation, N.H.; writing—original draft preparation, N.H.; writing—review and editing, I.-W.K.; visualization, N.H.; supervision, I.-W.K. and J.M.O.; funding acquisition, I.-W.K. and J.M.O. All authors have read and agreed to the published version of the manuscript.

Funding: This study was supported by the National Research Foundation of Korea grant funded by the Korean government (MSIT) (No. 2018R1A2B6001859 and 2019R1A2C1005211).

Institutional Review Board Statement: This study was exempt from the institutional review board of Seoul National University (IRB No. E1910/001-002).

Informed Consent Statement: The requirement for written informed consent from participants was waived because all participants were anonymized by National Biobank of Korea, the Centers for Disease Control and Prevention, Republic of Korea.

Data Availability Statement: The datasets generated during the current study are available from the corresponding authors on reasonable request.

Acknowledgments: This study was conducted with bioresources from the National Biobank of Korea, the Centers for Disease Control and Prevention, Republic of Korea (KBN-2019-065).

Conflicts of Interest: The authors declare no conflict of interest.

References

1. Lek, M.; Karczewski, K.J.; Minikel, E.V.; Samocha, K.E.; Banks, E.; Fennell, T.; O'Donnell-Luria, A.H.; Ware, J.S.; Hill, A.J.; Cummings, B.B.; et al. Analysis of protein-coding genetic variation in 60,706 humans. *Nature* **2016**, *536*, 285–291. [CrossRef] [PubMed]
2. Zhang, H.; Liu, R.; Yan, C.; Liu, L.; Tong, Z.; Jiang, W.; Yao, M.; Fang, W.; Chen, Z. Advantage of next-generation sequencing in dynamic monitoring of circulating tumor DNA over droplet digital PCR in cetuximab treated colorectal cancer patients. *Transl. Oncol.* **2019**, *12*, 426–431. [CrossRef] [PubMed]
3. Galvan-Femenia, I.; Obon-Santacana, M.; Pineyro, D.; Guindo-Martinez, M.; Duran, X.; Carreras, A.; Pluvinet, R.; Velasco, J.; Ramos, L.; Ausso, S.; et al. Multitrait genome association analysis identifies new susceptibility genes for human anthropometric variation in the GCAT cohort. *J. Med. Genet.* **2018**, *55*, 765–778. [CrossRef] [PubMed]
4. Tachmazidou, I.; Suveges, D.; Min, J.L.; Ritchie, G.R.S.; Steinberg, J.; Walter, K.; Iotchkova, V.; Schwartzentruber, J.; Huang, J.; Memari, Y.; et al. Whole-genome sequencing coupled to imputation discovers genetic signals for anthropometric traits. *Am. J. Hum. Genet.* **2017**, *100*, 865–884. [CrossRef] [PubMed]
5. Hellwege, J.N.; Velez Edwards, D.R.; Giri, A.; Qiu, C.; Park, J.; Torstenson, E.S.; Keaton, J.M.; Wilson, O.D.; Robinson-Cohen, C.; Chung, C.P.; et al. Mapping eGFR loci to the renal transcriptome and phenome in the VA Million Veteran Program. *Nat. Commun.* **2019**, *10*, 3842. [CrossRef]
6. Din, L.; Sheikh, M.; Kosaraju, N.; Smedby, K.E.; Bernatsky, S.; Berndt, S.I.; Skibola, C.F.; Nieters, A.; Wang, S.; McKay, J.D.; et al. Genetic overlap between autoimmune diseases and non-Hodgkin lymphoma subtypes. *Genet. Epidemiol.* **2019**, *43*, 844–863. [CrossRef]
7. Namjou, B.; Lingren, T.; Huang, Y.; Parameswaran, S.; Cobb, B.L.; Stanaway, I.B.; Connolly, J.J.; Mentch, F.D.; Benoit, B.; Niu, X.; et al. GWAS and enrichment analyses of non-alcoholic fatty liver disease identify new trait-associated genes and pathways across eMERGE Network. *BMC Med.* **2019**, *17*, 135. [CrossRef] [PubMed]
8. Popejoy, A.B. Diversity in precision medicine and pharmacogenetics: Methodological and conceptual considerations for broadening participation. *Pharmgenom. Pers. Med.* **2019**, *12*, 257–271. [CrossRef]
9. Massey, J.; Plant, D.; Hyrich, K.; Morgan, A.W.; Wilson, A.G.; Spiliopoulou, A.; Colombo, M.; McKeigue, P.; Isaacs, J.; Cordell, H.; et al. Genome-wide association study of response to tumour necrosis factor inhibitor therapy in rheumatoid arthritis. *Pharmacogenom. J.* **2018**, *18*, 657–664. [CrossRef] [PubMed]
10. Fabbri, C.; Tansey, K.E.; Perlis, R.H.; Hauser, J.; Henigsberg, N.; Maier, W.; Mors, O.; Placentino, A.; Rietschel, M.; Souery, D.; et al. New insights into the pharmacogenomics of antidepressant response from the GENDEP and STAR*D studies: Rare variant analysis and high-density imputation. *Pharmacogenom. J.* **2018**, *18*, 413–421. [CrossRef]
11. Yu, H.; Yan, H.; Wang, L.; Li, J.; Tan, L.; Deng, W.; Chen, Q.; Yang, G.; Zhang, F.; Lu, T.; et al. Five novel loci associated with antipsychotic treatment response in patients with schizophrenia: A genome-wide association study. *Lancet Psychiatry* **2018**, *5*, 327–338. [CrossRef]
12. Walker, G.J.; Harrison, J.W.; Heap, G.A.; Voskuil, M.D.; Andersen, V.; Anderson, C.A.; Ananthakrishnan, A.N.; Barrett, J.C.; Beaugerie, L.; Bewshea, C.M.; et al. Association of genetic variants in NUDT15 with thiopurine-induced myelosuppression in patients with inflammatory bowel disease. *JAMA* **2019**, *321*, 773–785. [CrossRef]
13. Carr, D.F.; Francis, B.; Jorgensen, A.L.; Zhang, E.; Chinoy, H.; Heckbert, S.R.; Bis, J.C.; Brody, J.A.; Floyd, J.S.; Psaty, B.M.; et al. Genomewide association study of statin-induced myopathy in patients recruited using the UK clinical practice research datalink. *Clin. Pharmacol. Ther.* **2019**, *106*, 1353–1361. [CrossRef] [PubMed]
14. Nicoletti, P.; Barrett, S.; McEvoy, L.; Daly, A.K.; Aithal, G.; Lucena, M.I.; Andrade, R.J.; Wadelius, M.; Hallberg, P.; Stephens, C.; et al. Shared genetic risk factors across carbamazepine-induced hypersensitivity reactions. *Clin. Pharmacol. Ther.* **2019**, *106*, 1028–1036. [CrossRef]
15. Ahmed, S.; Zhou, Z.; Zhou, J.; Chen, S.Q. Pharmacogenomics of drug metabolizing enzymes and transporters: Relevance to precision medicine. *Genom. Proteom. Bioinform.* **2016**, *14*, 298–313. [CrossRef]
16. Zarrei, M.; MacDonald, J.R.; Merico, D.; Scherer, S.W. A copy number variation map of the human genome. *Nat. Rev. Genet.* **2015**, *16*, 172–183. [CrossRef]
17. Pang, A.W.; MacDonald, J.R.; Pinto, D.; Wei, J.; Rafiq, M.A.; Conrad, D.F.; Park, H.; Hurles, M.E.; Lee, C.; Venter, J.C.; et al. Towards a comprehensive structural variation map of an individual human genome. *Genome. Biol.* **2010**, *11*, R52. [CrossRef] [PubMed]
18. Sudmant, P.H.; Mallick, S.; Nelson, B.J.; Hormozdiari, F.; Krumm, N.; Huddleston, J.; Coe, B.P.; Baker, C.; Nordenfelt, S.; Bamshad, M.; et al. Global diversity, population stratification, and selection of human copy-number variation. *Science* **2015**, *349*, aab3761. [CrossRef] [PubMed]
19. Arcella, A.; Limanaqi, F.; Ferese, R.; Biagioni, F.; Oliva, M.A.; Storto, M.; Fanelli, M.; Gambardella, S.; Fornai, F. Dissecting molecular features of gliomas: Genetic loci and validated biomarkers. *Int. J. Mol. Sci.* **2020**, *21*, 685. [CrossRef] [PubMed]
20. Gentile, G.; La Cognata, V.; Cavallaro, S. The contribution of CNVs to the most common aging-related neurodegenerative diseases. *Aging Clin. Exp. Res.* **2020**. [CrossRef] [PubMed]

21. Sullivan, P.F.; Owen, M.J. Increasing the clinical psychiatric knowledge base about pathogenic copy number variation. *Am. J. Psychiatry* **2020**, *177*, 204–209. [CrossRef] [PubMed]
22. Lauer, S.; Gresham, D. An evolving view of copy number variants. *Curr. Genet.* **2019**, *65*, 1287–1295. [CrossRef]
23. Kim, J.; Lee, S.Y.; Lee, K.A. Copy number variation and gene rearrangements in CYP2D6 genotyping using multiplex ligation-dependent probe amplification in Koreans. *Pharmacogenomics* **2012**, *13*, 963–973. [CrossRef]
24. Qiao, W.; Martis, S.; Mendiratta, G.; Shi, L.; Botton, M.R.; Yang, Y.; Gaedigk, A.; Vijzelaar, R.; Edelmann, L.; Kornreich, R.; et al. Integrated CYP2D6 interrogation for multiethnic copy number and tandem allele detection. *Pharmacogenomics* **2019**, *20*, 9–20. [CrossRef] [PubMed]
25. Santos, M.; Niemi, M.; Hiratsuka, M.; Kumondai, M.; Ingelman-Sundberg, M.; Lauschke, V.M.; Rodriguez-Antona, C. Novel copy-number variations in pharmacogenes contribute to interindividual differences in drug pharmacokinetics. *Genet. Med.* **2018**, *20*, 622–629. [CrossRef] [PubMed]
26. Han, J.; Shon, J.; Hwang, J.Y.; Park, Y.J. Effects of Coffee Intake on Dyslipidemia Risk According to Genetic Variants in the ADORA Gene Family among Korean Adults. *Nutrients* **2020**, *12*, 493. [CrossRef] [PubMed]
27. Kwon, Y.J.; Hong, K.W.; Park, B.J.; Jung, D.H. Serotonin receptor 3B polymorphisms are associated with type 2 diabetes: The Korean Genome and Epidemiology Study. *Diabetes Res. Clin. Pract.* **2019**, *153*, 76–85. [CrossRef]
28. Yang, Y.J.; Kim, J.; Kwock, C.K. Association of Genetic Variation in the Epithelial Sodium Channel Gene with Urinary Sodium Excretion and Blood Pressure. *Nutrients* **2018**, *10*, 612. [CrossRef]
29. Kim, Y.; Han, B.G. Cohort Profile: The Korean Genome and Epidemiology Study (KoGES) Consortium. *Int. J. Epidemiol.* **2017**, *46*, 1350. [CrossRef]
30. Thorn, C.F.; Klein, T.E.; Altman, R.B. PharmGKB: The Pharmacogenomics Knowledge Base. *Methods Mol. Biol.* **2013**, *1015*, 311–320.
31. Relling, M.V.; Klein, T.E. CPIC: Clinical Pharmacogenetics Implementation Consortium of the Pharmacogenomics Research Network. *Clin. Pharmacol. Ther.* **2011**, *89*, 464–467. [CrossRef] [PubMed]
32. Tutton, R. Pharmacogenomic biomarkers in drug labels: What do they tell us? *Pharmacogenomics* **2014**, *15*, 297–304. [CrossRef] [PubMed]
33. Moon, S.; Kim, Y.J.; Han, S.; Hwang, M.Y.; Shin, D.M.; Park, M.Y.; Lu, Y.; Yoon, K.; Jang, H.M.; Kim, Y.K.; et al. The Korea Biobank array: Design and identification of coding variants associated with blood biochemical traits. *Sci. Rep.* **2019**, *9*, 1382. [CrossRef] [PubMed]
34. Delaneau, O.; Marchini, J.; Zagury, J.F. A linear complexity phasing method for thousands of genomes. *Nat. Methods* **2011**, *9*, 179–181. [CrossRef]
35. Marchini, J.; Howie, B.; Myers, S.; McVean, G.; Donnelly, P. A new multipoint method for genome-wide association studies by imputation of genotypes. *Nat. Genet.* **2007**, *39*, 906–913. [CrossRef]
36. Durinck, S.; Moreau, Y.; Kasprzyk, A.; Davis, S.; De Moor, B.; Brazma, A.; Huber, W. BioMart and Bioconductor: A powerful link between biological databases and microarray data analysis. *Bioinformatics* **2005**, *21*, 3439–3440. [CrossRef]
37. Moon, S.; Kim, Y.J.; Hong, C.B.; Kim, D.J.; Lee, J.Y.; Kim, B.J. Data-driven approach to detect common copy-number variations and frequency profiles in a population-based Korean cohort. *Eur. J. Hum. Genet.* **2011**, *19*, 1167–1172. [CrossRef]
38. Sim, N.L.; Kumar, P.; Hu, J.; Henikoff, S.; Schneider, G.; Ng, P.C. SIFT web server: Predicting effects of amino acid substitutions on proteins. *Nucleic. Acids. Res.* **2012**, *40*, W452–W457. [CrossRef]
39. Adzhubei, I.A.; Schmidt, S.; Peshkin, L.; Ramensky, V.E.; Gerasimova, A.; Bork, P.; Kondrashov, A.S.; Sunyaev, S.R. A method and server for predicting damaging missense mutations. *Nat. Methods* **2010**, *7*, 248–249. [CrossRef]
40. Pique-Regi, R.; Caceres, A.; Gonzalez, J.R. R-Gada: A fast and flexible pipeline for copy number analysis in association studies. *BMC Bioinform.* **2010**, *11*, 380. [CrossRef]
41. Moon, S.; Kim, Y.J.; Kim, Y.K.; Kim, D.J.; Lee, J.Y.; Go, M.J.; Shin, Y.A.; Hong, C.B.; Kim, B.J. Genome-wide survey of copy number variants associated with blood pressure and body mass index in a Korean population. *Genom. Inform.* **2011**, *9*, 152–160. [CrossRef]
42. Bambury, R.M.; Bhatt, A.S.; Riester, M.; Pedamallu, C.S.; Duke, F.; Bellmunt, J.; Stack, E.C.; Werner, L.; Park, R.; Iyer, G.; et al. DNA copy number analysis of metastatic urothelial carcinoma with comparison to primary tumors. *BMC Cancer* **2015**, *15*, 242. [CrossRef] [PubMed]
43. Lindgren, D.; Sjodahl, G.; Lauss, M.; Staaf, J.; Chebil, G.; Lovgren, K.; Gudjonsson, S.; Liedberg, F.; Patschan, O.; Mansson, W.; et al. Integrated genomic and gene expression profiling identifies two major genomic circuits in urothelial carcinoma. *PLoS ONE* **2012**, *7*, e38863. [CrossRef]
44. Chang, C.C.; Chow, C.C.; Tellier, L.C.; Vattikuti, S.; Purcell, S.M.; Lee, J.J. Second-generation PLINK: Rising to the challenge of larger and richer datasets. *Gigascience* **2015**, *4*, 7. [CrossRef]
45. Barrett, J.C.; Fry, B.; Maller, J.; Daly, M.J. Haploview: Analysis and visualization of LD and haplotype maps. *Bioinformatics* **2005**, *21*, 263–265. [CrossRef]
46. Owen, R.P.; Gong, L.; Sagreiya, H.; Klein, T.E.; Altman, R.B. VKORC1 pharmacogenomics summary. *Pharm. Genom.* **2010**, *20*, 642–644. [CrossRef]
47. Sakuyama, K.; Sasaki, T.; Ujiie, S.; Obata, K.; Mizugaki, M.; Ishikawa, M.; Hiratsuka, M. Functional characterization of 17 CYP2D6 allelic variants (CYP2D6.2, 10, 14A-B, 18, 27, 36, 39, 47-51, 53-55, and 57). *Drug Metab. Dispos.* **2008**, *36*, 2460–2467. [CrossRef]

48. Kim, K.A.; Song, W.K.; Kim, K.R.; Park, J.Y. Assessment of CYP2C19 genetic polymorphisms in a Korean population using a simultaneous multiplex pyrosequencing method to simultaneously detect the CYP2C19*2, CYP2C19*3, and CYP2C19*17 alleles. *J. Clin. Pharm. Ther.* **2010**, *35*, 697–703. [CrossRef]
49. Scott, S.A.; Sangkuhl, K.; Stein, C.M.; Hulot, J.S.; Mega, J.L.; Roden, D.M.; Klein, T.E.; Sabatine, M.S.; Johnson, J.A.; Shuldiner, A.R.; et al. Clinical Pharmacogenetics Implementation Consortium guidelines for CYP2C19 genotype and clopidogrel therapy: 2013 update. *Clin. Pharmacol. Ther.* **2013**, *94*, 317–323. [CrossRef]
50. Carpenter, D.; Ringrose, C.; Leo, V.; Morris, A.; Robinson, R.L.; Halsall, P.J.; Hopkins, P.M.; Shaw, M.A. The role of CACNA1S in predisposition to malignant hyperthermia. *BMC Med. Genet.* **2009**, *10*, 104. [CrossRef]
51. Lee, J.H.; Choi, J.H.; Namkung, W.; Hanrahan, J.W.; Chang, J.; Song, S.Y.; Park, S.W.; Kim, D.S.; Yoon, J.H.; Suh, Y.; et al. A haplotype-based molecular analysis of CFTR mutations associated with respiratory and pancreatic diseases. *Hum. Mol. Genet.* **2003**, *12*, 2321–2332. [CrossRef] [PubMed]
52. Guan, S.; Huang, M.; Li, X.; Chen, X.; Chan, E.; Zhou, S.F. Intra- and inter-ethnic differences in the allele frequencies of cytochrome P450 2B6 gene in Chinese. *Pharm. Res.* **2006**, *23*, 1983–1990. [CrossRef]
53. Gadel, S.; Crafford, A.; Regina, K.; Kharasch, E.D. Methadone N-demethylation by the common CYP2B6 allelic variant CYP2B6.6. *Drug Metab. Dispos.* **2013**, *41*, 709–713. [CrossRef]
54. Paganotti, G.M.; Russo, G.; Sobze, M.S.; Mayaka, G.B.; Muthoga, C.W.; Tawe, L.; Martinelli, A.; Romano, R.; Vullo, V. CYP2B6 poor metaboliser alleles involved in efavirenz and nevirapine metabolism: CYP2B6*9 and CYP2B6*18 distribution in HIV-exposed subjects from Dschang, Western Cameroon. *Infect. Genet. Evol.* **2015**, *35*, 122–126. [CrossRef]
55. Ishmukhametova, A.; Chen, J.M.; Bernard, R.; de Massy, B.; Baudat, F.; Boyer, A.; Mechin, D.; Thorel, D.; Chabrol, B.; Vincent, M.C.; et al. Dissecting the structure and mechanism of a complex duplication-triplication rearrangement in the DMD gene. *Hum. Mutat.* **2013**, *34*, 1080–1084. [CrossRef]
56. Iskandar, K.; Dwianingsih, E.K.; Pratiwi, L.; Kalim, A.S.; Mardhiah, H.; Putranti, A.H.; Nurputra, D.K.; Triono, A.; Herini, E.S.; Malueka, R.G.; et al. The analysis of DMD gene deletions by multiplex PCR in Indonesian DMD/BMD patients: The era of personalized medicine. *BMC Res. Notes* **2019**, *12*, 704. [CrossRef]
57. Cho, A.; Seong, M.W.; Lim, B.C.; Lee, H.J.; Byeon, J.H.; Kim, S.S.; Kim, S.Y.; Choi, S.A.; Wong, A.L.; Lee, J.; et al. Consecutive Analysis of Mutation Spectrum in the Dystrophin Gene of 507 Korean Boys with Duchenne/Becker Muscular Dystrophy in a Single Center. *Muscle Nerve* **2017**, *55*, 727–734. [CrossRef]
58. Spire-Vayron de la Moureyre, C.; Debuysere, H.; Fazio, F.; Sergent, E.; Bernard, C.; Sabbagh, N.; Marez, D.; Lo Guidice, J.M.; D'Halluin, J.C. Characterization of a variable number tandem repeat region in the thiopurine S-methyltransferase gene promoter. *Pharmacogenetics* **1999**, *9*, 189–198.
59. Urbancic, D.; Smid, A.; Stocco, G.; Decorti, G.; Mlinaric-Rascan, I.; Karas Kuzelicki, N. Novel motif of variable number of tandem repeats in TPMT promoter region and evolutionary association of variable number of tandem repeats with TPMT*3 alleles. *Pharmacogenomics* **2018**, *19*, 1311–1322. [CrossRef]
60. Green, D.J.; Duong, S.Q.; Burckart, G.J.; Sissung, T.; Price, D.K.; Figg, W.D., Jr.; Brooks, M.M.; Chinnock, R.; Canter, C.; Addonizio, L.; et al. Association Between Thiopurine S-Methyltransferase (TPMT) Genetic Variants and Infection in Pediatric Heart Transplant Recipients Treated With Azathioprine: A Multi-Institutional Analysis. *J. Pediatr. Pharmacol. Ther.* **2018**, *23*, 106–110. [CrossRef]
61. Lee, S.S.; Kim, W.Y.; Jang, Y.J.; Shin, J.G. Duplex pyrosequencing of the TPMT*3C and TPMT*6 alleles in Korean and Vietnamese populations. *Clin. Chim. Acta* **2008**, *398*, 82–85. [CrossRef] [PubMed]
62. Yang, S.K.; Hong, M.; Baek, J.; Choi, H.; Zhao, W.; Jung, Y.; Haritunians, T.; Ye, B.D.; Kim, K.J.; Park, S.H.; et al. A common missense variant in NUDT15 confers susceptibility to thiopurine-induced leukopenia. *Nat. Genet.* **2014**, *46*, 1017–1020. [CrossRef] [PubMed]
63. Vijzelaar, R.; Botton, M.R.; Stolk, L.; Martis, S.; Desnick, R.J.; Scott, S.A. Multi-ethnic SULT1A1 copy number profiling with multiplex ligation-dependent probe amplification. *Pharmacogenomics* **2018**, *19*, 761–770. [CrossRef] [PubMed]
64. Guthrie, P.A.; Gaunt, T.R.; Abdollahi, M.R.; Rodriguez, S.; Lawlor, D.A.; Smith, G.D.; Day, I.N. Amplification ratio control system for copy number variation genotyping. *Nucleic. Acids. Res.* **2011**, *39*, e54. [CrossRef] [PubMed]
65. Haraksingh, R.R.; Snyder, M.P. Impacts of variation in the human genome on gene regulation. *J. Mol. Biol.* **2013**, *425*, 3970–3977. [CrossRef]

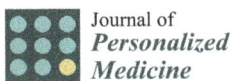

Article

Pharmacogenomics at the Point of Care: A Community Pharmacy Project in British Columbia

Samantha Breaux [1], Francis Arthur Derek Desrosiers [2], Mauricio Neira [1], Sunita Sinha [1,3] and Corey Nislow [1,*]

1. Pharmaceutical Sciences, University of British Columbia, Vancouver, BC V6T 1Z3, Canada; sbreaux@mail.ubc.ca (S.B.); maunei001@gmail.com (M.N.); sunita.sinha@ubc.ca (S.S.)
2. British Columbia Pharmacy Association, 430-1200 W. 73rd Avenue, Vancouver, BC V6P 6G5, Canada; derek@dessonconsulting.com
3. Sequencing and Bioinformatics Consortium, Office of the Vice-President, Research & Innovation (VPRI), University of British Columbia, Vancouver, BC V6T 1Z3, Canada
* Correspondence: corey.nislow@ubc.ca

Abstract: In this study 180 patients were consented and enrolled for pharmacogenomic testing based on current antidepressant/antipsychotic usage. Samples from patients were genotyped by PCR, MassArray, and targeted next generation sequencing. We also conducted a quantitative, frequency-based analysis of participants' perceptions using simple surveys. Pharmacogenomic information, including medication changes and altered dosing recommendations were returned to the pharmacists and used to direct patient therapy. Overwhelmingly, patients perceived pharmacists/pharmacies as an appropriate healthcare provider to deliver pharmacogenomic services. In total, 81 medication changes in 33 unique patients, representing 22% of all genotyped participants were recorded. We performed a simple drug cost analysis and found that medication adjustments and dosing changes across the entire cohort added $24.15CAD per patient per year for those that required an adjustment. Comparing different platforms, we uncovered a small number, 1.7%, of genotype discrepancies. We conclude that: (1). Pharmacists are competent providers of pharmacogenomic services. (2). The potential reduction in adverse drug responses and optimization of drug selection and dosing comes at a minimal cost to the health care system. (3). Changes in drug therapy, based on PGx tests, result in inconsequential changes in annual drug therapy cost with small cost increases just as likely as costs savings. (4). Pharmacogenomic services offered by pharmacists are ready for wide commercial implementation.

Keywords: community pharmacy; pharmacogenomic testing; pharmacogenetics; genetic privacy; pharmaco-economics

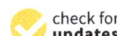

Citation: Breaux, S.; Desrosiers, F.A.D.; Neira, M.; Sinha, S.; Nislow, C. Pharmacogenomics at the Point of Care: A Community Pharmacy Project in British Columbia. J. Pers. Med. 2021, 11, 11. https://dx.doi.org/10.3390/jpm 11010011

Received: 9 November 2020
Accepted: 23 December 2020
Published: 24 December 2020

Publisher's Note: MDPI stays neutral with regard to jurisdictional claims in published maps and institutional affiliations.

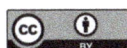

Copyright: © 2020 by the authors. Licensee MDPI, Basel, Switzerland. This article is an open access article distributed under the terms and conditions of the Creative Commons Attribution (CC BY) license (https://creativecommons.org/licenses/by/4.0/).

1. Introduction

Completion of the Human Genome Project in 2003 brought expectations that the information would revolutionize the practice of medicine and introduce new scientific, business, and medical models [1,2]. While many of those hopes are just beginning to be realized, the resulting discipline of pharmacogenomics (PGx) has matured considerably in the past decade. PGx uses genetic information to classify patients who may benefit from personalized medication or who may respond negatively to a particular treatment. PGx can help ensure that patients receive the most appropriate medication and dose, can reduce the number of adverse drug reactions (ADRs) and aid in medication adherence. The most appropriate provider of PGx testing, however, remains a subject of debate. In British Columbia (BC) Canada, pharmacists are the recognized drug experts [3]. Furthermore, over the past two decades their scope of practice has expanded to provide more aspects of comprehensive patient care [4]. These additions are a powerful way to address the fact that every year in BC over 200,000 people are admitted to hospitals due to adverse drug reactions of which 10,000–20,000 die; these patients' treatments cost an estimated

$49 million per year [5]. These numbers are likely to be higher because 95% of ADRs go unreported [6]. In 2011, the American Pharmacists Association acknowledged the importance and practicality of integrating genomics with medication therapy management programs to optimize patient drug therapy [7]. Such emphasis on a more patient-centered, individualized, and preventative approach to wellness is an antidote to the frustration of the one-size-fits-all paradigm of evidence-based medicine [8]. Implementation of PGx testing based on these benefits has, however, proven to be challenging. Causes include low acceptance of pharmacist recommendations by the physician and prescriber, mixed patient receptivity, low rates of reimbursement to pharmacists, inadequate human resources, and the physical layout of the pharmacy [9]. Our supposition for potentially unproductive interactions between pharmacists and physicians was due to the (self-reported) high levels of unfamiliarity with regards to genomics and by extension being uncomfortable with making drug therapy changes based on a participant's drug metabolism genotype [10]. An additional barrier is the cost of PGx testing which ranges from $200–$500, often left to the consumer because insurers have been hesitant to cover genetic testing for non-diagnostic purposes [11]. Fears include concerns over data security and actual clinical impact [12]. These barriers are surmountable and have been addressed in other contexts [13].

Building on earlier work in which we concluded that the community pharmacist is the appropriate healthcare expert for PGx deployment [14–16]; in this study we tested the hypothesis that medication changes as a result of PGx testing have a minimal impact on the overall cost of a patient's drug therapy. In today's market, there is a diversity of PGx-testing platform technologies [17]. DNA arrays and polymerase chain reaction (PCR)-based tests are commonly used methods for commercial genotype screening. An advantage of these two assays is that they are largely blind to detecting so-called incidental findings. Specifically, both arrays and PCR are used to confirm either the presence, absence, or duplication of specific known single nucleotide polymorphisms (SNPs) and as a result only information about those alleles under study can be gleaned from this process. Furthermore, the accuracy of these approaches has been validated [18–21] and they are simple and cost-effective, making them easy to implement in routine practice.

The objectives of this study were to; (1) test the feasibility and appropriateness of community pharmacists as a conduit for pharmacogenomics information, (2) to gauge the receptivity of patients in this setting and (3) assess the cost-effectiveness of this approach. Despite the limited size of the study, we satisfied these objectives and discuss how the lessons learned here can be applied.

2. Materials and Methods

See "Expanded Online Methods" in Supplementary Material files.

2.1. Pharmacy Selection

Community pharmacies were selected to reflect a diversity in geography and practice environments in BC. Pharmacies were required to have expressed interest in participating, a corporate membership with the BC Pharmacy Association, a sufficiently private counselling area and adequate staffing to ensure that the pharmacist could have uninterrupted time with participants during the education and consent process. Additional pharmacies were added as needed. Accounting for individual turnover, we ended up with 21 pharmacists recruiting patients at 17 participating community pharmacies in 13 locales across the province as shown in Map 1.

2.2. Pharmacist Training

In addition to the Tri-Council Policy Statement Ethical Conduct for Research Involving Humans Course on Research Ethics, the pharmacists had to complete a study training program done remotely via webinar and phone; (i) to ensure pharmacists followed all the requirements of the law and Research Ethics Board of the University of British Columbia

(UBC), especially with respect to patient privacy and (ii) to ensure that the patient experience was consistent regardless of the pharmacy type or location.

A study team member and the pharmacist discussed the project principles of informed consent, privacy requirements, patient education, obtaining consent, collecting patient information, and reviewed a consent checklist designed to guide the education and consent process. At the conclusion of this session, the pharmacist was asked a series of questions based on the training they received.

2.3. Operations Logistics & Report Interpretation

The details of sample collection, handling, return, and documentation were discussed with a study team leader. Pharmacists were required to complete the myDNA online pharmacist training program for PGx as well, providing an overview of pharmacogenomics as well as interpretation of the myDNA reports. The learning objectives for this training were (1) understand the basis of cytochrome (CYP) P450 genes/enzymes associated with CPIC guidelines, (2) understand how variants affect an individual's ability to metabolize medications, and (3) how to apply this knowledge in clinical practice to improve their patients' outcome.

2.4. Quality Control (QC)

Before the pharmacists enrolled patients in our study, a phone call to role play the registration and consent process with a study team member was conducted. The study team member completed the consent checklist (Supplement SI) during the process and at the end of the session reviewed the terminology, phrasing, and content with the pharmacist.

2.5. Participant Selection and Consent

To be enrolled in the study a potential participant must have been over 19, speak English, and needed to be taking a valid criteria drug at time of enrollment. Pharmacists were prohibited to search patient records to identify eligible participants. In a private area of the pharmacy, the pharmacist explained the project and summarized the Participant Information & Consent Form (Supplement SII). A checklist was completed for each potential participant. The potential participant was then shown a video specifically developed for this project. The video, (Supplement SIII–SIV), introduced the key concepts of PGx and the goals of the research project. The pharmacist watched the video with each patient to ensure that concepts were clear and to answer questions as necessary. The potential participant was then given the Patient Information & Consent Form to review, and was required to wait at least 24 h before committing to the study. This allowed patients time to reflect, to discuss the project with other family members or caregivers, and to obtain additional information to make an informed decision about their participation.

After a potential participant agreed to the study, the enrollment process started with the pharmacist answering questions generated in the contemplative (take-home) phase. Next, patients signed the consent form and were given a copy for their records. Following their consent, the patients provided a saliva sample (see Expanded Online Methods) and their pharmacist collected the required enrollment information. To avoid external incentives (or the appearance thereof) we specified that each pharmacist be limited to recruiting a maximum of 10 patients.

2.6. Data & Sample Collection

Mandatory information collected included date of birth, gender, current medications, history of ADRs as well as allergies and medical conditions. Disease and indication data were not collected from participants. Even though gender, age and drug therapy information were collected, the numbers in the study were too small to sufficiently address stratification by any of these data. The Genotek Oragene saliva collection kit was used according to manufacturer's protocol to collect patient sputum [22]. This process took 2–5 min in most cases, although there were participants who took longer and a small number who were unable to provide usable saliva samples. The reasons for this varied, but the common theme was that these participants complained of 'dry mouth'.

2.7. Experience Survey

A pharmacist and patient experience survey were mailed out with the recruitment kit (Supplement SV–SVI). The enrolling pharmacist ensured completion and return of the surveys at the end of the study. They were asked to indicate their level of agreement using a 4-point Likert scale, which was chosen over a 5-point scale [23], removing a "Neutral" option to require respondents to either agree or disagree with the statements.

2.8. Transport of Samples & Participant Information

After de-identification, the original copy of the patient enrollment documentation and the patient's saliva sample were sent via secure courier to UBC. A copy of the demographic information was kept and secured at the pharmacies. Saliva samples were received and catalogued and stored at our sequencing facility (https://sequencing.ubc.ca/). Participant information was used to update a key file linking identifying information to the participant code. All non-identifying information was transcribed and linked only to the participant code. Sample IDs were then subsequently linked to unique, randomized sample barcodes for downstream analysis and report tracking.

2.9. Sample Processing

DNA was extracted from 250 µL of saliva sample. Any remaining saliva was stored at room temperature for up to a week prior to long term storage at $-20\ °C$. The "prepIT.L2P" reagents were used according to the manufacturer's instructions (DNA Genotek). DNA was eluted in 50 µL molecular-grade water and DNA quality was assessed by gel electrophoresis and quantified by Nanodrop (Thermofisher Scientific, Waltham, MA, USA) and fluorometry using the Qubit dsDNA HS Assay Kit. The gel analysis provided a go/no-go step for the samples, in other words, if samples were extensively degraded at this QC step, we attempted a second extraction. DNA was stored at $-20\ °C$ until genotyping or TRS library preparation.

2.10. TargetRich Sequencing (TRS)

DNA was extracted as described above and processed according to the manufacturer (https://www.kailosgenetics.com/). Briefly, to prepare the sequencing library, guide oligos which contain the sequences to be amplified are annealed, followed by a restriction enzyme digestion, after which Illumina adapter sequences are annealed along with the unique identifier (barcode) for the library sample. The samples are then enzymatically cleaned via magnetic beads before being amplified and cleaned a final time. Samples were QC'd by agarose gel electrophoresis and quantified with Qubit. Pooled amplicons were sequenced on an Illumina Miseq platform, generating paired-end 78 bp reads [24]. Long range PCR was used to determine duplication as described by the manufacturer [25].

2.11. Genotyping

We worked with myDNA—https://www.mydna.life/en-ca/to perform SNP analysis using the iPLEX MassArray System, a non-fluorescent platform utilizing MALDI-TOF (matrix-assisted laser desorption/ionization—time of flight) mass spectrometry, coupled with end point PCR to measure PCR-derived amplicons in multiplexed reactions. Briefly, polymorphic sites were detected by primer extension where the targeted region is amplified; remaining dNTPs are neutralized and then a terminating extension reaction using a promoter that binds immediately upstream of the polymorphic site as a 'mass modified' nucleotide lacking the 3′-hydroxyl extends the product by a single base [19–21,26]. The number of CYP2D6 gene copies was detected by qPCR using a 7900HT PCR system [27].

2.12. Data Reporting

Patient reports were generated using myDNA's PGx software (https://www.mydna.life/en-ca/). These reports were uploaded to a secure website accessible to the primary project team by the PI (CN), the User Partner Lead (FADD), and the project's Research Assistant (SB). Data was encrypted and only de-identified to the appropriate pharmacist after review by the project team. Genomic reports and patient IDs were sent separately in encrypted Excel spreadsheets. GitHub (https://github.com/) was used to store all analysis routines and to ensure version control.

In addition to genotyping 150 samples, 46 were subjected to Kailos TRS or "target rich sequencing protocol". The NGS data and the final TRS reports were not returned to the pharmacists and restricted to internal comparisons.

2.13. Patient Consults at the Pharmacy

Every patient enrolled in the study who was able to be genotyped received a copy of their myDNA report. Neither the patient nor the pharmacist was returned a copy of the TRS report, which was used for our own reference to further validate the myDNA results as well as do a basic comparison of the functionality of sequencing over an array-based analysis. The reports were released directly to CN and FADD at which point we would review them before informing the pharmacist. Reports were reviewed with each participant in a face-to-face appointment with the pharmacist following a standardized script. The pharmacist delivered results, discussed possible therapy change recommendations, and asked if the participant wanted the report shared with the patient's physician. Participants had the option of sharing the report directly themselves or having the pharmacist send a copy. Pharmacists were responsible for recording medication changes. All medication changes were made the patient's physician or general practitioner and all participants were asked to complete a qualitative survey.

2.14. Data Collection & Analysis

To process the myDNA reports for our meta-analysis, each participant's medical considerations and genotypes were extracted from PDFs using tabula [28]. Files were then manually edited to include a patient ID and any potential drug-drug interaction information. Genotype information from the TRS reports were manually entered into a .csv file and further tidied, such as conversion from wide to long data, using R (version 3.6.1), a programming language for data analysis [29]. To compare genotype calls between TRS and myDNA, only shared alleles were analyzed. A file containing every unique myDNA call was matched with the corresponding TRS genotype. Population frequencies for the genotypes CYP2D6, CYP2C19, CYP2C9, and VKORC1 were taken from an analysis of an Australian population [27]. The frequency of CYP2D6 *36 was taken from an American population [30]. The population frequencies of the SLCO1B1, CYP1A2, CYP3A4, CYP3A5, and OPRM1 genotypes were calculated from the global SNP frequency. Global Frequency of the SNPs were gathered from the Genome Aggregation Database (gnomAD) (https://gnomad.broadinstitute.org/) [31]. Hardy-Weinberg equilibrium [32] was used to calculate the genotype frequencies in an ideal population.

All genotype data manipulation and analyses were completed in R version 3.6.1 (Supplement SVII). Analysis depended on R packages: Tidyverse, data.table, reshape2, compare, plyr, and rowr [33–38]. Cost-benefit analysis and tabulation of survey results was completed in Excel. Drug prices were retrieved from the McKesson Canada wholesale drug price list in effect at that time.

2.15. Research Ethics Board Approval & Legal Compliance

In developing our Research Ethics Board (REB) procedure, we considered the following Canadian and British Columbian legislation:

1. The Personal Information Protection Act, The Freedom of Information and Protection of Privacy Act, The Health Professions Act and its Bylaws, The Health Care (Consent)

and Care Facility (Admission) Act, and The Pharmacy Operations and Drug Scheduling Act. These laws lay out the obligations of the pharmacist, the pharmacy and the University of British Columbia with respect to personal and health information.
2. The Health Professions Act and its Bylaws and The Personal Information Protection Act. These laws governed the pharmacist with respect to the collection, use, disclosure and security of personal and health information.
3. The Freedom of Information and Protection of Privacy Act and the policies of UBC and its Research Ethics Board.

2.16. Timeline

Starting in mid-2017, our project ran until January of 2018. Most aspects of the project were completed in tandem as opposed to sequentially. In the first six months we prepared the pharmacist training material and updated patient recruitment kits. During this time, we initiated patient marketing and recruitment. While the bulk of these activities was completed in the first 6 months, recruitment persisted until completion of sequencing. Enrollment began after pharmacist training was complete and patients had to be taking at least 1 of the mental health drugs listed in Table 1. We used a batch approach to sample processing, beginning 6 months after project initiation and persisted for an additional 9 months. Data analysis began after first results were returned in quarter 3. The last activity we accomplished were the pharmacist consultations where we returned reports and completed the final aspect of our data analysis. These activities persisted for 9 months.

3. Results

In this study we built on our and others work to further test feasibility of community pharmacogenomic testing, in addition to assessing pharmacist and community comfort with pharmacogenomic services and to conduct a simple drug cost analysis [14,16,39]. To accomplish this, 21 pharmacists at 17 pharmacies, Figure 1, were enlisted to recruit 150–200 patients for genotyping (or genotyping and TRS) when they filled or renewed a prescription for an antidepressant/antipsychotic, Table 1. MyDNA genotyping analysis (https://www.mydna.life/en-ca/) was used to assess patient responses to a wide variety of medications with a focus on mental health medications.

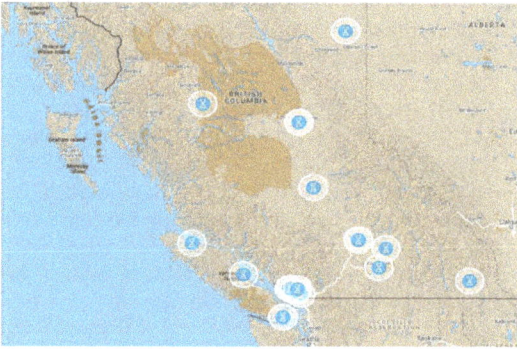

Figure 1. Map of participating pharmacies by their locations. For table of locations and pharmacies see Supplement SIX.

Table 1. Study compounds. Patients had to be currently taking at least one of the medications in the table to be included in the study. Included are usage frequency of each drug. Some patients were taking multiple compounds.

Antidepressants	Usage	Antidepressants	Usage	Antipsychotics	Usage
Agomelatine	0	Mianserin	0	Aripiprazole	9
Amitriptyline	12	Mirtazapine	12	Clozapine	0
Citalopram	26	Moclobemide	2	Haloperidol	0
Clomipramine	0	Nortriptyline	6	Olanzapine	5
Dothiepin	0	Paroxetine	2	Quetiapine	24
Duloxetine	10	Sertraline	17	Risperidone	4
Escitalopram	27	Trimipramine	0	Zuclopenthixol	0
Fluoxetine	12	Vanlafaxine	23		
Fluvoxamine	1	Vortioxetine	2		
Imipramine	1				Total: 195

Antidepressants and antipsychotics are metabolized by diverse enzymes. The cytochrome p450 isoforms CYP2C19 and CYP2D6 are responsible for metabolism of more than two-thirds of the currently available psychiatric drugs; these genes are also highly polymorphic with a variety of stable alleles and mutations, including whole and partial duplications and deletions [40–42]. As a consequence, the range of enzyme activity and downstream phenotypes is large [40]. Indeed, the amount of clinically relevant mutations in these genes appears to be above 50% for most populations [40]. Additionally, the rate of initial response to antidepressant treatment was only 49.6% [41]. The additional costs incurred for management of these non-responders is ~$10,000USD/yr./patient [43]. This combination of factors; (1) a large pool of diverse alleles, (2) high degrees variation in drug metabolism and the high costs of productive patient prescribing highlight the importance and usefulness of personalized treatment for these medications [42]. Actionable results (based on up-to-date guidelines from the Clinical Pharmacogenetics Implementation Consortium (CPIC) [44] were returned to the pharmacist for review (see a sample report-Supplement SVIII) with the patient and the prescriber (if appropriate). Net costs were calculated for all therapy changes made to a patient's current medications. Patient and pharmacist experience surveys were used to judge the participant's thoughts on the services and experience. We also assessed if the medication was discontinued/changed/dosage altered, the overall financial impact of the changes on drug therapy costs, and the reliability and quality of genotyping results.

Sample collection and genotyping was accomplished in two main batches. Batch one comprised 130 samples, 116 of which passed QC. In batch two 48 samples were collected, 42 of which passed QC. We also received 19 samples as a retest, in total generating 150 myDNA and 37 TRS genetic reports, with 47 samples that did not pass QC. For example, some patient's sputum simply did not provide adequate DNA as re-extraction only continued to produce insufficient or degraded samples. This may be due to an inability to produce the appropriate amount of sputum, natural variations in cheek shedding, or effects of medications.

3.1. Comparison of Genotypes

We found 9 total differences in genotype calls between those that underwent both TRS and myDNA genotyping (for a total of 592 SNPS), Table 2. Between the two datasets there were 296 comparable genotypes giving a discordance of 1.7%. One gene could not be called by TRS. This may have been due to the region being degraded or problems with amplification for the patient. TRS also called two additional alleles that myDNA does not, CYP2D6 *35A and CYP3A4 *8. *35A is a subset of the *2 allele. *2 contains SNPs 2851: c > t and 4181: g > c, while *35A contains the additional SNP 31 g > a. *35A has the same normal metabolizer phenotype [45]. As such, the two calls containing *35A can be considered the same as that by myDNA. The CYP3A4 *8 allele has been associated with decreased function of the CYP3A4 protein, although PharmGKB lists this as a level 3 (i.e., low evidence) claim [46]. Regardless, this genotype is absent in the myDNA report resulting in a normal metaboliser call. The remaining differences were minor, suggesting a small number of SNP-specific variables for each platform.

Table 2. Differences found between genes shared in the TRS and myDNA datasets.

GENE	TRS Genotype	myDNA Genotype	Comparison
CYP2C19	*XX/*XX	*1/*17	Kailos no call
CYP2C19	CYP2C19 *1/*2	*2/*2	different
CYP2C9	*1/*3	*3/*3	different
CYP2D6	*2/*2	*2/*5	different
CYP2D6	*35A/*5	*2/*5	Kailos only allele *35A
CYP2D6	*35A/*4	*2/*4	Kailos only allele *35A
CYP3A4	*1/*8	*1/*1	Kailos only allele *8
SLCO1B1	T/C Het	T/T Wild	different
SLCO1B1	T/C Het	T/T Wild	different

*: allele.

Next, we compared the frequency of a subset of genotypes that were part of both the TRS and myDNA reports. Genotypes were compared both to each other and to the population average. Population averages, comprising of Australian, American, and global ethic data [27,30,31] closely matched those from within the study at both sites, Table 3. The averages between myDNA and TRS were similar, showing little variance between the two data types.

Table 3. Sample of a table comparing the frequency of myDNA calls and Kailos calls to population averages of those genotypes. Full table contains 62 genetic variations. See Appendix A.

GENE	myDNA Genotype	TRS Genotype	Phenotype	myDNA Genotype Frequency % $n = 150$	TRS Genotype Frequency % $n = 37$	Population Level Frequency %
CYP2C19	*1/*1	*1/*1	Normal metabolizer	35.33	27	39.7
CYP2C19	*1/*17	*1/*17	Rapid metabolizer	33.33	37.8	25.80%
CYP2C19	*1/*2	*1/*2	Intermediate metabolizer	14	18.9	20.70%
CYP2C19	*17/*17	*17/*17	Ultrarapid metabolizer	2.67	2.7	0
CYP2C19	*2/*17	*2/*17	High intermediate metabolizer	8	8.1	6.20%
CYP2C19	*2/*2	*2/*2	Poor metabolizer	6.67	2.7	2.90%
CYP2C19	NA	*XX/*XX	NA	NA	2.7	NA
CYP2C9	*1/*1	*1/*1	Normal metabolizer	69.33	62.2	64.84%
CYP2C9	*1/*2	*1/*2	High intermediate metabolizer	15.33	21.6	20.38%
CYP2C9	*1/*3	*1/*3	Intermediate metabolizer	10	10.8	10.60%

*: allele.

3.2. Community Acceptance

To gauge the scope and scale of community acceptance a simple two-pronged quantitative, frequency-based analysis of patient and pharmacist attitudes and thoughts was conducted via simple surveys. Each participating patient was asked to complete a short seven question survey in which they ranked their response to statements about the project. Similarly, each participating pharmacist was asked to complete a survey in which they ranked their response to statements about the training and support they received throughout the project. We received 20/21 pharmacists' experience surveys and 111 patient experience surveys with a response rate of 62%. Some patients were not able to be reached at the end of the study and one pharmacist dropped from the study. The patients strongly agreed with the seven statements and also agreed that pharmacists are the appropriate providers of pharmacogenomic services as well as pharmacies being an ideal location to collect samples, Figure 2.

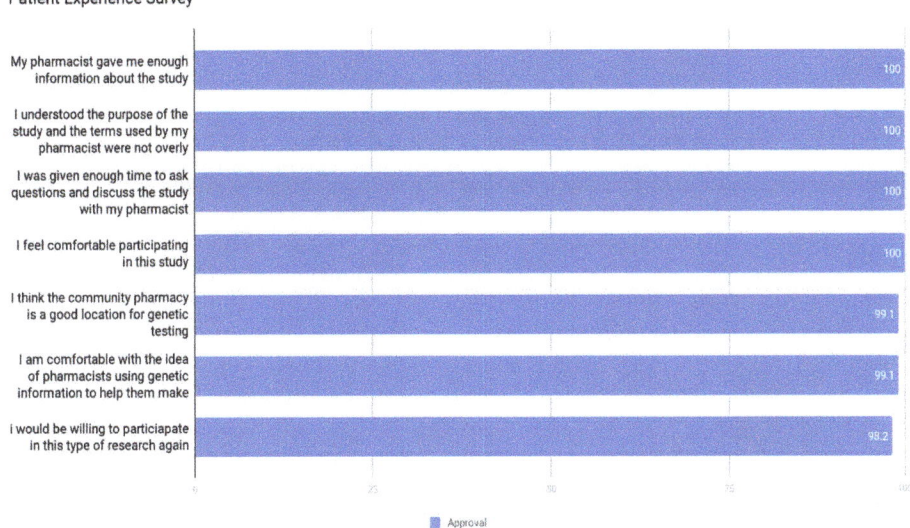

Figure 2. Patient experience survey. All results, 98.2–100% strongly agree/agree, $N = 111$.

Pharmacists' opinions were generally very positive as well, Figure 3. The biggest pharmacist's concern was communication with our research team. This is a fair criticism and likely reflects two constraints of the experimental design; (i) because samples were batched, an overly long time (up to six months) between sample collection and report returns was experienced for the samples collected earliest in the project, and (ii) the project team strove to maintain an arm's length distance for any prescribing decisions.

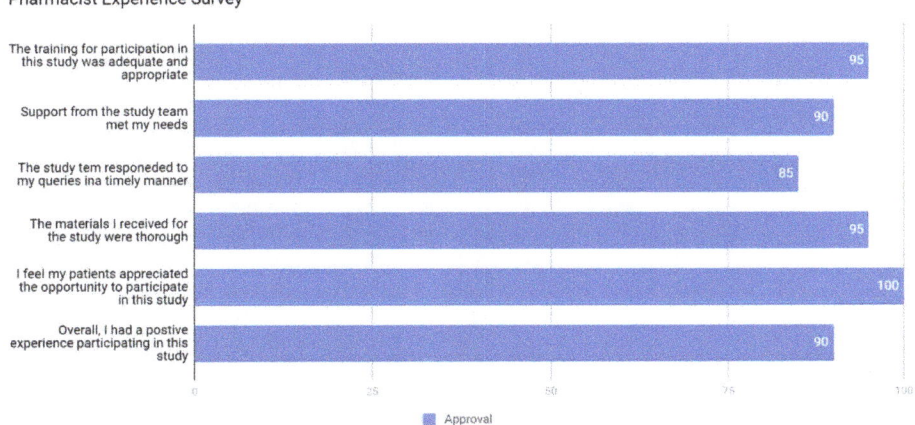

Figure 3. Pharmacist experience survey, 85–100% strongly agree or agree, $N = 20$.

3.3. Drug Cost Analysis

The myDNA reports returned to the pharmacists were used to produce the data in the drug cost analysis. Reports offered three prescribing considerations: 'usual—normal label use of compound'; 'minor- consider test results, as results may be significant'; and 'major—significant results, medication should be reviewed'. The restriction to mental health drugs was only for the eligibility to participate. Once a participant was enrolled, we reviewed all their drugs and many of the drug therapy changes that were made were for drugs other than mental health drugs. All drug changes, regardless of therapeutic category, were included in the simple drug costs analysis. In a small number of cases (16), reports could not be returned as some pharmacists had lost contact with study participants. Additionally, some doctors either felt uncomfortable changing prescribing considerations based on the report results or did not think it was necessary for some patients. For medications that patients were currently taking, 92 were found to have at least one minor prescribing consideration, 39 had at least one major consideration, and an additional 139 participants were taking a medication with usual prescribing considerations, Figure 4. In comparison to a PGx study examining 3 genes using a WES data set, 20% of study participants had immediately actionable results, comparable to the 26% that we found with a major prescribing concern [47].

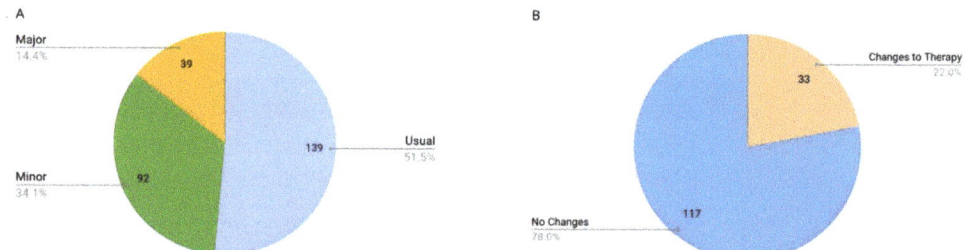

Figure 4. (**A**) Visualization of major, minor, and usual drug considerations discovered, $N = 150$; (**B**) Visualization of medication changes in response to the study, $N = 150$.

Taken together, the aggregate medication changes translated into therapy interventions in 33 patients, representing 22% of all genotyped patients in the project. In addition, the report interpretation with the pharmacist and participant often prompted closer review of patient medications by physicians. There was a total of 81 changes. The changes included dose increases in 11 patients, dose decreases in 5 patients, new drugs added to the therapy of 20 patients, and 22 patients having drugs discontinued. There were instances of multiple changes for an individual patient, Figure 5. Based on this data, we calculate that a year's worth of modified medication therapy for all participants collectively was $797CAD. This represents a per patient cost of $24.15CAD (annual drug cost based on patient specific dosages and net of all changes including discontinued drugs, new drugs added and/or dosage changes) considering only those patients who had a medication change (not including the initial non-recurring testing cost of $199 which was covered by the project budget and should be amortized over the life of each patient). Note that costs in this simple drug cost analysis are all based on annual ongoing treatment costs and are not limited to the actual prescription over the study period. That is to say, the per patient cost of $24.15 represents the average total annual cost increase for each patient's therapy after implementing the changes. It is not restricted to only the cost of each patient's therapy for the study period. Study participants were not followed at all beyond the consultation with the pharmacist to review results and implement any suggested drug therapy changes. This was a time and budgetary limitation of the study.

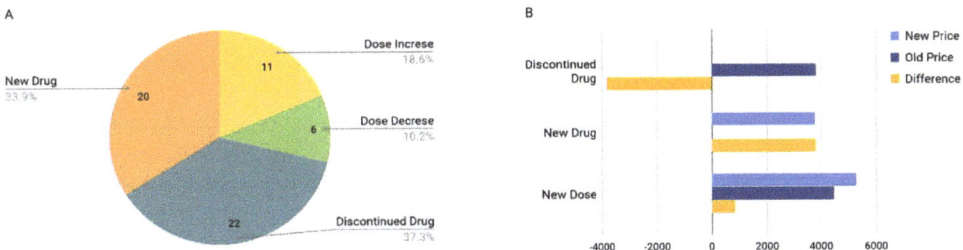

Figure 5. (**A**) Breakdown of therapy changes made by type of change, N = 59; (**B**) Cost-benefit of drug changes—shows drug cost changes by type of therapy change. Bars represent total cost in CAD.

4. Discussion

PGx testing is a cost-effective service valued by the participants. More work should be pursued to further educate physicians and drug/insurance providers on the benefits and potential improvement to patient treatment outcomes and well-being to enhance acceptance and implementation in BC. Additionally, prescribers need further education on PGx concepts. While with relatively simple courses our pharmacist felt confident in their understanding of the science and rational behind PGx testing—Doctors may feel uneducated to make prescribing changes based off of PGx information [10,48]. This information may contain contradictory or poorly validated results that could lead to denial of treatment [49]. However, integrating pharmacists as the drug experts to guide PGx prescribing, creating standardized reporting guidelines, and educating clinicians promises to improve the reliability of PGx dosing.

While the results that have come from this project might allow us to extrapolate to a large number of very specific conclusions related to PGx testing in the community by pharmacists, we have limited our conclusions to the following six statements:

1. The public perceives pharmacists/pharmacies as a very appropriate healthcare professional/venue to deliver pharmacogenomic services.
2. Frequencies of alleles, interactions, and clinically actionable results are consistent with other studies published in the scientific literature.
3. Changes in drug therapy based on PGx test results represent an inconsequential change in annual drug therapy cost. While drug therapy changes may result in a small cost increase, it is just as likely that costs may decrease.
4. Any cost increase due to drug therapy changes is likely to be small and is justified on the basis that the patient will be taking the most appropriate drug and dose for them as an individual based on their phenotype.
5. Pharmacogenomic testing is appropriate and affordable for certain patient populations.
6. Pharmacogenomic services offered by pharmacists are ready for primetime wide commercial implementation.

4.1. Selection of Antidepressants/Antipsychotics as Inclusion Criteria

In consultation with one of our funders, Green Shield Canada, we decided to focus on mental health drugs. Two out of three people will need to try multiple/different antidepressants until they find one that works for them [50]. While this may not match the amount of medication changes, we found (22%) we don't know how long the patient has been taking their psychiatric medication and if they are satisfied with the results of them. Antidepressant/antipsychotic usage was a criterion for the study patients may have had their own personal reasons for choosing to enroll. We also don't know how many different antidepressants they've been on previously. Additionally, they may not be taking them for their major indication but rather an off-label effect. The most common reason for needing to switch was due to side effects, which can leave a person physically debilitated and even worsen their mood disorder [50]. Additionally, antidepressant use is linked with age, with the elderly (those over 60) being 40.2% more likely to use an antidepressant than the rest of the population [51]. The elderly also take multiple classes of drugs with 51.6% of seniors in Canada taking 1–4 drugs of different classes chronically and an additional 35.3% taking 5 or more [52]. Some of these drugs are used to mitigate ADR symptoms from their other medications. Identifying problematic medications can reduce the drug cost if other medications can be discontinued if they are no longer needed to manage ADRs.

4.2. Pharmacist- & Pharmacy-Specific Considerations

We erred on the side of caution in making sure that the pharmacists had a high level of familiarity with PGx (equivalent to a 1st year graduate course), including its potential and its limitations. The quality, quantity, and level of detail of information provided in the individual patient reports generated in this project allowed pharmacists to easily interpret results and make drug therapy recommendations with little to no additional training. In BC, pharmacies are operated as private businesses with the ability to bill the public healthcare system for services. Using pharmacies as study sites required compliance with the privacy regulations specific to private businesses. In some instances, this was a higher threshold than that required by a public university research project. As the focus of this study was to develop and test a protocol that could be commercialized, we focused on ensuring compliance with the highest standards of privacy and informed consent. The underlying premise was that compliance, if introduced and explained at the outset with a clear rationale and requirements, would mitigate the potential for non-compliance. This was coupled with the idea that standardizing the process from the outset, would allow identification of any barriers present in each individual pharmacy practice setting. Participating pharmacists reported that the detailed training resulted in no difficulty in complying with the SOPs developed in Phase 1.

4.3. Potential Impact of S-201 and Other Pending Legislation

Patients were less concerned with privacy and confidentiality issues than we anticipated. Patients generally believed that pharmacists have access to their confidential health information, including their full medical record that exists with their physician. While this is not the case, pharmacists in the project were careful to ensure that patients understood the implications of sharing personal confidential medical information about themselves. Patients showed considerable trust in their pharmacists in handling this information and were pleased with the level of detail included in the project consent form. When this study was launched, there were no legal protections of a patient's genetic information data. This changed in 2016 with the passage of bill S-201, the Genetic Non-Discrimination Act which provides robust, albeit untested, protections against discrimination based in genetic information [53]. In practice, we did not encounter resistance to participation but additional work will be required to assess the impact of these protections on patient behavior with regard to testing.

4.4. Drug Cost Consequences

Although the additional yearly per-patient cost is ~$25CAD, PGx testing represents a saving to the community as we maximize the therapeutic efficiency of treatments. In fact, other studies have shown cost saving benefits of PGx testing [54,55]. While opportunities in PGx are clear- reduction in ADRs, elimination of medication trial and error, and more accurate dosing of prescribed medications, data to support the economic argument of drug cost savings are limited. However, it is not a stretch to hypothesize and make an effective argument that an additional value of PGx testing is the avoidance of weeks to months of costly trial and error when prescribing multiple drugs, especially in the mental health realm. Thus, using PGx testing to get a patient on the right drug at the right dose has the potential to generate long-term savings relative to that patient's overall healthcare costs. Furthermore, it could be argued that the wrong drug and/or wrong dose for a patient may contribute to poor adherence, further contributing to unnecessary costs. Using PGx could and probably does contribute to improved adherence, which in turn improves cost effectiveness of therapy. Longer-term economic implications related to reduced physician and urgent care (e.g., emergency room) visits, reduced absenteeism, and improved productivity require further study and analysis.

5. Limitations of the Study

While our study demonstrated the feasibility of pharmacist-led, community pharmacy-based pharmacogenomic testing there are several limitations. Although we attempted to, whenever possible, make the methodology suitable across Canada, there are province-specific considerations that will likely need to be considered. We also note that the size of this study is not sufficient to draw general conclusions regarding particular gene-drug interactions. It is also worth noting that although eligibility criteria included a limitation to being on at least one mental health drug, the gene-drug interactions reviewed in the reports included all relevant gene-drug interactions for each patient and not just their mental health drugs. Also, our decision to batch samples for processing slowed the return of results. Finally, in an effort to avoid potential privacy concerns, we did not collect detailed demographic data, nor did we follow the patients once the study was completed.

Supplementary Materials: The data that support the findings of this study is available upon request to the corresponding author. The following are available online at https://www.mdpi.com/2075-4426/11/1/11/s1, Expanded Online Methods, Supplement SI: Recruitment_Checklist, Supplement SII: Information_&_Consent, Supplement SIII: Informational_Video, Supplement SIV: Video_Script Supplement SV: Pharmacist_Survey. Supplement SVI: Patient_Survey. Supplement SVII: R_Analysis. Supplement SVIII: Example_Report. Supplement SIX: Pharmacy_Locations.

Author Contributions: Conceptualization, C.N. and F.A.D.D.; methodology, C.N. and F.A.D.D.; software, S.B.; validation, S.S., M.N., S.B., C.N. and F.A.D.D.; formal analysis, S.B. and F.A.D.D.; investigation, S.B.; resources, C.N. and F.A.D.D.; data curation, S.B. and F.A.D.D.; writing—original draft preparation, S.B.; writing—review and editing, C.N., S.S., and F.A.D.D.; visualization, S.B. and F.A.D.D.; supervision, C.N. and F.A.D.D.; project administration, C.N. and F.A.D.D.; funding acquisition, C.N. and F.A.D.D. All authors have read and agreed to the published version of the manuscript.

Funding: Funding for this project was received from Green Shield Canada, grant number UPP-031; Pfizer Canada; the BC Pharmacy Association; and Genome BC.

Acknowledgments: Both phases of the project would not have been possible without the financial support of Genome BC through their User Partnership Program and the generous financial and in-kind support of the British Columbia Pharmacy Association as the User Partner. We are also grateful for the generous financial support received for the Phase 2 project from Green Shield Canada and Pfizer Canada. CN has been supported by the CRC as a Tier 1 chair in Translational genomics. The authors would like to thank the entire staff of the BCPhA and especially Geraldine Vance and Cyril Lopez. The College of Pharmacists of British Columbia provided support and advice in the early phases of this project. John Spinelli and Treena McDonald of the BC Generations project provided access to control samples. Finally, we thank all the participating patients and pharmacists for their essential contributions to this study.

Conflicts of Interest: The authors declare no conflict of interest.

Appendix A

Full table comparing the frequency of myDNA calls and TRS calls to population averages of those genotype.

GENE	myDNA Genotype	TRS Genotype	Phenotype	myDNA Genotype Frequency	TRS Genotype Frequency	myDNA Genotype Frequency % n = 150	TRS Genotype Frequency %, n = 37	Population Level
CYP2C19	*1/*1	CYP2C19 *1/*1	Normal metaboliser	53	10	35.33	27	39.7
CYP2C19	*1/*17	CYP2C19 *1/*17	Rapid metaboliser	50	14	33.33	37.8	25.80%
CYP2C19	*1/*2	CYP2C19 *1/*2	Intermediate metaboliser	21	7	14	18.9	20.70%
CYP2C19	*17/*17	CYP2C19 *17/*17	Ultrarapid metaboliser	4	1	2.67	2.7	0
CYP2C19	*2/*17	CYP2C19 *2/*17	High intermediate metaboliser	12	3	8	8.1	6.20%
CYP2C19	*2/*2	CYP2C19 *2/*2	Poor metaboliser	10	1	6.67	2.7	2.90%
CYP2C19	NA	CYP2C19 *XX/*XX	NA	NA	1	NA	2.7	NA
CYP2C9	*1/*1	CYP2C9 *1/*1	Normal metaboliser	104	23	69.33	62.2	64.84%
CYP2C9	*1/*2	CYP2C9 *1/*2	High intermediate metaboliser	23	8	15.33	21.6	20.38%
CYP2C9	*1/*3	CYP2C9 *1/*3	Intermediate metaboliser	15	4	10	10.8	10.60%
CYP2C9	*2/*2	CYP2C9 *2/*2	Poor metaboliser	4	1	2.67	2.7	1.65%
CYP2C9	*2/*3	CYP2C9 *2/*3	Poor metaboliser	3	1	2	2.7	1.87%
CYP2C9	*3/*3	CYP2C9 *3/*3	Poor metaboliser	1	NA	0.67	NA	0.67%
CYP2D6	*1/*1	CYP2D6 *1/*1	Normal metaboliser	23	4	15.33	10.8	14.37%
CYP2D6	*1/*10	CYP2D6 *1/*10	Normal metaboliser	3	NA	2	NA	2.02%
CYP2D6	*1/*1 × 2	CYP2D6 *1/*1 × 2	Ultrarapid metaboliser	1	NA	0.67	NA	0.54%
CYP2D6	*1/*2	CYP2D6 *1/*2	Normal metaboliser	32	9	21.33	24.3	14.76%
CYP2D6	*1/*2 × 3	CYP2D6 *1/*2 × 3	Ultrarapid metaboliser	1	NA	0.67	NA	0.89%
CYP2D6	*1/*3	CYP2D6 *1/*3	Low normal metaboliser	2	1	1.33	2.7	1.24%
CYP2D6	*1/*36	CYP2D6 *1/*36	Low normal metaboliser	1	NA	0.67	NA	0.04%
CYP2D6	*1/*4	CYP2D6 *1/*4	Low normal metaboliser	17	3	11.33	8.1	13.79%
CYP2D6	*1/*41	CYP2D6 *1/*41	Normal metaboliser	12	2	8	5.4	7.93%
CYP2D6	*1/*5	CYP2D6 *1/*5	Low normal metaboliser	3	1	2	2.7	2.22%
CYP2D6	*1/*6	CYP2D6 *1/*6	Low normal metaboliser	1	NA	0.67	NA	0.46%

Gene	Allele	Genotype	Phenotype				
CYP2D6	*1/*9	CYP2D6 *1/*9	Normal metaboliser	1	1	0.67	2.7	1.70%
CYP2D6	*10/*10	CYP2D6 *10/*10	Intermediate metaboliser	1	NA	0.67	NA	0.92%
CYP2D6	*2/*10	CYP2D6 *2/*10	Normal metaboliser	2	1	1.33	2.7	0.91%
CYP2D6	*2/*2	CYP2D6 *2/*2	Normal metaboliser	9	3	6	8.1	5.09%
CYP2D6	*2/*2 × 2	CYP2D6 *2/*2 × 2	Ultrarapid metaboliser	1	NA	0.67	NA	0.02%
CYP2D6	*2/*3	CYP2D6 *2/*3	Low normal metaboliser	1	NA	0.67	NA	0.67%
CYP2D6	*2/*4	CYP2D6 *2/*4	Low normal metaboliser	11	1	7.33	2.7	7.23%
CYP2D6	*2/*41	CYP2D6 *2/*41	Normal metaboliser	5	1	3.33	2.7	4.46%
CYP2D6	*2/*5	CYP2D6 *2/*5	Low normal metaboliser	4	1	2.67	2.7	1.24%
CYP2D6	*2/*6	CYP2D6 *2/*6	Low normal metaboliser	1	1	0.67	2.7	0.41%
CYP2D6	*3/*3	CYP2D6 *3/*3	Poor metaboliser	1	NA	0.67	NA	0.02%
CYP2D6	*3/*41	CYP2D6 *3/*41	Intermediate metaboliser	1	NA	0.67	NA	0.33%
CYP2D6	NA	CYP2D6 *35/*5	NA	NA	1	NA	2.7	NA
CYP2D6	*4/*10	CYP2D6 *4/*10	Intermediate metaboliser	2	NA	1.33	NA	0.70%
CYP2D6	NA	CYP2D6 *4/*35A	NA	NA	1	NA	2.7	NA
CYP2D6	*4/*4	CYP2D6 *4/*4	Poor metaboliser	4	3	2.67	8.1	3.42%
CYP2D6	*4/*41	CYP2D6 *4/*41	Intermediate metaboliser	5	2	3.33	5.4	3.59%
CYP2D6	*4/*6	CYP2D6 *4/*6	Poor metaboliser	1	NA	0.67	NA	0.28%
CYP2D6	*4/*9	CYP2D6 *4/*9	Intermediate metaboliser	1	NA	0.67	NA	0.76%
CYP2D6	*5/*41	CYP2D6 *5/*41	Intermediate metaboliser	1	NA	0.67	NA	0.48%
CYP2D6	*9/*41	CYP2D6 *9/*41	Intermediate metaboliser	2	1	1.33	2.7	0.50%
CYP3A4	*1/*1	CYP3A4 *1/*1	Normal metaboliser	141	33	94	89.2	93.70%
CYP3A4	*1/*22	CYP3A4 *1/*22	Normal metaboliser	8	3	5.33	8.1	6.20%
CYP3A4	NA	CYP3A4 *1/*8	NA	NA	1	NA	2.7	0
CYP3A5	*1/*3	CYP3A5 *1/*3	Low normal metaboliser	14	1	9.33	2.7	38.80%
CYP3A5	*3/*3	CYP3A5 *3/*3	Poor metaboliser	136	36	90.67	97.3	54.30%
OPRM1	AA	NA	Normal metaboliser	107	NA	71.33	NA	77.10%
OPRM1	AG	NA	Low normal metaboliser	35	NA	23.33	NA	21.40%
OPRM1	GG	NA	Reduced metaboliser	8	NA	5.33	NA	1.50%

SLCO1B1	CC	rs4149056:C/C Hom	Reduced metaboliser	3	NA	2	NA	1.80%
SLCO1B1	TC	rs4149056:T/C Het	Low normal metaboliser	37	10	24.67	27	23.10%
SLCO1B1	TT	rs4149056:T/T Wild	Normal metaboliser	110	27	73.33	73	75.20%
CYP1A2	*1F/*1F	rs762551:A/A Hom	Rapid metaboliser	69	12	46	32.4	45%
CYP1A2	*1A/*1F	rs762551:C/A Het	Normal metaboliser	69	23	46	62.2	44.20%
CYP1A2	*1A/*1A	rs762551:C/C Wild	Normal metaboliser	12	2	8	5.4	10.80%
VKORC1	GG	rs9923231:C/C Wild	Normal warfarin sensitivity	57	15	38	40.5	35.80%
VKORC1	AG	rs9923231:C/T Het	Increased warfarin sensitivity	59	13	39.33	35.1	47.90%
VKORC1	AA	rs9923231:T/T Hom	High warfarin sensitivity	34	9	22.67	24.3	16.30%

*: allele.

References

1. Tolstoi, L.G.; Smith, C.L. Human genome project and cystic fibrosis-a symbiotic relationship. *J. Am. Diet. Assoc.* **1999**, *99*, 1421–1427. [CrossRef]
2. Van Ommen, G.; Bakker, E.; den Dunnen, J. The human genome project and the future of diagnostics, treatment, and prevention. *Lancet* **1999**, *354*, S5–S10. [CrossRef]
3. Dobson, R.T.; Taylor, J.G.; Henry, C.J.; Lachaine, J.; Zello, G.A.; Keegan, D.L.; Forbes, D.A. Taking the lead: Community pharmacists' perception of their role potential within the primary care team. *Res. Soc. Adm. Pharm.* **2009**, *5*, 327–336. [CrossRef]
4. Smith, S.R.; Clancy, C.M. Medication therapy management programs: Forming a new cornerstone for quality and safety in medicare. *Am. J. Med. Qual.* **2006**, *21*, 276–279. [CrossRef] [PubMed]
5. University of British Columbia. Adverse Drug Events Costly to Health Care System, Canadian Study Shows. 2011. Available online: https://www.sciencedaily.com/releases/2011/02/110225082932.htm (accessed on 4 June 2020).
6. Hazell, L.; Shakir, S.A.W. Under-reporting of adverse drug reactions: A systematic review. *Drug Saf.* **2006**, *29*, 385–396. [CrossRef]
7. Owen, J.A. Integrating pharmacogenomics into pharmacy practice via medication therapy management. *J. Am. Pharm. Assoc.* **2011**, *51*, e64–e74. [CrossRef]
8. Goldberger, J.J.; Buxton, A.E. Personalized medicine vs. guideline-based medicine. *JAMA* **2013**, *309*, 2559. [CrossRef]
9. Blalock, S.J.; Roberts, A.W.; Lauffenburger, J.C.; Thompson, T.; O'Connor, S.K. The effect of community pharmacy-based interventions on patient health outcomes: A systematic review. *Med. Care Res. Rev.* **2013**, *70*, 235–266. [CrossRef]
10. Korf, B.R.; Berry, A.B.; Limson, M.; Marian, A.J.; Murray, M.F.; O'Rourke, P.P.; Passamani, E.R.; Relling, M.V.; Tooker, J.; Tsongalis, G.J.; et al. Framework for development of physician competencies in genomic medicine: Report of the Competencies Working Group of the Inter-Society Coordinating Committee for Physician Education in Genomics. *Genet. Med.* **2014**, *16*, 804–809. [CrossRef]
11. Shin, J.; Kayser, S.R.; Langaee, T.Y. Pharmacogenetics: From discovery to patient care. *Am. J. Health Syst. Pharm.* **2009**, *66*, 625–637. [CrossRef]
12. Klein, M.E.; Parvez, M.M.; Shin, J.-G. Clinical implementation of pharmacogenomics for personalized precision medicine: Barriers and solutions. *J. Pharm. Sci.* **2017**, *106*, 2368–2379. [CrossRef] [PubMed]
13. O'Connor, S.K.; Ferreri, S.P.; Michaels, N.M.; Chater, R.W.; Viera, A.J.; Faruki, H.; McLeod, H.L.; Roederer, M. Making pharmacogenetic testing a reality in a community pharmacy. *J. Am. Pharm. Assoc.* **2012**, *52*, e259–e265. [CrossRef] [PubMed]
14. Padgett, L.; O'Connor, S.; Roederer, M.; McLeod, H.; Ferreri, S. Pharmacogenomics in a community pharmacy: ACT now. *J. Am. Pharm. Assoc.* **2011**, *51*, 189–193. [CrossRef] [PubMed]
15. Valgus, J.; Weitzel, K.W.; Peterson, J.F.; Crona, D.J.; Formea, C.M. Current practices in the delivery of pharmacogenomics: Impact of the recommendations of the Pharmacy Practice Model Summit. *Am. J. Health. Syst. Pharm.* **2019**, *76*, 521–529. [CrossRef]
16. Nislow, C.; Kunzli, M.; Spinelli, J.; Neira, M.; Sinha, S. Desrosiers D. Pharmacogenomics at the point of care: Phase 1. Unpublished.
17. Hippman, C.; Nislow, C. Pharmacogenomic Testing: Clinical Evidence and Implementation Challenges. *J. Pers. Med.* **2019**, *9*, 40. [CrossRef]

18. Agena Bioscience. Clinical Approval. Agenabio. Agena Bioscience. 2014. Available online: https://agenabio.com/company/clinical-approval/ (accessed on 4 June 2020).
19. Johansen, P.; Andersen, J.D.; Børsting, C.; Morling, N. Evaluation of the iPLEX® Sample ID Plus Panel designed for the Sequenom MassARRAY® system. A SNP typing assay developed for human identification and sample tracking based on the SNPforID panel. *Forensic Sci. Int. Genet.* **2013**, *7*, 482–487. [CrossRef]
20. Syrmis, M.W.; Moser, R.J.; Whiley, D.M.; Vaska, V.; Coombs, G.W.; Nissen, M.D.; Sloots, T.P.; Nimmo, G.R. Comparison of a multiplexed MassARRAY system with real-time allele-specific PCR technology for genotyping of methicillin-resistant Staphylococcus aureus. *Clin. Microbiol. Infect.* **2011**, *17*, 1804–1810. [CrossRef]
21. Bray, M.S.; Boerwinkle, E.; Doris, P.A. High-throughput multiplex SNP genotyping with MALDI-TOF mass spectrometry: Practice, problems and promise. *Hum. Mutat.* **2001**, *17*, 296–304. [CrossRef]
22. Nunes, A.P.; Oliveira, I.O.; Santos, B.R.; Millech, C.; Silva, L.P.; González, D.A.; Hallal, P.C.; Menezes, A.M.B.; Araújo, C.L.; Barros, F.C. Quality of DNA extracted from saliva samples collected with the Oragene™ DNA self-collection kit. *BMC Med. Res. Methodol.* **2012**, *12*, 65. [CrossRef]
23. Sullivan, G.M.; Artino, A.R. Analyzing and interpreting data from likert-type scales. *J. Grad. Med. Educ.* **2013**, *5*, 541–542. [CrossRef]
24. Kailos Genetics. TargetRichTM UMI/IndexAdapters & Sequencing User Manual for PGX. 2017. Available online: https://d10u8wcbc2zotv.cloudfront.net/media/Kailos_TargetRich_UMI-Sample_Adapter_PGX_Seq_Protocol_August2017.pdf (accessed on 4 June 2020).
25. Kailos Genetics. Long-Range PCR for CYP2D6 CNV Analysis. Supplementary procedure for TargetRichTM PGx Assay. 2017. Available online: https://d10u8wcbc2zotv.cloudfront.net/media/Kailos_2D6CNV_LR-PCR_Protocol2017-RevB.pdf (accessed on 4 June 2020).
26. Ellis, J.A.; Ong, B. The Massarray® System for Targeted Snp Genotyping. 2017. Available online: http://link.springer.com/10.1007/978-1-4939-6442-0_5 (accessed on 4 June 2020).
27. Mostafa, S.; Kirkpatrick, C.M.J.; Byron, K.; Sheffield, L. An analysis of allele, genotype and phenotype frequencies, actionable pharmacogenomic (Pgx) variants and phenoconversion in 5408 Australian patients genotyped for CYP2D6, CYP2C19, CYP2C9 and VKORC1 genes. *J. Neural Transm.* **2019**, *126*, 5–18. [CrossRef] [PubMed]
28. Aristarán, M.; Tigas, M. Introducing Tabula. Available online: https://source.opennews.org/articles/introducing-tabula/ (accessed on 4 June 2020).
29. R Core Team. R: A Language and Environment for Statistical Computing. Available online: https://www.R-project.org/ (accessed on 4 June 2020).
30. Del Tredici, A.L.; Malhotra, A.; Dedek, M.; Espin, F.; Roach, D.; Zhu, G.U.; Voland, J.; Moreno, T.A. Frequency of cyp2d6 alleles including structural variants in the united states. *Front. Pharmacol.* **2018**, *9*, 305. [CrossRef] [PubMed]
31. Karczewski, K.J.; Francioli, L.C.; Tiao, G.; Cummings, B.B.; Alföldi, J.; Wang, Q.; Collins, R.L.; Laricchia, K.M.; Ganna, A.; Birnbaum, D.P.; et al. The Mutational Constraint Spectrum Quantified from Variation in 141,456 Humans. 2019. Available online: http://biorxiv.org/lookup/doi/10.1101/531210 (accessed on 4 June 2020).
32. Hardy, G.H. Mendelian proportions in a mixed population. *Science* **1908**, *28*, 49–50. [CrossRef] [PubMed]
33. Wickham, H.; Averick, M.; Bryan, J.; Chang, W.; McGowan, L.D.; François, R.; Grolemund, G.; Hayes, A.; Henry, L.; Hester, J.; et al. Welcome to the tidyverse. *JOSS* **2019**, *4*, 1686. [CrossRef]
34. Dowle, M.; Srinivasan, A.; Gorecki, J.; Chirico, M.; Stetsenko, P.; Short, T.; Lianoglou, S.; Antonyan, E.; Bonsch, M.; Parsonage, H. Data. Table: Extension of "Data. Frame". 2019. Available online: https://CRAN.R-project.org/package=data.table (accessed on 4 June 2020).
35. Wickham, H. Reshaping Data with the reshape Package. *J. Stat. Softw.* **2007**, *21*, 1–20. [CrossRef]
36. Murrell, P. Compare: Comparing Objects for Differences. 2015. Available online: https://CRAN.R-project.org/package=compare (accessed on 4 June 2020).
37. Wickham, H. The split-apply-combine strategy for data analysis. *J. Stat. Softw.* **2011**, *40*, 1–29. [CrossRef]
38. Varrichio, C. Rowr: Row-Based Functions for R Objects. 2016. Available online: https://cran.r-project.org/web/packages/rowr/index.html (accessed on 4 June 2020).
39. Van der Wouden, C.H.; Bank, P.C.D.; Özokcu, K.; Swen, J.J.; Guchelaar, H.J. Pharmacist-Initiated Pre-Emptive Pharmacogenetic Panel Testing with Clinical Decision Support in Primary Care: Record of PGx Results and Real-World Impact. *Genes* **2019**, *10*, 416. [CrossRef]
40. Hiemke, C.; Bergemann, N.; Clement, H.W.; Conca, A.; Deckert, J.; Domschke, K.; Eckermann, G.; Egberts, K.; Gerlach, M.; Greiner, C.; et al. Consensus Guidelines for Therapeutic Drug Monitoring in Neuropsychopharmacology: Update 2017. *Pharmacopsychiatry* **2018**, *51*, 9–62. [CrossRef]
41. Van Westrhenen, R.; Aitchison, K.J.; Ingelman-Sundberg, M.; Jukić, M.M. Pharmacogenomics of Antidepressant and Antipsychotic Treatment: How Far Have We Got and Where Are We Going? *Front. Psychiatry* **2020**, *11*, 94. [CrossRef]
42. Corponi, F.; Fabbri, C.; Serretti, A. Pharmacogenetics in Psychiatry. *Adv. Pharmacol.* **2018**, *83*, 297–331.
43. Rush, A.J.; Trivedi, M.H.; Wisniewski, S.R.; Nierenberg, A.A.; Stewart, J.W.; Warden, D.; Niederehe, G.; Thase, M.E.; Lavori, P.W.; Lebowitz, B.D.; et al. Acute and longer-term outcomes in depressed outpatients requiring one or several treatment steps: A STAR*D report. *Am. J. Psychiatry* **2006**, *163*, 1901–1917. [CrossRef] [PubMed]

44. Hoffman, J.M.; Dunnenberger, H.M.; Hicks, J.K.; Caudle, K.E.; Carrillo, M.W.; Freimuth, R.R.; Williams, M.S.; Klein, T.E.; Peterson, J.F. Developing knowledge resources to support precision medicine: Principles from the Clinical Pharmacogenetics Implementation Consortium (Cpic). *J. Am. Med. Inform. Assoc.* **2016**, *23*, 796–801. [CrossRef] [PubMed]
45. Buermans, H.P.; Vossen, R.H.; Anvar, S.Y.; Allard, W.G.; Guchelaar, H.J.; White, S.J.; van der Straaten, T. Flexible and Scalable Full-Length CYP2D6 Long Amplicon PacBio Sequencing. *Hum. Mutat.* **2017**, *38*, 310–316. [CrossRef] [PubMed]
46. Clinical Annotation for CYP3A4*1, CYP3A4*20, CYP3A4*8; Paclitaxel; Breast Neoplasms and Ovarian Neoplasms (Level 3 Toxicity/ADR). 2015. Available online: https://www.pharmgkb.org/variant/PA166157507/clinicalAnnotation/1444666533 (accessed on 4 June 2020).
47. Cousin, M.A.; Matey, E.T.; Blackburn, P.R.; Boczek, N.J.; McAllister, T.M.; Kruisselbrink, T.M.; Babovic-Vuksanovic, D.; Lazaridis, K.N.; Klee, E.W. Pharmacogenomic findings from clinical whole exome sequencing of diagnostic odyssey patients. *Mol. Genet. Genom. Med.* **2017**, *5*, 269–279. [CrossRef]
48. Krebs, K.; Milani, L. Translating pharmacogenomics into clinical decisions: Do not let the perfect be the enemy of the good. *Hum. Genom.* **2019**, *13*, 39. [CrossRef]
49. Rahman, T.; Ash, D.M.; Lauriello, J.; Rawlani, R. Misleading Guidance from Pharmacogenomic Testing. *Am. J. Psychiatry* **2017**, *174*, 922–924. [CrossRef]
50. Keks, N.; Hope, J.; Keogh, S. Switching and stopping antidepressants. *Aust. Prescr.* **2016**, *39*, 76–83.
51. Pratt, L.A.; Brody, D.J.; Gu, Q. Antidepressant use among persons aged 12 and over: United States, 2011–2014. *NCHS Data Brief* **2017**, *283*, 1–8.
52. Proulx, J. Drug use among seniors in Canada, 2016. *Value Health* **2018**, *21*, S146. [CrossRef]
53. Walker, J. Legislative Summary of Bill S-201: An Act to Prohibit and Prevent Genetic Discrimination. 2016. Available online: https://lop.parl.ca/sites/PublicWebsite/default/en_CA/ResearchPublications/LegislativeSummaries/421S201E (accessed on 4 June 2020).
54. Winner, J.G.; Carhart, J.M.; Altar, C.A.; Goldfarb, S.; Allen, J.D.; Lavezzari, G.; Parsons, K.K.; Marshak, A.G.; Garavaglia, S.; Dechairo, B.M. Combinatorial pharmacogenomic guidance for psychiatric medications reduces overall pharmacy costs in a 1 year prospective evaluation. *Curr. Med. Res. Opin.* **2015**, *31*, 1633–1643. [CrossRef]
55. Tanner, J.-A.; Brown, L.C.; Yu, K.; Li, J.; Dechairo, B.M. Canadian medication cost savings associated with combinatorial pharmacogenomic guidance for psychiatric medications. *Clin. Outcomes Res.* **2019**, *11*, 779–787. [CrossRef] [PubMed]

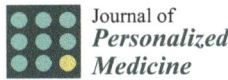

Article

Practical Barriers and Facilitators Experienced by Patients, Pharmacists and Physicians to the Implementation of Pharmacogenomic Screening in Dutch Outpatient Hospital Care—An Explorative Pilot Study

Pauline Lanting [1,*], Evelien Drenth [1], Ludolf Boven [1], Amanda van Hoek [1], Annemiek Hijlkema [1], Ellen Poot [1], Gerben van der Vries [1], Robert Schoevers [2], Ernst Horwitz [2], Reinold Gans [3], Jos Kosterink [4,5], Mirjam Plantinga [1], Irene van Langen [1], Adelita Ranchor [6], Cisca Wijmenga [1], Lude Franke [1], Bob Wilffert [4,5] and Rolf Sijmons [1]

[1] Department of Genetics, University Medical Center Groningen, University of Groningen, 9713 GZ Groningen, The Netherlands; w.h.drenth@umcg.nl (E.D.); l.g.boven@umcg.nl (L.B.); amandavanhoek@home.nl (A.v.H.); annemiekhijlkema@hotmail.nl (A.H.); ellenpoot@hotmail.com (E.P.); g.b.van.der.vries@umcg.nl (G.v.d.V.); m.plantinga@umcg.nl (M.P.); i.m.van.langen@umcg.nl (I.v.L.); c.wijmenga@rug.nl (C.W.); l.h.franke@umcg.nl (L.F.); r.h.sijmons@umcg.nl (R.S.)

[2] Department of Psychiatry, University Medical Center Groningen, University of Groningen, 9713 GZ Groningen, The Netherlands; r.a.schoevers@umcg.nl (R.S.); Ernst.Horwitz@ggzfriesland.nl (E.H.)

[3] Department of Internal Medicine, University Medical Center Groningen, University of Groningen, 9713 GZ Groningen, The Netherlands; r.o.b.gans@umcg.nl

[4] Department of Clinical Pharmacy and Pharmacology, University Medical Center Groningen, University of Groningen, 9713 GZ Groningen, The Netherlands; j.g.w.kosterink@umcg.nl (J.K.); b.wilffert@rug.nl (B.W.)

[5] Unit of PharmacoTherapy, Epidemiology & Economics, Groningen Research Institute of Pharmacy, University of Groningen, 9713 AV Groningen, The Netherlands

[6] Department of Health Psychology, University Medical Center Groningen, University of Groningen, 9713 GZ Groningen, The Netherlands; a.v.ranchor@umcg.nl

* Correspondence: p.lanting@umcg.nl; Tel.: +31-50-3617100

Received: 18 November 2020; Accepted: 18 December 2020; Published: 21 December 2020

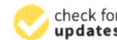

Abstract: Pharmacogenomics (PGx) can provide optimized treatment to individual patients while potentially reducing healthcare costs. However, widespread implementation remains absent. We performed a pilot study of PGx screening in Dutch outpatient hospital care to identify the barriers and facilitators to implementation experienced by patients ($n = 165$), pharmacists ($n = 58$) and physicians ($n = 21$). Our results indeed suggest that the current practical experience of healthcare practitioners with PGx is limited, that proper education is necessary, that patients want to know the exact implications of the results, that healthcare practitioners heavily rely on their computer systems, that healthcare practitioners encounter practical problems in the systems used, and a new barrier was identified, namely that there is an unclear allocation of responsibilities between healthcare practitioners about who should discuss PGx with patients and apply PGx results in healthcare. We observed a positive attitude toward PGx among all the stakeholders in our study, and among patients, this was independent of the occurrence of drug-gene interactions during their treatment. Facilitators included the availability of and adherence to Dutch Pharmacogenetics Working Group guidelines. While clinical decision support (CDS) is available and valued in our medical center, the lack of availability of CDS may be an important barrier within Dutch healthcare in general.

Keywords: pharmacogenetics; pharmacogenomics; implementation; screening; pre-emptive; personalized medicine; precision medicine

---

1. Introduction

Pharmacogenomics (PGx) studies the interplay between variation in the human genome and drug response. Knowledge about PGx can help predict which medication will be most effective and safe in individual patients while potentially reducing healthcare costs [1,2]. Different approaches to apply PGx knowledge in patient care exist. On one hand, PGx testing can be performed in a reactive manner to find an explanation for a low therapeutic response or the occurrence of adverse drug reactions (ADRs). On the other hand, ideally, an individual's PGx profile is already known before drug prescription, so treatment can be tailored to the individual's genome without awaiting potential treatment failure or the occurrence of ADRs. This approach is known as pre-emptive PGx testing or PGx screening.

The potential benefits of introducing PGx screening into a routine healthcare setting include reduced hospitalizations and cost and improved safety, adherence and efficacy [3]. Dutch national guidelines on the practical application of PGx for drug prescription of 95 drugs, developed by the Dutch Pharmacogenetics Working Group (DPWG), are available through the Dutch drug database, referred to as the G-standard [4,5]. Based on these DPWG guidelines, it is estimated that an alternative dosage or drug would be recommended for 1 in 20 drug prescriptions in primary care if PGx screening became the standard-of-care in the Netherlands [6]. Nevertheless, PGx is rarely applied in current clinical practice [2,7].

A number of barriers to PGx implementation have been identified so far. These include unclear procedures, insufficient evidence, inefficient infrastructure, lack of a standardized format for reporting results, lack of ICT support tools, and lack of knowledge, training and experience among healthcare practitioners. Reported facilitators include recognition of clinical utility, pharmacist's feelings of responsibility for delivering PGx to patients, and the availability of professional guidelines for interpreting test results [1,8–13]. To the best of our knowledge, no study has identified barriers and facilitators from the perspective of all the relevant stakeholders in an actual implementation setting. Therefore, we carried out an explorative pilot study to identify such barriers and facilitators while offering PGx screening in two outpatient clinics of the University Medical Center of Groningen (UMCG) in the Netherlands.

2. Materials and Methods

This study was designed as an explorative pilot study with mixed methods. The study timeline is shown in Figure 1A, and an overview of the study design in Figure 1B. Additional background information is provided in Supplementary Methods Section S1.

2.1. Recruitment of Participants

The outpatient clinics of Internal Medicine and Psychiatry and the hospital pharmacy of the UMCG were approached to participate in this study. Information about the study's aim was provided during an introductory meeting with each department. Physicians who took part recruited participants from their own patients on a first-come-first-served basis until the study test capacity of 165 PGx individuals was reached. Inclusion criteria were: 18 years or older, cognitively competent, able to read and speak Dutch, and able to provide a blood sample. Eligible patients received printed information about the project goal, procedures for testing, reporting of results and links to resources with additional information (project website and animated video). Copies of these materials (in Dutch) are available upon request.

Community pharmacists listed in the patient's electronic health record (EHR) were invited to fill out questionnaires by mail simultaneously with the reporting of PGx screening results (T1).

UMCG physicians at the two clinics and hospital pharmacists involved in patient care were invited to fill out study questionnaires by email at the end of follow-up (T2, Figure 1A). See Supplementary Methods Section S3 for additional details.

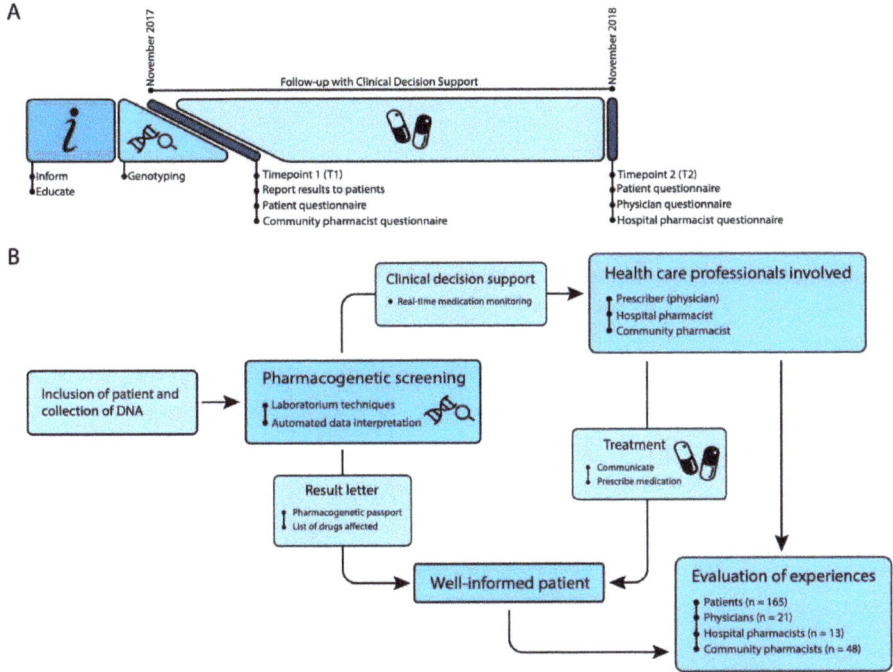

Figure 1. Study timeline and design (**A**). Study timeline (**B**). Study design.

2.2. Genotyping and Reporting of PGx Screening Results

After providing written informed consent, patients underwent genotyping with a custom panel of 14 genes (Table S1). Next, patients received a letter with their PGx screening results and an explanation in layman's terms (see Supplementary Material 1). Copies were also stored in their hospital EHR and sent to their community pharmacist and general practitioner (GP) (Figure 1B). See Supplementary Methods Section S4 for additional details.

Custom clinical decision support (CDS) software developed prior to the study was used to provide hospital prescribers with relevant DPWG recommendations in real time during drug prescription (Figure 1). See Supplementary Methods Section S5 for additional details.

2.3. Data Collection

PGx screening results, predicted drug-gene interactions (DGIs), and CDS use, including user comments and actions that were taken based on recommendations, were stored in the study database. Relevant medical information, including patient drug use during the follow-up period November 2017–November 2018, was manually extracted from EHRs (see Supplementary Methods Section S6 for additional details). Follow-up started from the time the results were reported and therefore varied between patients, up to a maximum of a year (Figure 1A). We conducted five questionnaires to evaluate the experiences of patients, physicians, and pharmacists via open- and closed-ended questions at the time of result reporting (T1) and after follow-up (T2, Figure 1A). The survey study was designed by a multidisciplinary team using input from an explorative qualitative interview and focus group study with 13 prescribers from the participating outpatient clinics, 13 patients and

7 pharmacists (see Supplementary Methods Section S2). The questionnaires included items on various themes: sociodemographics, knowledge and education about PGx, attitude towards PGx screening, application of PGx, provision of information about PGx, and result reporting (Table S2). The attitude questions originate from the theory of planned behavior framework [14]. All other questions were self-constructed. The two patient questionnaires were sent out on paper, with the option to respond digitally, at the time of results reporting (T1) and after follow-up (T2). If necessary, patients were reminded by mail and again by telephone to respond. Community pharmacists were invited to respond to the survey on paper, with the option to respond digitally at the time results were reported (T1). The outpatient clinic physicians and hospital pharmacists received an invitation for a digital survey by email after follow-up (T2, Figure 1A). Digital survey responses were collected using the routine outcome monitoring application RoQua [15]. Responses on paper were registered in RoQua by the researchers.

2.4. Data Analysis

CDS searches and survey responses to open-ended questions were independently categorized by two researchers (AvH, AMAH), and discrepancies were resolved by a third independent researcher (PL). All data collected was pseudonymized and analyzed per theme using R [16]. For survey responses, the Shapiro–Wilk test was used to assess normality. Subsequent subgroup comparisons were performed using a t-test or Wilcoxon test. Cronbach's alpha was used to assess the internal consistency of survey questions.

2.5. Ethical Approval

This study was approved by the Medical Ethics Review Board of the UMCG (reference: 2017.266).

3. Results

3.1. Participants

This study included 165 patients, 21 physicians, 13 hospital pharmacists, and 48 community pharmacists (Figure 1B) and explored various themes around practical barriers and facilitators. Response rates to the patient questionnaires were 84% (($n = 138$, T1) and 74% (($n = 122$, T2). Response rates to the healthcare practitioner questionnaires were 19% (physicians, T2), 28% (hospital pharmacists, T2), and 77% (community pharmacists, T1). Response rates per survey item varied since not all respondents have answered all items. Median patient follow-up was 244 days (range: 117–365). See Table S3 for the full demographics of study participants.

3.2. Screening Results, Drug Use and DGIs

Out of the study population, 158 patients (96% of the study population) carried at least one actionable PGx haplotype or predicted PGx phenotype (Table S4 lists frequencies of PGx haplotypes and predicted PGx phenotypes). During follow-up, 60 patients received drug treatment (36%). Following DPWG guidelines, DGIs were observed in 21 patients (13%): 18 with one DGI, one with two DGIs and two with three DGIs. Actionable DGIs were observed in 20 patients (12%): 18 with one actionable DGI and two-with-two actionable DGIs. In total, 120 unique drugs were used during follow-up, including 18 with a known DGI (15%), of which 15 were actionable in the study population. During follow-up, patients used two drugs (range: 0–13 drugs) on average, and 27 patients (23% of T2 respondents) reported being prescribed at least one new drug. Patients reported that prescriptions originated from their GP's office (83% of T2 respondents) or hospital physician (17% of T2 respondents). See Supplementary Results Section S1 for survey results on the review of patient drug use in response to PGx screening results.

3.3. CDS Searches and Output during Follow-Up

During follow-up, CDS was used to consult the DPWG guidelines 59 times for 20 patients. A CDS search was performed for eight patients who received drug treatment, and four had DGIs. CDS searches were categorized into six subgroups using treatment information from the EHR: prescribing situation (5%), cascade (search in response to the previous search) (2%), potential future treatment (29%), current treatment (47%), past treatment (5%), and other (12%). Of the CDS searches, 27 (45.8%) yielded recommendations requiring an action by the prescriber, 14 (23.7%) did not require an action, 10 (16.9%) found no available recommendations (e.g., in case of normal metabolizers), and 8 (13.6%) had inconclusive test results. Of the actionable recommendations, 12 (44%) advised adhering to an adjusted maximum (daily) dose or prescribing an alternative, 5 (19%) advised prescribing an alternative, 5 (19%) advised lowering the dose and monitoring plasma concentrations, 2 (7%) advised adjusting the dose based on the effect observed, 2 (7%) advised lowering the maintenance dose, and 1 (4%) advised increasing the dose. Details of the DGIs involved and an evaluation of DPWG guidelines are presented in Supplementary Results Sections S2 and S3.

3.4. Prior Experience of Healthcare Practitioners with PGx

Twenty-one community pharmacists (44% of respondents), one hospital pharmacist (8%), and five physicians (24%) reported that this study was their first experience with PGx test results. One in eight community pharmacists, six hospital pharmacists (46%) and half of the physicians (52%) reported having taken the initiative to conduct PGx testing at least once in the past. These results highlight that the current practical experience is limited.

3.5. Knowledge and Education of Healthcare Practitioners

In all professions, half the healthcare practitioners participating in this study reported having received postgraduate education about PGx. The self-graded knowledge level was significantly higher in these subgroups (Table 1). Pharmacists reported a need for further education, both for themselves ($n = 47$, 77%) and for pharmacy staff ($n = 52$, 87%), whereas physicians did not report this need.

Table 1. Self-graded knowledge and application level of healthcare practitioners.

Healthcare Practitioner		Self-Graded Knowledge Level		Self-Graded Application Level	
Community pharmacists	with postgraduate education	6.5 (4–8)	$p = 0.011$	7 (5–10)	$p = 0.005$
	without postgraduate education	6 (2–7)		5 (2–8)	
Hospital pharmacists	with postgraduate education	7.7 (7–9)	$p = 0.01$	7.5 (7–9)	$p = 0.016$
	without postgraduate education	6.3 (5–7)		6 (2–7)	
Physicians	with postgraduate education	7 (1–9)	$p = 0.002$	7 (6–8)	$p = 0.203$
	without postgraduate education	4 (6–8)		6 (3–9)	

3.6. Patient Attitudes towards PGx Screening after Follow-Up (T2)

Most patients reported that genetic testing in general ($n = 89$, 77% of T2 respondents) or PGx testing ($n = 102$, 88%) did not frighten them. Knowing their PGx profile was considered comforting ($n = 106$, 89%) and useful ($n = 111$, 92%), and patients thought that it has added value when their pharmacotherapy is adjusted using PGx ($n = 107$, 91%). No significant difference was found in the attitude of patients with or without observed DGIs.

3.7. Healthcare Practitioner Attitudes towards PGx Screening

Nearly all healthcare practitioners were positive about the usefulness of PGx information for their patients (useful to have $n = 69$, 84% of respondents; would like to use more in daily practice: $n = 72$, 88%; added value: $n = 71$, 87%). However, nine community pharmacists (19%), two hospital pharmacists (15%) and four physicians (20%) did not feel ready to apply PGx information in daily practice.

3.8. Practical Application of PGx

Community pharmacists graded their expected application level (T1), whereas hospital pharmacists and physicians graded their perceived application level (T2). The self-graded application level is significantly higher in the education subgroups for both community and hospital pharmacists, but not for physicians (Table 1). Prominent arguments provided to explain higher self-graded application levels were that application of PGx was possible with the use of the pharmacy or hospital computer system ($n = 12$) and that healthcare practitioners had come across PGx more often (during education or in practice) ($n = 8$). Notable arguments to explain lower self-graded application levels were that healthcare practitioners perceived insufficient knowledge themselves ($n = 8$) and reported practical barriers present within computer systems, for example, that not all PGx results could be registered ($n = 5$). In summary, healthcare practitioners relied heavily on their computer system for the application of PGx, perceived a need for education on PGx application, and experienced practical barriers within computer systems that hindered PGx application. Supplementary Results Section S4 describes an event that occurred during follow-up that illustrates the importance of educating and informing all healthcare practitioners involved in the practical application of PGx.

3.9. Patients' Needs for Information about Their PGx Screening Results

After receiving the PGx screening results, 15 patients (11% of T1 respondents) reported still having questions with respect to these results, most often wanting to know the exact implications, e.g., the level of dose adjustment or suitable alternative drugs ($n = 6$). Patients generally consulted their treating physician in the hospital during follow-up to gain additional information. After follow-up, the number of patients having questions about their PGx screening results has increased to 23 (19% of T2 respondents). They still primarily wanted to know the implications of the results for them ($n = 7$). Thirty-six patients (30% of T2 respondents) reported that improvements could be made in the information provided, most importantly in explaining the exact implications of the results for them ($n = 9$), providing better explanation in general ($n = 7$), and better educating healthcare practitioners ($n = 4$).

A detailed evaluation of the PGx result letter is presented in Supplementary Results Section S5. In summary, some patients wished to receive more and different information than provided in this study.

3.10. Discussing PGx Screening Results with Patients: Patient Surveys

After receiving the PGx screening results, 47 patients (35% of T1 respondents) believed a healthcare practitioner should always discuss these results with them, 29 (21%) only if patients express the need, and 33 (24%) only if the results have consequences. Twenty-six (19%) thought the results should not be discussed with them at all. According to patients, the preferred healthcare practitioners to discuss PGx screening results are the treating physician in the hospital ($n = 80$, 44%), GP ($n = 47$, 26%), clinical geneticist ($n = 30$, 16%), or pharmacist ($n = 22$, 12%).

After receiving the PGx screening results, 101 patients (74% of T1 respondents) planned to discuss them with their treating physician, with 44 patients (37% of T2 respondents) reporting having done so after follow-up in a regular appointment and 6 (5%) reporting having done so in a separate appointment. In total, 101 conversations about PGx screening results between patients and healthcare practitioners were scored by patients (46% physician, 21% community pharmacist, 21% GP, 8% physician from another hospital, 2% home nurse, 2% thrombosis care, and 1% nursing home). Seventy-one percent of these conversations were scored as "(very) good". In one case, the conversation was scored as "good", but the patient reported that the healthcare practitioner did not (fully) understand the results. Thirteen percent of conversations were scored as "(very) bad". In two cases, the conversation as such was scored as "(very) bad" even though, on a positive note, the healthcare practitioner had started using the PGx results (Figure 2).

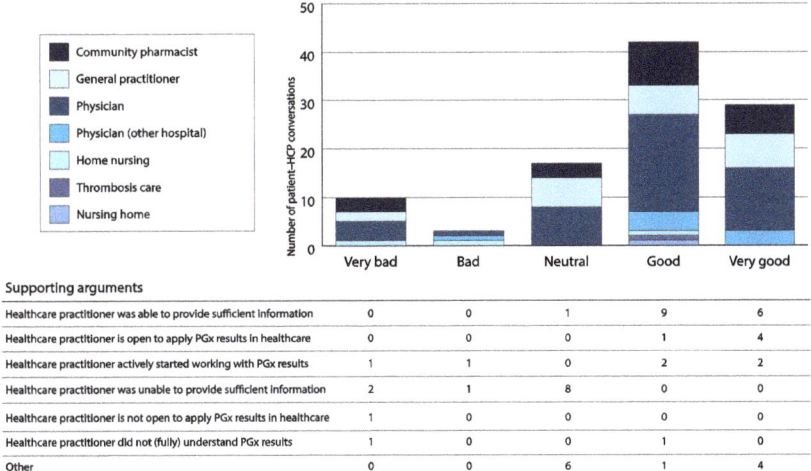

Figure 2. Conversation scores for the discussion of pharmacogenomic test results with healthcare practitioners. The number of conversations between patients and different healthcare practitioners, the score patients gave to those conversations, and the supporting arguments for the score given.

3.11. Discussing PGx Screening Results with Patients: Healthcare Practitioner Surveys

Sixteen community pharmacists (36% of respondents), eight hospital pharmacists (62%) and 13 physicians (62%) believed that PGx screening results should always be discussed with patients by a healthcare practitioner, with eight (18%), two (15%) and five (24%), respectively, believing it should only be done if a patient expresses the need and 19 (42%), three (23%) and three (14%), respectively, only if the results have consequences. Two community pharmacists (4%) did not believe results should be discussed with patients at all. Community pharmacists primarily placed the responsibility for discussing PGx screening results with patients in the hands of the treating physician in the hospital ($n = 26, 38\%$) or pharmacist ($n = 21, 31\%$), and to a lesser extent with the clinical geneticist ($n = 13, 19\%$). Hospital pharmacists also primarily placed this responsibility in the hands of the treating physician in the hospital ($n = 11, 39\%$) or pharmacist ($n = 8, 29\%$), and to a lesser extent with the GP ($n = 4, 14\%$) or clinical geneticist ($n = 4, 14\%$). Physicians primarily indicated that they, as treating physicians in the hospital, should discuss PGx screening results with patients ($n = 19, 59\%$), followed by the pharmacist ($n = 7, 22\%$) and the GP ($n = 3, 9\%$).

Community pharmacists were asked what they planned to do with the PGx screening results they had received (T1). All plans reported for PGx screening results are shown in Figure 3. Although four community pharmacists reported that PGx screening results should always be discussed with the patient by a healthcare practitioner, preferably the pharmacist, none of these four pharmacists reported that they themselves intended to discuss the results with their patients.

Five out of six hospital pharmacists, and all eight physicians who discussed PGx screening results with patients and/or other healthcare practitioners felt they had sufficient knowledge to do so. None of them reported questions about PGx that they were unable to answer.

3.12. Responsibility for Application of PGx Screening Results in Patient Care

Healthcare practitioners were also asked about whom they regarded as having the final responsibility for the application of PGx screening results in patient care. The results are presented in Table 2 and show that the majority of physicians reported that this responsibility lies with the prescriber. Hospital pharmacists largely agreed with this, although a notable group also reported the pharmacist as responsible. Community pharmacists were more divided and specifically indicated that there is a shared responsibility. In summary, the allocation of responsibility for the application of PGx screening results in patient care is currently unclear.

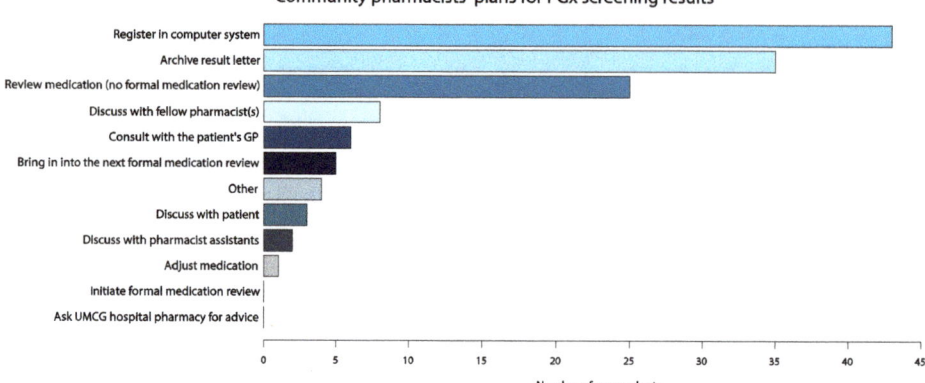

Figure 3. The steps which community pharmacists reported they would take after having received pharmacogenomic screening results.

Table 2. Final responsibility for the application of pharmacogenomic screening results in patient care.

Responsible Person	Community Pharmacists	Hospital Pharmacists	Physicians
Pharmacist	18 (39%)	5 (38%)	2 (9.5%)
Prescriber	10 (22%)	8 (62%)	16 (76%)
Clinical geneticist	7 (15%)	-	2 (9.5%)
General practitioner	-	-	-
Other		-	
Shared responsibility in general	5 (11%)		
Pharmacist and prescriber are jointly responsible	4 (9%)		
Pharmacist, providing sufficient information transfer	1 (2%)		
Depending on drugs prescribed	-		1 (5%)
Other	1 (2%)		

3.13. Identified Practical Barriers and Facilitators

An overview of the identified practical barriers and facilitators within the various themes discussed above, as perceived by healthcare practitioners and patients, is presented in Table 3.

Table 3. Barriers and facilitators to pharmacogenomic screening implementation.

	Perceived by Stakeholder			
	Patient	Community Pharmacist	Hospital Pharmacist	Physician
Barriers				
Practical experience is limited	No	Yes	Yes	Yes
Need for further postgraduate education	No	Yes	Yes	No
Rely on computer systems for application	No	Yes	Yes	Yes
Need for education about PGx application	No	Yes	Yes	Yes
Practical barriers within computer systems	No	Yes	Yes	Yes

Table 3. *Cont.*

	Perceived by Stakeholder			
	Patient	Community Pharmacist	Hospital Pharmacist	Physician
Lack of information, specifically about exact implications of PGx screening results	Yes	No	No	No
Unclear allocation of responsibilities among healthcare practitioners	Yes	Yes	Yes	Yes
Facilitators				
Positive attitude towards PGx	Yes	Yes	Yes	Yes
DPWG guidelines are generally well adhered to	No	No	No	Yes

4. Discussion

This study identified practical barriers and facilitators within various themes, as perceived by healthcare practitioners and patients, to the use of PGx screening results and associated DPWG recommendations in a Dutch outpatient hospital care setting (Table 3). As some of the survey questions dealt with the actual outcome of PGx testing, we discuss these first.

4.1. Frequencies of PGx Variants and DGIs

We confirmed that actionable PGx variants are present in the majority of the patient population of outpatient clinics in frequencies comparable to those reported in the literature (Table S4). Since the majority of new prescriptions during follow-up originated from the GP, and drugs prescribed by GPs were not considered in our study, the number of DGIs we report is likely an underestimation. It is important that the number of DGIs is determined in more detail for a variety of patient populations in order to assess the value of PGx for individual patients.

CDS searches were performed in only four patients with a DGI, but recommendations were shown for more patients. This is explained by the fact that an alternative drug without a DGI was prescribed following the recommendation shown or because drugs were not prescribed directly following the search. The latter is illustrated by the search types we could distinguish. Some searches concerned past or future treatment, and prescribers also checked drugs they did not want to prescribe at that moment, for example, commonly used treatment alternatives or drugs that were suggested in a recommendation. Furthermore, it is likely that prescribers started to remember the recommendations for DGIs they had encountered previously and did not perform a CDS search every time. The number of CDS searches reported is therefore likely to be an underestimation of the actual number of times prescribers dealt with PGx results.

From the actionable recommendations evaluated, we conclude that DPWG guidelines are generally well adhered to, although the practical application can transcend guideline recommendations, and application is thus not always straightforward.

4.2. Practical Barriers and Facilitators

In agreement with the literature, our results show that current practical experience with PGx is limited, even though DPWG guidelines have been available nationwide since 2006 [2,4,7]. A lack of knowledge and training among healthcare practitioners has previously been reported as a barrier to PGx implementation [1,8–10,12,13]. The community and hospital pharmacists in our study reported wanting more education about PGx for themselves and pharmacy staff. Physicians in our study did not report this, which does not directly imply that they have enough knowledge or skills, given that some also reported not feeling ready to apply PGx in daily practice. While physicians themselves perceived the general introduction and presentation of DPWG guideline recommendations provided in this study as sufficient, some patients wanted physicians to be better informed. According to these patients, some physicians were unable to provide sufficient explanation or did not fully understand the results. Our findings suggest that postgraduate education could increase the ability of healthcare practitioners to apply PGx in practice. Due to the explorative nature of our study, we can only speculate that the currently available training may not correspond well with practical needs (specifically on the topic of communication with patients), that training may not be optimized for physicians, that physicians may be unaware of their lack of knowledge and skills, or that physicians may have a lower demand for in-depth knowledge about PGx in general compared to pharmacists. Further research is needed to investigate the details underlying this barrier.

Literature reports that recognition of the clinical utility of PGx is a facilitator for implementation and that disbelief is a barrier [8–10,12,13]. In our study, patients were positive about PGx, including its expected clinical utility, regardless of the occurrence of DGIs during their treatment, whereas healthcare practitioners were generally positive about the clinical utility, although some did not feel ready to apply it in daily practice. These results should, however, be interpreted with caution because patients and healthcare practitioners who recognized the clinical utility were more likely to participate in this study and our study size was limited. In addition, patients and physicians were recruited from only two outpatient clinics, Psychiatry and Internal Medicine, and this may have influenced the outcome, for example, because practical use of reactive PGx testing is relatively common in psychiatry compared to other medical fields.

In our study, PGx screening results were reported directly to patients by mail without the presence of a healthcare practitioner. In the absence of a standardized reporting format for PGx testing results, which has previously been reported as a barrier [9], we drafted a patient result letter with a brief explanation of the results in laymen's terms and suggested actions, e.g., that the patient discusses their results with their current healthcare practitioners and share results with any new ones. Considering that pharmacotherapy is often a complex balance between treatment options, effectiveness, (risk of) ADRs, co-morbidities, and co-medication, it is our view that communicating the implications should be up to the individual healthcare practitioner and should be tailored to the individual patient at the time it is relevant. Patients should only have to know when to share the PGx screening results with their healthcare practitioner, e.g., in those cases where that information is not routinely included in their EHR. While the patient result letter was developed based on feedback from patients in focus groups prior to the study, our results indicate that some patients wanted to receive more and different information than provided. Most importantly, patients repeatedly reported wanting to know the exact implication of the PGx screening results for them, e.g., the level of dose adjustment or suitable alternative drugs. However, not all patients desired this depth of information, implying that one format for reporting PGx results to all patients would not suffice. An electronic personal health environment could present information to patients about their PGx screening results while containing multiple layers of information that enable them to receive the depth of information they desire, while also providing a standardized reporting format for PGx results and a way for patients to easily share their results with their healthcare practitioners.

A new barrier emerged from our study: the unclear allocation of responsibilities among healthcare practitioners. The majority of patients reported that PGx screening results should be discussed with them by a healthcare practitioner but had differing preferences for which healthcare practitioner should be responsible. We also found that healthcare practitioners themselves perceived they had a shared, and therefore still unclear, responsibility for discussing PGx screening results with patients. It was also unclear to both patients and healthcare practitioners at what point in the treatment process PGx screening results and their implications should be discussed, if ever. It is also unclear which healthcare practitioner is ultimately responsible for the application of PGx screening results in different patient care situations. Furthermore, a group of patients reported their current drugs were not reviewed by a healthcare practitioner even though they desired this (data presented in Supplementary Results Section S1). Although some patient's drugs may have been reviewed without their knowledge, these results underline the importance of clear communication with patients and expectation management. In addition, we should be aware of the risk of suboptimal pharmacotherapy in situations where patients are unassertive or have a more "wait-and-see" attitude because it is unclear which healthcare practitioner is responsible for discussing and applying PGx in practice. In our opinion, it should never be the patient's responsibility to make sure PGx screening results are discussed and/or applied. Overall, this newly identified barrier needs to be addressed to facilitate the responsible implementation of PGx screening. However, this may not be easily done nationally or internationally, as the interactions between healthcare practitioners can be highly variable between countries, regions, and even healthcare organizations or healthcare practitioners. As we identified this barrier in our limited local setting, additional research is needed to identify whether an unclear allocation of responsibilities is also a national/international barrier.

For logistical reasons, CDS software was only available as a separate tool outside the EHR in which the drugs are prescribed during our study, which presented a barrier for physicians to consider PGx screening results during prescription. This approach was taken because the availability of CDS software was deemed crucial in our pre-pilot study (see Supplementary Methods Section S2), which is supported by the literature [7,12,13]. In response to our explorative pilot study, PGx-based medication surveillance has now been incorporated into our hospital EHR (since July 2020) in order to facilitate the application of DPWG guidelines for every patient, both those admitted and those treated in outpatient clinics. The availability of CDS within our EHR is an important and crucial step towards the use of PGx-based medication surveillance in routine healthcare. However, not all computer systems used by healthcare practitioners outside of our hospital can handle (all) PGx screening results. Since healthcare practitioners rely heavily on their computer system for insight into DPWG guidelines during drug prescription and medication surveillance, the lack of availability of CDS may be an important barrier within Dutch healthcare in general.

In the Netherlands, PGx testing is currently only reimbursed by the insurer to investigate the cause of an ADR or as part of an optional reimbursement package. In anticipation of resolving this financial barrier to the broad implementation of PGx testing and screening, we provided physicians with the opportunity to perform PGx screening for their patients free-of-charge and with minimal selection criteria. This study did not address which patients should be screened and at what time point in their treatment; the costs of PGx screening would be best justified. Further research, including health technology assessment, should inform policy decision-making on these aspects.

To conclude, our exploratory pilot study confirmed known practical barriers and facilitators and suggested a new barrier to the implementation of PGx screening, namely an unclear allocation of responsibilities among healthcare practitioners. With this knowledge, we have more insight into which facilitators can be leveraged and which barriers need to be overcome to successfully implement PGx screening in Dutch outpatient hospital care. This study also provides a foundation for more detailed novel research that will hopefully further aid PGx implementation and contribute to unlocking the full potential of genome-guided drug prescription to enable personalized medication schemes with optimized treatment tolerance and response.

Supplementary Materials: The following are available online at http://www.mdpi.com/2075-4426/10/4/293/s1, Supplementary Material 1: Patient result letter (English translation); Supplementary Methods; Supplementary Results; Table S1: Details on custom genotyping panel; Table S2: Overview of the questions included in the surveys; Table S3: Demographics of participating patients, community pharmacists, hospital pharmacists and physicians; Table S4: Frequencies of PGx haplotypes and predicted phenotypes. Table S5: Alphabetical list of abbreviations.

Author Contributions: Conceptualization, P.L., R.S. (Robert Schoevers), R.G., J.K., M.P., I.v.L., A.R., C.W., B.W. and R.S. (Rolf Sijmons); data curation, P.L., A.v.H., A.H. and E.P.; formal analysis, P.L., A.v.H., A.H. and E.P.; funding acquisition, R.G., J.K., I.v.L., A.R., C.W., B.W. and R.S. (Rolf Sijmons); investigation, P.L., E.D., L.B., A.v.H. and E.P.; methodology, P.L., M.P., I.v.L., A.R. and B.W.; project administration, P.L. and E.H.; resources, P.L., E.D., G.v.d.V., R.S. (Robert Schoevers), E.H., R.G. and R.S. (Rolf Sijmons); software, P.L. and G.v.d.V.; supervision, C.W., L.F., B.W. and R.S. (Rolf Sijmons); validation, P.L.; visualization, P.L. and L.F.; writing—original draft, P.L.; writing—review and editing, E.D., R.G., J.K., M.P., I.v.L., A.R., L.F., B.W. and R.S. (Rolf Sijmons). All authors have read and agreed to the published version of the manuscript.

Funding: This research was funded by a University Medical Center Groningen (UMCG) Healthy Aging Pilot fund (CDO15.0022) and by a Netherlands Organization for Scientific Research Spinoza Prize (SPI 92-266 to C.W.).

Acknowledgments: The authors thank Kate Mc Intyre for editing the manuscript, the UMCG Department of Genetics Integral Sample Management for processing DNA samples, and the UMCG Departments of Internal Medicine, Psychiatry and Clinical Pharmacy and Pharmacology, community pharmacists and patients for participating in this research. We thank the UMCG Genomics Coordination Center, the UG Center for Information Technology, and their sponsors BBMRI-NL and TarGet for storage and compute infrastructure.

Conflicts of Interest: The authors declare no conflict of interest.

References

1. Bartlett, M.J.; Green, D.W.; Shephard, E.A. Pharmacogenetic testing in the UK clinical setting. *Lancet* **2013**, *381*, 1903. [CrossRef]
2. Rigter, T.; Jansen, M.E.; de Groot, J.M.; Janssen, S.W.J.; Rodenburg, W.; Cornel, M.C. Implementation of Pharmacogenetics in Primary Care: A Multi-Stakeholder Perspective. *Front. Genet.* **2020**, *11*, 10. [CrossRef] [PubMed]
3. Krebs, K.; Milani, L. Translating pharmacogenomics into clinical decisions: Do not let the perfect be the enemy of the good. *Hum. Genom.* **2019**, *13*, 39. [CrossRef] [PubMed]
4. Swen, J.J.; Wilting, I.; de Goede, A.L.; Grandia, L.; Mulder, H.; Touw, D.J.; de Boer, A.; Conemans, J.M.; Egberts, T.C.; Klungel, O.H.; et al. Pharmacogenetics: From bench to byte. *Clin. Pharmacol. Ther.* **2008**, *83*, 781–787. [CrossRef] [PubMed]
5. Swen, J.J.; Nijenhuis, M.; de Boer, A.; Grandia, L.; Maitland-van der Zee, A.H.; Mulder, H.; Rongen, G.A.; van Schaik, R.H.; Schalekamp, T.; Touw, D.J.; et al. Pharmacogenetics: From bench to byte—An update of guidelines. *Clin. Pharmacol. Ther.* **2011**, *89*, 662–673. [CrossRef] [PubMed]
6. Bank, P.C.D.; Swen, J.J.; Guchelaar, H.J. Estimated nationwide impact of implementing a preemptive pharmacogenetic panel approach to guide drug prescribing in primary care in The Netherlands. *BMC Med.* **2019**, *17*, 110. [CrossRef] [PubMed]
7. van Gelder, T.; van Schaik, R.H.N. Pharmacogenetics in daily practice. *Ned. Tijdschr. Geneeskd.* **2020**, *164*, D4191. [PubMed]
8. van der Wouden, C.H.; Paasman, E.; Teichert, M.; Crone, M.R.; Guchelaar, H.-J.; Swen, J.J. Assessing the Implementation of Pharmacogenomic Panel-Testing in Primary Care in the Netherlands Utilizing a Theoretical Framework. *JCM* **2020**, *9*, 814. [CrossRef] [PubMed]
9. Shuldiner, A.R.; Relling, M.V.; Peterson, J.F.; Hicks, K.; Freimuth, R.R.; Sadee, W.; Pereira, N.L.; Roden, D.M.; Johnson, J.A.; Klein, T.E. The Pharmacogenomics Research Network Translational Pharmacogenetics Program: Overcoming Challenges of Real-World Implementation. *Clin. Pharmacol. Ther.* **2013**, *94*, 207–210. [CrossRef] [PubMed]
10. Stanek, E.J.; Sanders, C.L.; Taber, K.A.J.; Khalid, M.; Patel, A.; Verbrugge, R.R.; Agatep, B.C.; Aubert, R.E.; Epstein, R.S.; Frueh, F.W. Adoption of Pharmacogenomic Testing by US Physicians: Results of a Nationwide Survey. *Clin. Pharmacol. Ther.* **2012**, *91*, 450–458. [CrossRef] [PubMed]
11. Van Driest, S.; Shi, Y.; Bowton, E.; Schildcrout, J.; Peterson, J.; Pulley, J.; Denny, J.; Roden, D. Clinically Actionable Genotypes among 10,000 Patients with Preemptive Pharmacogenomic Testing. *Clin. Pharmacol. Ther.* **2014**, *95*, 423–431. [CrossRef] [PubMed]
12. Horgan, D.; Jansen, M.; Leyens, L.; Lal, J.A.; Sudbrak, R.; Hackenitz, E.; Bußhoff, U.; Ballensiefen, W.; Brand, A. An Index of Barriers for the Implementation of Personalised Medicine and Pharmacogenomics in Europe. *Public Health Genom.* **2014**, *17*, 287–298. [CrossRef] [PubMed]

13. Dunnenberger, H.M.; Crews, K.R.; Hoffman, J.M.; Caudle, K.E.; Broeckel, U.; Howard, S.C.; Hunkler, R.J.; Klein, T.E.; Evans, W.E.; Relling, M.V. Preemptive Clinical Pharmacogenetics Implementation: Current Programs in Five US Medical Centers. *Annu. Rev. Pharmacol. Toxicol.* **2015**, *55*, 89–106. [CrossRef] [PubMed]
14. Ajzen, I. The theory of planned behavior. *Organ. Behav. Hum. Decis. Process.* **1991**, *50*, 179–211. [CrossRef]
15. Sytema, S.; van der Krieke, L. Routine outcome monitoring: A tool to improve the quality of mental health care? In *Improving Mental Health Care*; Thornicroft, G., Ruggeri, M., Goldberg, D., Eds.; John Wiley & Sons: Chichester, UK, 2013; pp. 246–263. ISBN 978-1-118-33798-1.
16. R Core Team. *R: A Language and Environment for Statistical Computing*; R Foundation for Statistical Computing: Vienna, Austria, 2018.

Publisher's Note: MDPI stays neutral with regard to jurisdictional claims in published maps and institutional affiliations.

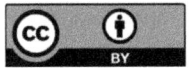

© 2020 by the authors. Licensee MDPI, Basel, Switzerland. This article is an open access article distributed under the terms and conditions of the Creative Commons Attribution (CC BY) license (http://creativecommons.org/licenses/by/4.0/).

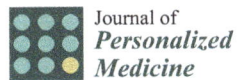 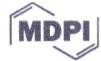

Article

Establishment of a Pharmacogenetics Service Focused on Optimizing Existing Pharmacogenetic Testing at a Large Academic Health Center

Amy L. Pasternak *, Kristen M. Ward, Mohammad B. Ateya, Hae Mi Choe, Amy N. Thompson, John S. Clark and Vicki Ellingrod

Department of Clinical Pharmacy, University of Michigan College of Pharmacy, Ann Arbor, MI 48109, USA; kmwiese@med.umich.edu (K.M.W.); Mohammad.Ateya@pfizer.com (M.B.A.); haemi@med.umich.edu (H.M.C.); amynt@med.umich.edu (A.N.T.); johnclar@med.umich.edu (J.S.C.); vellingr@med.umich.edu (V.E.)
* Correspondence: amylp@med.umich.edu; Tel.: +734-647-1590; Fax: +734-763-4480

Received: 9 September 2020; Accepted: 27 September 2020; Published: 3 October 2020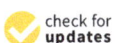

Abstract: Multiple groups have described strategies for clinical implementation of pharmacogenetics (PGx) that often include internal laboratory tests that are specifically developed for their implementation needs. However, many institutions are not able to follow this practice and instead must utilize external laboratories to obtain PGx testing results. As each external laboratory might have different ordering and reporting workflows, consistent reporting and storing of PGx results within the medical record can be a challenge. This might result in patient safety concerns as important PGx information might not be easily identifiable at the point of current or future prescribing. Herein, we describe initial PGx clinical implementation efforts at a large academic medical center, focusing on optimizing three different test ordering workflows and two distinct result reporting strategies. From this, we identified common issues such as variable reporting location and structure of PGx results, as well as duplicate PGx testing. We identified several opportunities to optimize our current processes, including—(1) PGx laboratory stewardship, (2) increasing visibility of PGx tests, and (3) clinician and patient education. Key to the success was the importance of engaging clinician, informatics, and pathology stakeholders, as we developed interventions to improve our PGX implementation processes.

Keywords: pharmacogenetics; pharmacogenomics; implementation; pharmacogenetics service

1. Introduction

Pharmacogenetics (PGx) is a pillar of precision medicine that aims to improve healthcare by using genetics to guide prescribing towards safer, more effective medication outcomes. Examples of PGx include testing for genetic variants in human leukocyte antigen (HLA) presenting genes, to decrease the risk of serious adverse drug reactions associated with drugs like abacavir and carbamazepine, and testing for genetic variability in drug metabolizing enzymes, to guide antidepressant dosing. Despite clinical guidelines and Food and Drug Administration-approved package labeling that provides recommendations for select medications based on genotype, pharmacogenetic implementation efforts across the United States are varied in depth and scope [1,2]. Pharmacogenetic implementation pioneers frequently developed research-based programs where patients consent to broad panel-based testing that is integrated into electronic systems, to guide drug prescribing [3–6]. Others developed inpatient clinical programs where single drug-gene pairs were selected and implemented within a specific practice setting, such as CYP2C19 testing for percutaneous coronary intervention [7–9]. Some organizations also developed ambulatory pharmacogenetics services where patients are referred to pharmacogenetics clinics to help guide and interpret pharmacogenetic testing [10,11]. In the majority of cases of these early adopters, the institutions identified a single source for PGx testing, such as internal PGx testing panels, which were customized to the needs of their project, institution, and population.

However, it is unlikely that all health systems will have the capability to establish an internal pharmacogenetics laboratory, and therefore the majority of clinicians will likely utilize commercial laboratories, where pharmacogenetic test offerings are increasing [12]. Without dedicated pharmacogenetics oversight, each clinical specialty within the institution might select a different laboratory and develop their own test, ordering and reporting the workflow for pharmacogenetic results in the electronic medical record (EMR). Multiple independent processes confound the integration of pharmacogenetics into prescribing decisions, and these independent processes might cause decreased visibility of relevant test results to all clinicians providing care to the patient, especially when the results are returned as unstructured text documents, such as Portable Document Format (PDF) files. Multiple groups are creating resources to enable uniform discrete reporting of genetic results in the EMR, however, widespread adoption is not yet achieved [13–15]. Consistent result visibility is critical to ensuring appropriate and safe medication use.

Our institution began a pharmacogenetics service in 2018, with the hiring of two clinical pharmacist specialists focused in PGx implementation. However, prior to the initiation of this service several clinical service lines already utilized pharmacogenetic testing. We chose to use an evidence-based approach to determine initial PGx interventions. Therefore, our service focused on developing standardized strategies for incorporating existing PGx results into the EMR, for all relevant patient care decisions for gene-drug pairs, with established recommendations for dosing or use, based on Clinical Pharmacogenetics Implementation Consortium (CPIC) guidelines or Food and Drug Administration (FDA) package insert information. The description of these implementation efforts are unique because the strategies for evaluating and integrating existing PGx results are less well described than implementation of a new PGx-service that sets the testing criteria [16]. We believe that describing our PGx implementation strategy will be informative for clinicians at institutions that are encountering external PGx testing. Our processes might help guide opportunities for PGx result integration when their institution might not have the infrastructure to develop their own pharmacogenetic testing platforms or large-scale informatics efforts. Herein, we describe our initial processes to identify and execute PGx-focused interventions, through the optimization of existing pharmacogenetic testing strategies, implemented at a large academic medical center.

2. Materials and Methods

A retrospective review of pharmacogenetics utilization across the health system was designed to assist the team with identifying areas where interventions could be made to optimize or expand existing workflows, improve patient safety, or identify areas for increased education to clinicians. Our goals were to—(1) identify what PGx tests were being ordered within the institution, (2) determine the ordering and return location of the PGx results, and (3) identify what clinical specialties utilized PGx tests.

After obtaining approval from the institution's internal review board (HUM00143486), the EMR was queried for PGx test results from 1 June 2014–31 December 2018. Discrete variables were identified through DataDirect, an internal, electronic data repository that extracts discrete information from the institutional EMR [17]. The Electronic Medical Record Search Engine (EMERSE), a free-text search engine of the EMR, was used to extract additional data of interest that could not be captured as a discrete variable (e.g., clinical note documentation or text reported lab results) [18]. In both systems, preliminary searches of laboratory tests, problem list entries, and clinical notes began by using names of germline pharmacogenes, with guidelines from CPIC or germline genes included in the FDA Pharmacogenomic Biomarkers table. Searches were then expanded to include names of pharmacogenetic testing panels, such as Genesight®, to further identify cases of commercial pharmacogenetic tests, ordered as a panel.

Once a PGx result was identified in the medical record, additional data were gathered for each result, such as, ordering workflow, testing laboratory (internal vs. external), location of result storage in EMR, and format of result in EMR (i.e., discrete vs. text).

In addition to the retrospective chart review, the pharmacogenetics team began informally surveying providers about their use and perceptions of pharmacogenetics, to determine what services would be beneficial to clinicians and identify opportunities for education. A pharmacogenetic consult service was also established and advertised to providers at our institution. This service is available for any questions related to pharmacogenetics from providers and their patients. Direct consults with patients can be requested by the provider for either pre- or post-PGx testing and are complete via telephone. Clinicians can also request post-result interpretations of pharmacogenetics tests ordered for patients. These interpretations are completed by a clinical pharmacy specialist and returned via a standard pharmacogenetic note template that includes genotype and CPIC phenotype interpretation, in addition to patient-specific considerations for prescribing.

3. Results

3.1. Retrospective Chart Review

Between 1 June 2014 and 31 December 2018, 6302 pharmacogenetic test results were identified for 5663 patients. Thirteen unique pharmacogenes and 16 unique pharmacogenetic test orders were identified in the EMR (Table 1). Thiopurine methyltransferase (*TPMT*) was the most commonly tested pharmacogene, accounting for 50.6% of all PGx tests ordered. *TPMT* also had the most test order options, with three distinct tests orderable in the EMR, two enzyme activity assays and one genotype test.

Table 1. Pharmacogenetic tests identified in electronic medical record from 1 June 2014–31 December 2018.

Test	N (%)	Laboratory	Order Process	Result Location	Result Format
TPMT enzyme assay	2694 (42.7)	External	Discrete	EMR Results	Text
G6PD activity	2122 (33.7)	Internal	Discrete	EMR Results	Discrete
HLA-B*57:01	579 (9.2)	Internal	Discrete	EMR Results	Text
TPMT Genotype	496 (7.9)	External	Discrete	EMR Results	Text
Genesight®	200 (3.2)	External	External	Clinical Note/Media	NA
UGT1A1 Genotype	178 (2.8)	Internal	Discrete	EMR Results	Text
IL28B Genotype	15 (0.2)	External	Discrete	EMR Results	Discrete
HLA-B*15:02	5 (0.08)	Internal	Discrete	EMR Results	Text
DPYD Genotype	5 (0.08)	External	Non-discrete	EMR Results	Text
CYP2D6 Genotype	4 (0.06)	External	Non-discrete	EMR Results	Text
CYP2C9/VKORC1 genotype	2 (0.03)	External	Non-discrete	EMR Results	Text
HLA-B*58:01	1 (0.02)	External	Non-discrete	EMR Results	Text
Drug metabolizing enzyme panel	1 (0.02)	External	Non-discrete	EMR Results	Text

EMR—electronic medical record, discrete—reportable and measurable data in EMR, and non-discrete—non-measurable data in EMR.

Three unique test ordering processes were identified—(1) discrete order in EMR, meaning the test order could be searched in the EMR, (2) non-discrete order in EMR, meaning the test result was within the EMR but the test was placed as a "miscellaneous" order, and (3) external-to-EMR orders, where the test order was placed directly through the commercial laboratory. Ten of the 16 PGx tests were available as discrete orders in the EMR, 5 were available as non-discrete orders in the EMR, and one was ordered external to the EMR.

Of the 15 PGx tests that could be ordered in the EMR, four were performed by an internal laboratory and all were discrete orders. The remaining EMR-orderable PGx tests, whether discrete or non-discrete, were sent to external laboratories. All tests that were ordered within the EMR had the test results displayed within the results section of the EMR. Two of the PGx test results were reported as a discrete genotype or phenotype (*IL28B* and G6PD), while all other PGx test results were reported in the laboratory results, as text comments based on the original laboratory report.

The only way to identify that an external-to-EMR PGx test was completed for a patient was to search for clinician documentation in an encounter note. All identified cases were for a pharmacogenetic panel test that was focused on psychotropic prescribing, and searching for the name of the test panel was the most efficient way to identify cases. In 58% of the identified cases, the genotype result for the patient was identifiable, most commonly through a scanned PDF of the laboratory report that was uploaded into the EMR. Although clinicians mentioned testing was performed in clinical notes, they rarely reported the genotype results for the patient in the associated documentation.

The overall volume of PGx tests did not vary from year to year, although the proportion of *IL28B* tests decreased over the study period, while the proportion of Genesight® panel tests increased over the study period, likely reflecting practice changes over the study period.

3.1.1. Duplicate Test Results

Although the median number of pharmacogenetic tests per subject was 1, the range of tests per subject was 1–8. Therefore, we evaluated the prevalence of duplicate pharmacogenetic tests.

Overall, 12% of patients ($n = 680$) had >1 result for the same pharmacogenetic test in the EMR, during our study time frame. This was most common for patients with TPMT testing (15%), followed by those with G6PD testing (6.8%), then *HLA-B*57:01* (3%), and *UGT1A1* genotype testing (2.2%). The median number of duplicate tests per patient was 2 (range 2–8). For *HLA-B*57:01*, and *UGT1A1* genotypes, 100% of the duplicate orders occurred during unique patient appointments. For TPMT, 73% of duplicate test orders occurred in unique appointments, while the remainder of duplicate tests were ordered at the same appointment. Sixty percent ($n = 319$) of patients with > 1 TPMT test had multiple TPMT enzyme assay tests, 33% had an enzyme assay and genotype test, and the remainder had multiple TPMT enzyme assays and a genotype test. The large proportion of testing repeated at separate patient appointments suggests the first test result might have been missed by the ordering clinician.

3.1.2. Pharmacogenetic Problem List Entries

Seventy-seven subjects had pharmacogenetic problem list entries for 13 different pharmacogenes (Table 2). A corresponding pharmacogenetic test result was identified in the EMR for 54 (70%) of these PGx problem list entries. The majority of the problem list entries provided information about the gene that was tested, but limited the information about the identified genetic variant or phenotype to allow for clinical application.

Table 2. Pharmacogenetic problem listing the entries identified in electronic medical record (EMR).

Gene	Problem List Entry	N
TPMT	Intermediate TPMT activity	33
	TPMT intermediate metabolizer	1
	Poor metabolizer of azathioprine	1
	Thiopurine methytransferase deficiency	1
RYR1	Monoallelic mutation of RYR1	14
	Biallelic mutation of RYR1	2
CYP2D6	CYP2D6 deficiency	2
	Cytochrome p450 2D6 enzyme deficiency	2
	Poor drug metabolizer due to cytochrome p450 CYP2D6 variant	2
DPD	DPD Deficiency	6
CYP2C9	Monoallelic mutation of CYP2C9 gene	1
	CYP2C9 deficiency	2
CYP3A4	Ultra-rapid metabolizer associated with CYP3A4	2
	Cytochrome p450 3A4 enzyme deficiency	1
CACN1S	Monoallelic mutation in CACN1S	2
CYP1A2	CYP1A2 gene mutation	2
CYP2C19	CYP2C19 intermediate metabolizer	1
	Cytochrome p450 2C19 enzyme deficiency	1
CYP mutation	CYP gene mutation – unknown type	1
	Mutation of liver cytochrome that can lead to impaired drug metabolism	1
MTHFR	Biallelic mutation of MTHFR gene	1
CYP2B6	CYP2B6 intermediate metabolizer	1
CYP3A5	CYP3A5 gene mutation	1

3.2. Clinical Services

Based on the findings of the retrospective evaluation, we developed additional pharmacogenetic services in the form of clinical decision support to improve PGx-associated workflows. To improve result visibility, we added the relevant pharmacogenetic test result to the medication order screens for abacavir and thiopurines. To address the high rates of duplicate testing, we began the development of clinical decision support, which was implemented for *HLA-B*57:01* and *TPMT*. Both passive and active clinical decision support (CDS) strategies were used to notify clinicians that a pharmacogenetic test result was either missing for a relevant medication order, or was already available for a duplicate laboratory order (Figure 1). CDS was also developed to notify clinicians of a high-risk result for the *HLA-B*57:01* genotype, which was reported as an unstructured text comment in the EMR. Using custom structured query language, test results were extracted and were subsequently stored in the EMR as discrete data elements. We compared the rate of patients with a duplicate TPMT test order for 6 months pre- and post-CDS implementation. In the pre-CDS period (1 April 2019–1 October 2019), for 17.6% of patients, the TPMT test order placed in this time period was a duplicate test; in the post-CDS period only 9.6% of patients had a duplicate TPMT order placed. No duplicate test alerts fired for *HLA-B*57:01* in the post-CDS time period.

A. *Passive BPA for abcavir and HLA-B*57:01*

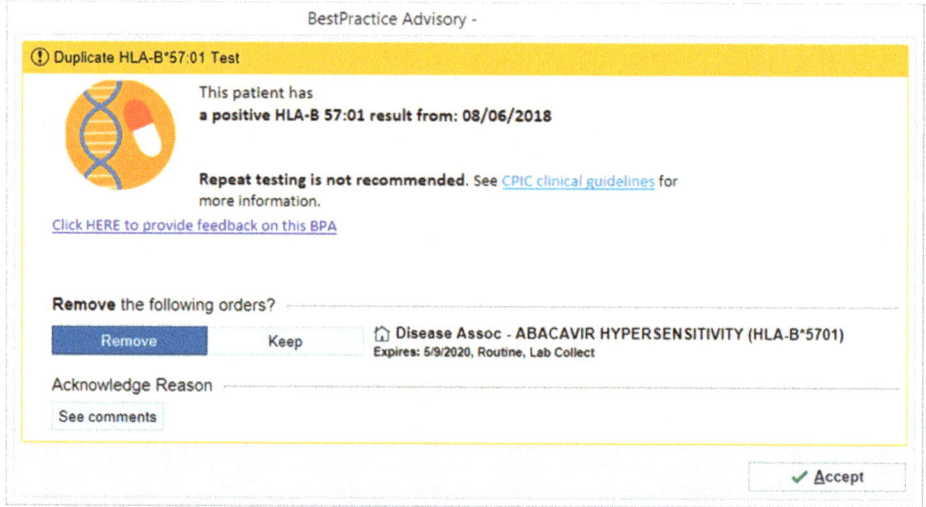

B. *Active BPA for duplicate HLA-B*57:01 test*

Figure 1. Sample screenshots of pharmacogenetic best practice advisory (BPA) alerts. © 2020 Epic Systems Corporation.

While evaluating the discrete test orders, we also identified there was a cost difference between the two available TPMT enzyme assays, with no strong clinical indication to prefer one test from the other. We therefore worked with the laboratory formulary committee and clinicians who utilized this testing to decrease the number of TPMT enzyme assay orders in the EMR, to decrease the overall costs of testing. The overall estimated cost savings for the institution based on these interventions was approximately $47,000 annually.

In addition to clinical decision support, the pharmacogenetics service provided both education and clinical consultation, based on the findings of our initial inquiries. In terms of educational efforts, a grand rounds presentation was provided to the department of pharmacy, as well as small group education with pharmacists on the CDS interventions discussed above. Education and outreach efforts with non-pharmacists were primarily focused on services that utilized the external-to-EMR test orders. The education sessions varied, but frequently covered a review of pharmacogenetics, introduction to pharmacogenetics resources such as the Clinical Pharmacogenetics Implementation Consortium, discussion on how to interpret PGx test results, and potential limitations of pharmacogenetics. Approximately 200 clinical pharmacogenetic consults were completed to date via the consult service, primarily in ambulatory psychiatry, for assistance with the interpretation of commercial laboratory psychotropic pharmacogenetic panels.

4. Discussion

Through this investigation, our team identified multiple opportunities for pharmacogenetic interventions to optimize pharmacogenetic testing strategies that already existed within our institution, and to increase the integration of these results into prescribing decisions. There was substantial heterogeneity in terms of both the test ordering and test resulting procedures within our institution. Additionally, we unexpectedly discovered that many patients had duplicate pharmacogenetic testing performed. These findings were not previously described in the pharmacogenetics implementation literature, but are likely true at many institutions where the clinical service lines developed independent strategies for using PGx testing. All of these discoveries present opportunities for pharmacist-led, PGx-focused interventions that have the potential to decrease costs and improve patient safety.

Laboratory stewardship is the process of improving patient safety by ensuring that appropriate tests are ordered, returned, and interpreted correctly for patients, while maintaining and developing testing protocols that are fiscally responsible [19]. Pharmacists, and other PGx-trained clinicians, can play a significant role in PGx laboratory stewardship within their institutions, by helping to identify inappropriate testing, as well as comparing different testing strategies. This could present opportunities to improve test ordering and resulting workflows, as well as identify cost-saving opportunities, such as our intervention to remove a more expensive, but clinically comparable, TPMT enzyme assay. Although this process does not directly impact the daily pharmacist workflows, it helped to develop and establish mutually beneficial projects for pharmacy, pathology, and clinicians.

Ideally, all PGx results would be available in a discrete format in one location in the EMR, however, there are substantial barriers to deploying this strategy that might not make it feasible at all institutions. Use of pharmacogenetics is likely to increase and so pharmacists should work to develop strategies to document pharmacogenetic results into the EMR, regardless of the testing source, to improve result visibility and ease communication of test implications. Our initial strategy for improving documentation is a standardized note template that includes the genotype result and uses standardized CPIC phenotype terminology. One primary goal of the result interpretation was to specifically address issues related to psychotropic panel testing. First, the products currently used by our providers only describe pharmacogenetic guided recommendations for psychotropic medications, when the PGx result might be applicable to other drug classes. An example is *CYP2C19* testing, where clinical recommendations currently exist for psychotropic, cardiovascular, and antifungal agents [20–23]. Providers might not be aware of the non-psychotropic implications of the PGx result and these potentially significant drug–gene interactions might be missed. Secondly, the laboratory interpretations do not consider other patient-specific factors that might impact result interpretation of pharmacogenetics, such as renal and hepatic function and drug–drug interactions. Finally, many of the genetic results are not consistently interpreted into pharmacogenetic phenotypes by different labs [24]. This results in variable interpretations that are sometimes at odds with recommendations from pharmacogenetic guidelines. As our consultation translates the genotype result into a phenotype, based on the CPIC standardized phenotype definitions, results for all patients with consultations show a consistent interpretation. Although this process has limitations, it overcomes many barriers to the traditional storage of PDF lab reports, in that, it is searchable in the EMR, improves the visibility of the genetic results, and overcomes the barrier of variable phenotype interpretations by commercial laboratories that could be inconsistent with interpretations from pharmacogenetic guideline organizations [24].

As described by others, when implementing new clinical services, each of these interventions required the engagement and buy-in of relevant stakeholders. The first step of clinician engagement was educating them on the current state of testing in their practices and presenting potential interventions to optimize the existing process. Once clinician buy-in was achieved, we then engaged pathology and health informatics to further evaluate and approve these interventions. Many PGx programs described establishing pharmacogenetics oversight committees that include stakeholders and provide approvals for all PGx-related testing and interventions [3,25]. The development of this type of oversight committee might represent a barrier to PGx implementation for some institutions, as it might not fit in the existing committee structure or might have too much overlap with other existing committees. We demonstrated that pharmacogenetic interventions can be successfully deployed without establishing a PGx-focused oversight committee, as long as all relevant stakeholders are involved in the development of the interventions.

There are some limitations to the approach we took to conduct our retrospective review of pharmacogenetics at our institution. Although the queries were completed with extensive terminology in multiple data tracking systems, cases of PGx testing might still have been missed. The EMERSE system helps to minimize this risk, by allowing for "synonym" searches for common alternative or misspellings of the query word, however, some terms might still have been missed in the clinician documentation [18]. Additionally, external results are frequently stored as scanned PDFs in the EMR and there is currently no query method to evaluate this PDF data at our institution. This complication implies that it is likely that additional cases of both single-gene and panel-pgx tests could have been missed in this preliminary search, if they were not also reported in the clinical note format. As this is a challenge many institutions likely face, it highlights how clinicians need to be proactive in identifying what PGx testing is occurring within their practice areas and across their institution to ensure they can be incorporated into relevant patient-care decisions.

Until pharmacogenetic tests are reported as discrete results from all laboratories into all EMRs, interim strategies for capturing pharmacogenetic results will be needed. Clinicians have, and likely will continue, to independently integrate relevant PGx tests into their practices as new PGx associations are discovered. Pharmacists and other PGx-focused clinicians can have a significant impact in optimizing the use of pharmacogenetic tests within their institutions, by contributing to laboratory stewardship, providing education, and providing support for patients and providers on PGx result interpretation.

5. Conclusions

Herein, we described the initial processes we developed to establish a PGx-service focused on optimizing the workflows and visibility of existing PGx test orders within our institution. We were able to establish a consult service, with a standard documentation strategy to improve result visibility and develop CDS tools within the EMR, to identify patients who might require PGx testing and prevent duplicate PGx test orders. Successful implementation of services required an assessment of PGx utilization, engagement, and support of relevant stakeholders, and collaboration with informatics. Ideally further integration of test results into the EMR as discrete data would allow for additional CDS development, particularly for results from external laboratories.

Author Contributions: Conceptualization, A.L.P., K.M.W., H.M.C., A.N.T., J.S.C., and V.E.; Methodology, A.L.P., K.M.W., and M.B.A.; Formal Analysis, A.L.P. and K.M.W.; Investigation, A.L.P., K.M.W., and M.B.A.; Writing—Original Draft Preparation, A.L.P. and K.M.W.; Writing—Review & Editing, M.B.A., H.M.C., A.N.T., J.S.C., and V.E. All authors have read and agreed to the published version of the manuscript.

Funding: This research received no external funding.

Acknowledgments: The authors acknowledge the Michigan Genomic Initiative participants, the University of Michigan Medical School Research Data Warehouse/DataDirect, and Precision Health for providing data aggregation, management, and distribution services in support of the research reported in this publication. No funding was received for this study.

Conflicts of Interest: The authors declare no conflict of interest.

References

1. Relling, M.V.; Klein, T.E.; Gammal, R.S.; Whirl-Carrillo, M.; Hoffman, J.M.; Caudle, K.E. The Clinical Pharmacogenetics Implementation Consortium: 10 Years Later. *Clin. Pharmacol. Ther.* **2019**, *107*, 171–175. [CrossRef]
2. FDA. Table of Pharmacogenomic Biomarkers in Drug Labeling. 2020. Available online: https://www.fda.gov/drugs/science-and-research-drugs/table-pharmacogenomic-biomarkers-drug-labeling (accessed on 8 September 2020).
3. Hoffman, J.M.; Haidar, C.E.; Wilkinson, M.R.; Crews, K.R.; Baker, D.K.; Kornegay, N.M.; Yang, W.; Pui, C.-H.; Reiss, U.M.; Gaur, A.H.; et al. PG4KDS: A model for the clinical implementation of pre-emptive pharmacogenetics. *Am. J. Med Genet. Part C Semin. Med Genet.* **2014**, *166*, 45–55. [CrossRef]
4. Bielinski, S.J.; Olson, J.E.; Pathak, J.; Weinshilboum, R.M.; Wang, L.; Lyke, K.J.; Ryu, E.; Targonski, P.V.; Van Norstrand, M.D.; Hathcock, M.A.; et al. Preemptive genotyping for personalized medicine: Design of the right drug, right dose, right time-using genomic data to individualize treatment protocol. *Mayo Clin. Proc.* **2014**, *89*, 25–33. [CrossRef]
5. Pulley, J.M.; Denny, J.C.; Peterson, J.F.; Bernard, G.R.; Vnencak-Jones, C.L.; Ramirez, A.H.; Delaney, J.T.; Bowton, E.; Brothers, K.; Johnson, K.; et al. Operational Implementation of Prospective Genotyping for Personalized Medicine: The Design of the Vanderbilt PREDICT Project. *Clin. Pharmacol. Ther.* **2012**, *92*, 87–95. [CrossRef]
6. O'Donnell, P.H.; Bush, A.; Spitz, J.; Danahey, K.; Saner, D.; Das, S.; Cox, N.J.; Ratain, M.J. The 1200 patients project: Creating a new medical model system for clinical implementation of pharmacogenomics. *Clin. Pharmacol. Ther.* **2012**, *92*, 446–469. [CrossRef]
7. Shuldiner, A.R.; Palmer, K.; Pakyz, R.E.; Alestock, T.D.; Maloney, K.A.; O'Neill, C.; Bhatty, S.; Schub, J.; Overby, C.L.; Horenstein, R.B.; et al. Implementation of pharmacogenetics: The University of Maryland Personalized Anti-platelet Pharmacogenetics Program. *Am. J. Med Genet. Part C Semin. Med Genet.* **2014**, *166*, 76–84. [CrossRef]
8. Harada, S.; Zhou, Y.; Duncan, S.; Armstead, A.R.; Coshatt, G.M.; Dillon, C.; Brott, B.C.; Willig, J.; Alsip, J.A.; Hillegass, W.B.; et al. Precision Medicine at the University of Alabama at Birmingham: Laying the Foundational Processes Through Implementation of Genotype-Guided Antiplatelet Therapy. *Clin. Pharmacol. Ther.* **2017**, *102*, 493–501. [CrossRef]
9. Cavallari, L.H.; Weitzel, K.W.; Elsey, A.R.; Liu, X.; A Mosley, S.; Smith, D.M.; Staley, B.J.; Winterstein, A.G.; Mathews, C.A.; Franchi, F.; et al. Institutional profile: University of Florida Health Personalized Medicine Program. *Pharmacogenomics* **2017**, *18*, 421–426. [CrossRef]
10. Dunnenberger, H.M.; Biszewski, M.; Bell, G.C.; Sereika, A.; May, H.; Johnson, S.G.; Hulick, P.J.; Khandekar, J. Implementation of a multidisciplinary pharmacogenomics clinic in a community health system. *Am. J. Heal. Pharm.* **2016**, *73*, 1956–1966. [CrossRef]
11. Arwood, M.J.; Dietrich, E.; Duong, B.Q.; Smith, D.M.; Cook, K.; Elchynski, A.; Rosenberg, E.I.; Huber, K.N.; Nagoshi, Y.L.; Wright, A.; et al. Design and Early Implementation Successes and Challenges of a Pharmacogenetics Consult Clinic. *J. Clin. Med.* **2020**, *9*, 2274. [CrossRef]
12. Haga, S.B.; Kantor, A. Horizon Scan of Clinical Laboratories Offering Pharmacogenetic Testing. *Heal. Aff.* **2018**, *37*, 717–723. [CrossRef]
13. Hoffman, J.M.; Dunnenberger, H.M.; Hicks, J.K.; E Caudle, K.; Whirl-Carrillo, M.; Freimuth, R.; Williams, M.S.; E Klein, T.; Peterson, J.F. Developing knowledge resources to support precision medicine: Principles from the Clinical Pharmacogenetics Implementation Consortium (CPIC). *J. Am. Med. Inform. Assoc.* **2016**, *23*, 796–801. [CrossRef]
14. National Academies of Sciences Engineering and Medicine. DIGITizE: Displaying and Integrating Genetic Information through the EHR. 2020. Available online: http://www.nationalacademies.org/hmd/Activities/Research/GenomicBasedResearch/Innovation-Collaboratives/EHR.aspx (accessed on 8 September 2020).
15. Alterovitz, G.; Heale, B.; Jones, J.; Kreda, D.; Lin, F.; Liu, L.; Liu, X.; Mandl, K.D.; Poloway, D.W.; Ramoni, R.; et al. FHIR Genomics: Enabling standardization for precision medicine use cases. *NPJ Genom. Med.* **2020**, *5*, 13–14. [CrossRef]
16. Weitzel, K.W.; Smith, D.M.; Elsey, A.R.; Duong, B.Q.; Burkley, B.; Clare-Salzler, M.; Gong, Y.; Higgins, T.A.; Kong, B.; Langaee, T.; et al. Implementation of Standardized Clinical Processes for TPMT Testing in a

Diverse Multidisciplinary Population: Challenges and Lessons Learned. *Clin. Transl. Sci.* **2018**, *11*, 175–181. [CrossRef]
17. Kheterpal, S. RDW/DataDirect: A Self-Serve Tool for Data Retrieval. 2015. Available online: https://datadirect.med.umich.edu/ (accessed on 8 September 2020).
18. Hanauer, D.A.; Mei, Q.; Law, J.; Khanna, R.; Zheng, K. Supporting information retrieval from electronic health records: A report of University of Michigan's nine-year experience in developing and using the Electronic Medical Record Search Engine (EMERSE). *J. Biomed. Inform.* **2015**, *55*, 290–300. [CrossRef]
19. Dickerson, J.A.; Fletcher, A.H.; Procop, G.; Keren, D.F.; Singh, I.R.; Garcia, J.J.; Carpenter, R.B.; Miles, J.; Jackson, B.; Astion, M.L. Transforming Laboratory Utilization Review into Laboratory Stewardship: Guidelines by the PLUGS National Committee for Laboratory Stewardship. *J. Appl. Lab. Med.* **2017**, *2*, 259–268. [CrossRef]
20. Hicks, J.K.; Sangkuhl, K.; Swen, J.J.; Ellingrod, V.L.; Müller, D.J.; Shimoda, K.; Bishop, J.R.; Kharasch, E.D.; Skaar, T.C.; Gaedigk, A.; et al. Clinical pharmacogenetics implementation consortium guideline (CPIC) for CYP2D6 and CYP2C19 genotypes and dosing of tricyclic antidepressants: 2016 update. *Clin. Pharmacol. Ther.* **2017**, *102*, 37–44. [CrossRef]
21. Moriyama, B.; Obeng, A.O.; Barbarino, J.; Penzak, S.R.; Henning, S.A.; Scott, S.A.; Agúndez, J.A.; Wingard, J.R.; McLeod, H.L.; Klein, T.E.; et al. Clinical Pharmacogenetics Implementation Consortium (CPIC) Guidelines for CYP2C19 and Voriconazole Therapy. *Clin. Pharmacol. Ther.* **2017**, *102*, 45–51. [CrossRef]
22. Hicks, J.K.; Bishop, J.R.; Sangkuhl, K.; Muller, D.J.; Ji, Y.; Leckband, S.G.; Leeder, J.S.; Graham, R.L.; Chiulli, D.L.; Llerena, A.; et al. Clinical Pharmacogenetics Implementation Consortium (CPIC) Guideline for CYP2D6 and CYP2C19 Genotypes and Dosing of Selective Serotonin Reuptake Inhibitors. *Clin. Pharmacol. Ther.* **2015**, *98*, 127–134. [CrossRef]
23. Scott, S.A.; Sangkuhl, K.; Stein, C.M.; Hulot, J.-S.; Mega, J.L.; Roden, D.M.; Klein, T.E.; Sabatine, M.S.; Johnson, J.A.; Shuldiner, A.R. Clinical Pharmacogenetics Implementation Consortium Guidelines for CYP2C19 Genotype and Clopidogrel Therapy: 2013 Update. *Clin. Pharmacol. Ther.* **2013**, *94*, 317–323. [CrossRef]
24. Bousman, C.A.; Dunlop, B.W. Genotype, phenotype, and medication recommendation agreement among commercial pharmacogenetic-based decision support tools. *Pharmacogenomics J.* **2018**, *18*, 613–622. [CrossRef]
25. Empey, P.E.; Stevenson, J.M.; Tuteja, S.; Weitzel, K.W.; Angiolillo, D.J.; Beitelshees, A.L.; Coons, J.C.; Duarte, J.D.; Franchi, F.; Jeng, L.J.; et al. Multisite Investigation of Strategies for the Implementation of CYP2C19 Genotype-Guided Antiplatelet Therapy. *Clin. Pharmacol. Ther.* **2018**, *104*, 664–674. [CrossRef]

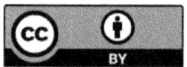

© 2020 by the authors. Licensee MDPI, Basel, Switzerland. This article is an open access article distributed under the terms and conditions of the Creative Commons Attribution (CC BY) license (http://creativecommons.org/licenses/by/4.0/).

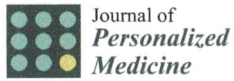

Article

Pharmacogenomic (PGx) Counseling: Exploring Participant Questions about PGx Test Results

Tara Schmidlen [1,2,*], Amy C. Sturm [2] and Laura B. Scheinfeldt [1,*]

1 Coriell Institute for Medical Research, Camden, NJ 08003, USA
2 Genomic Medicine Institute, Geisinger, Danville, PA 17822, USA; asturm@geisinger.edu
* Correspondence: tjschmidlen@geisinger.edu (T.S.); lscheinfeldt@coriell.org (L.B.S.)

Received: 25 March 2020; Accepted: 19 April 2020; Published: 23 April 2020

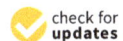

Abstract: As pharmacogenomic (PGx) use in healthcare increases, a better understanding of patient needs will be necessary to guide PGx result delivery. The Coriell Personalized Medicine Collaborative (CPMC) is a prospective study investigating the utility of personalized medicine. Participants received online genetic risk reports for 27 potentially actionable complex diseases and 7 drug–gene pairs and could request free, telephone-based genetic counseling (GC). To explore the needs of individuals receiving PGx results, we conducted a retrospective qualitative review of inquiries from CPMC participants who requested counseling from March 2009 to February 2017. Eighty out of 690 (12%) total GC inquiries were focused on the discussion of PGx results, and six salient themes emerged: "general help", "issues with drugs", "relevant disease experience", "what do I do now?", "sharing results", and "other drugs". The number of reported medications with a corresponding PGx result and participant engagement were significantly associated with PGx GC requests ($p < 0.01$ and $p < 0.02$, respectively). Our work illustrates a range of questions raised by study participants receiving PGx test results, most of which were addressed by a genetic counselor with few requiring referrals to prescribing providers or pharmacists. These results further support a role for genetic counselors in the team-based approach to optimal PGx result delivery.

Keywords: pharmacogenomics; return of results; genetic counseling; qualitative

1. Introduction

Pharmacogenomics (PGxs) is a rapidly growing segment of precision medicine projected to reach a market size of USD 9.9 billion globally by 2025 (https://www.researchandmarkets.com/reports/4801556/global-pharmacogenomics-market-2019-2025). There are over 250 drugs approved by the United States Food and Drug Administration (FDA), with labels containing pharmacogenetic information (https://www.fda.gov/drugs/science-and-research-drugs/table-pharmacogenomic-biomarkers-drug-labeling; accessed on 22 January 2020). In October 2018, the FDA granted 23andMe the first and only authorization to sell a PGx test that reports on 33 pharmacogenetic variants directly to consumers [1]. Aside from 23andMe, a growing number of clinical laboratories currently offer PGx testing, with many allowing consumers to initiate testing via an independent ordering provider rather than their personal physician. Outside of the consumer-driven genetic testing marketplace, there are large research initiatives like the National Institutes of Health's *All of Us* Research Program that is planning to return pharmacogenomic test results to as many as one million participants (https://news.nnlm.gov/psr-latitudes/nih-all-of-us-research-program-plans-genome-sequencing-and-genetic-counseling-for-participants/; posted on 21 August 2019). As the availability and use of pharmacogenomic (PGx) information in healthcare increases, a better understanding of the informational needs of individuals receiving this information will be necessary to help guide PGx result delivery.

There is relatively little information published on the extent to which patients understand PGx test results. Lemke and colleagues [2] surveyed 57 patients from NorthShore University Health System in suburban Chicago, Illinois, USA, who had undergone a 19-gene panel PGx test through either a PGx clinic or by direct access in-home testing. Participants were mostly female (72%), Caucasian (98%), and educated (93% with some college or more). Clinic patients received a discussion of benefits, risks, and limitations of PGx testing from a PGx specialist prior to sample collection in the clinic. Direct access patients watched a 4 min video covering the same topics prior to sample collection in their home. Results were returned to patients and placed in the electronic health record with the PGx clinic team available to answer questions. When surveyed 4 to 8 weeks after result receipt, the majority (63%) of these patients reported that they strongly agreed or somewhat agreed with the statement "I have a clear understanding of my test results from PGx testing". About 25% markedly disagree or strongly disagreed in response to this statement. Forty percent reported feeling confused by their PGx test results "often" or "sometimes". Forty percent indicated that they "looked up additional information" about their PGx results after discussing them with a provider, and 36% said that they wanted more follow-up discussion on their PGx results with their healthcare provider. The only difference in findings between the clinic and direct access was that clinic patients had a higher self-perceived understanding of their PGx test results than direct access patients (77.3 vs. 51.5%; $p = 0.06$). A third of patients commented in the open text at the end of the survey, and the need for additional education in results explanation was a key issue raised.

Haga and Liu [3] conducted an online survey of 99 individuals who had subscribed to a newsletter offered by Genelex, a United States-based commercial PGx laboratory. Respondents were mostly female (76%), Caucasian (93%), educated (60% with Bachelor's degree or higher), and older (majority 50–59 years, range 18–80+). Most (91%) had PGx testing through Genelex, and 48% had tested more than one year from survey completion. Most (87%) had received their results in-person with the remainder by phone or by email. Approximately half of the respondents reported viewing one or more of four Genelex educational web pages. Forty-three percent felt that they understood their PGx test results very well, 39% indicated that they "somewhat" understood their PGx results, and 11% reported that they did not really understand their PGx results. No significant association between education level or educational web page viewing and understanding of PGx test results was observed.

The Mayo Clinic Right Drug, Right Dose, Right Time Protocol (RIGHT Protocol) is a preemptive PGx study of 1013 individuals selected from the Mayo Clinic Biobank based on age, sex, and race. Olson et al. [4] surveyed 869 participants who had received *CYP2D6* metabolizer statuses via the RIGHT Protocol. Respondents were mostly Caucasian (98%), female (55%), educated (57%—4 or more years post-secondary), and aged 58.9 ± 5.5 years on average. Study participants received a result summary letter via mail along with an educational brochure with one page of information on how to sign in to the Mayo Clinic Patient Portal to access results, two pages of education on PGx testing and *CYP2D6*, a 9-page survey and a postage-paid envelope to return the survey. The majority (67%) of study participants responded that they either completely or mostly understood their *CYP2D6* result when asked, "How well do you feel you understand or don't understand your *CYP2D6* test result?" About a third (33%) responded that they either only somewhat understood (26%) or did not understand their result at all (7%). Education was the only relevant predictor, with those reporting high school or less or some college being 1.6 times as likely to report understanding somewhat or not at all compared with those who had a four-year college degree or greater education level. Over half (53%) of the 499 participants who logged in to view their result on the patient portal agreed with the statement, "It was easy to understand my pharmacogenomic result in the Patient Portal", while 33% disagreed. When asked to comment on confidence level in their ability to explain their *CYP2D6* result to a friend or family member, 38% responded "somewhat confident". Responses varied by education level with 13% of high school or less and 23% graduate/professional degree holders reporting that they were "extremely confident", while 30% of high school or less and 18% of graduate/professional degree holders reported being "not at all confident" in their ability to explain results to others.

Limited studies to date have commented on patient understanding of PGx test results. Several have found that even among well-educated patients, there remain significant gaps, and, therefore, opportunities for improvement upon PGx result return approaches. Here we describe the informational needs of individuals receiving PGx test results through an online web portal as part of their participation in the Coriell Personalized Medicine Collaborative (CPMC), a large prospective precision medicine study.

2. Materials and Methods

We conducted a retrospective qualitative review of genetic counseling session summaries from participants who requested counseling to discuss their CPMC PGx results. The Coriell Institute for Medical Research Institutional Review Board reviewed and approved this study. As a retrospective review of existing CPMC participant records, no additional participant consent was required.

The CPMC, described in detail in Keller et al. [5], is a prospective research study that assesses the impact of personalized genetic information on disease risk and medication management [6] on health behaviors and outcomes. CPMC participants must be at least 18 years of age, have a valid, personal email address, and attend or view a 45 min long informed consent PowerPoint presentation. The informed consent presentation provides an explanation of personalized medicine, study design and participation requirements, risks and benefits, examples of potentially actionable health conditions and drug-gene pairs reported to participants (e.g., coronary artery disease; CYP2C19, and Plavix), and examples of excluded health conditions (rare, single-gene Mendelian diseases and conditions with no available medical or behavioral risk reduction). The CPMC defines a "potentially actionable" condition as a condition for which the risk is likely to be mitigated by either behavior or lifestyle modifications (diet and exercise, smoking cessation) or by medical actions such as changing a drug or drug dose, increased screening, preventative treatment, or early intervention [5,6].

Participants provide a saliva sample for genomic analysis (Affymetrix™ Genome-Wide Human SNP Array 6.0 and DMET Plus Array genotyping chips). The DMET Plus Array assays over 1900 genetic markers located in genes involved in drug absorption, distribution, metabolism, and elimination (ADME) [7]. Participants also complete mandatory online questionnaires about their medical history, family history, medication use, demographics, and lifestyle. Those who complete all required questionnaires are invited to view their results through a secure web-based portal. During the 6-year time frame captured by this study, participants received the following PGx results: warfarin (CYP2C9, VKORC1, CYP4F2), clopidogrel (CYP2C19), proton pump inhibitors (CYP2C19), thiopurines (TPMT), simvastatin (SLCO1B1), metformin (ATM), and celecoxib (CYP2C9). Example reports for clopidogrel and simvastatin are displayed in Figure 1.

2.1. Participants

The CPMC is comprised of several cohorts [5,8–13]: a CPMC community cohort recruited from the general population, a cancer (breast and prostate) cohort recruited through oncologists at Fox Chase Cancer Center, a chronic disease (congestive heart failure and hypertension) cohort recruited through primary care physicians or cardiologists at Ohio State University Medical Center, a community cohort recruited through Ohio State University, and a cohort recruited through the United States Air Force. All participants are at least 18 years of age and have given written, informed consent to enroll in the study. No participants were excluded based on comorbidities. In total, information from 690 participant requests for genetic counseling support was included in the current analysis.

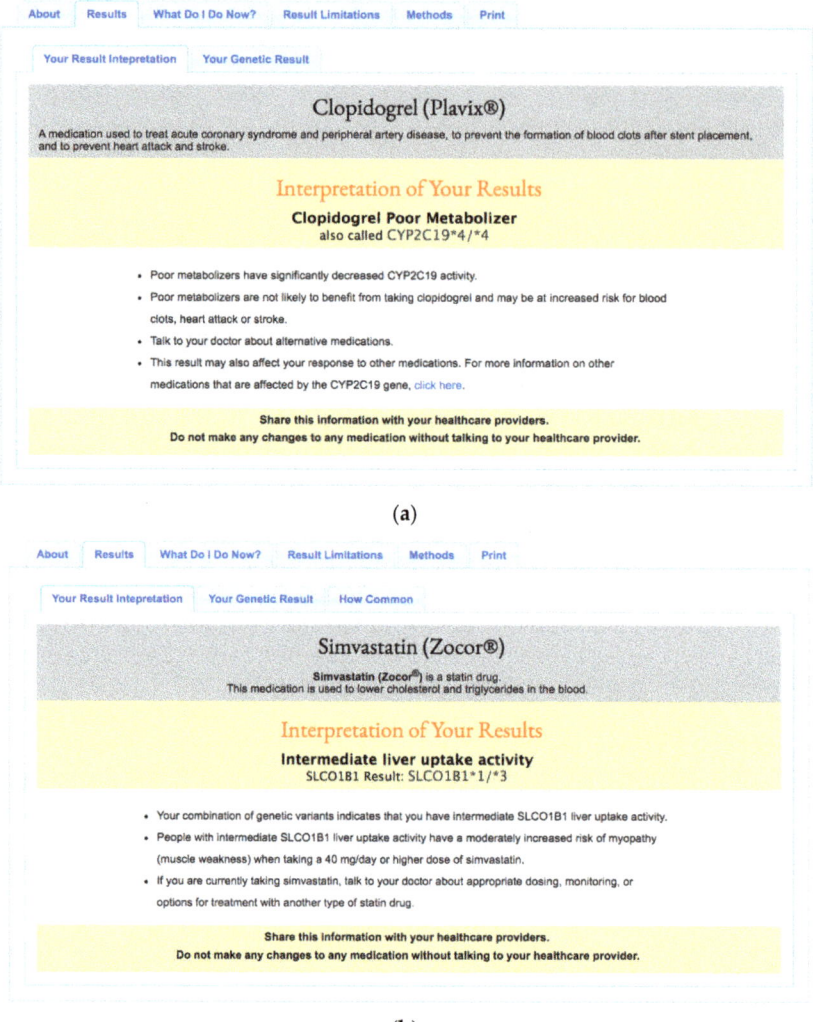

Figure 1. Example Coriell Personalized Medicine Collaborative (CPMC) pharmacogenomic (PGx) reports. Figure 1 displays example PGx reports for (**a**) clopidogrel and (**b**) simvastatin.

2.2. Procedures

Participants included in the current analysis received email invitations to view online genetic risk reports for up to 27 actionable complex diseases and 7 drug-gene pairs. Participants could elect to view or not view each report and were encouraged, but not required, to share and discuss their results with a healthcare provider. Participants had the option to request a telephone genetic counseling session paid for by the study via email, by phone, or through a secure web portal. All written requests for counseling (email or web portal requests) and subsequent written communications were stored verbatim, while the content of telephone genetic counseling sessions was captured in the form of detailed session summaries which identified participant questions, issues, and information provided. Counseling notes for 30 telephone genetic counseling sessions and email transcripts for 50 email inquiries made by CPMC participants between April 2009 and February 2017 were included in this analysis. All genetic counseling sessions included in this study were conducted by two licensed board-certified genetic counselors employed by the Coriell Institute for Medical Research.

2.3. Data Analysis

Genetic counseling session summaries were coded and analyzed via a general inductive approach to identify themes related to the research questions and study aims. Study investigators compared coded genetic counseling session summaries, modified codes as needed, and developed rules and definitions to ensure coding consistency. Codes from this finalized codebook were then applied to each of the 80 genetic counseling session summaries by two study investigators (TS, AS) with an inter-coder reliability of 91%. Line-by-line codes were compared for all session summaries, and all instances of disagreement were resolved by consensus.

We used logistic regression to model whether a participant was more likely to request PGx genetic counseling as the outcome, with recruitment cohort, gender, education, income, occupation, and age as demographic covariates, and number of medications, number of medications with CPMC risk reports, and number of viewed CPMC risk reports as independent variables. We used the step function in R to choose the demographic model with the lowest AIC: request_PGx_GC~ age + cohort, and then tested each independent variable with this model.

3. Results

We conducted a retrospective qualitative review of genetic counseling session summaries from participants who requested counseling to discuss their CPMC PGx results. As of 30 September 2015, 5021 had completed the required baseline surveys, had their sample genotyped, and were provided with at least 1 PGx result report. Of those 5021 participants with available PGx results, 4779 participants (95%) chose to view at least one risk report, and 3247 participants (65%) chose to view at least one PGx result. Of those 4779 who chose to view at least one report, 569 (12%) participants submitted at least 1 request for genetic counseling to a CPMC genetic counselor. Of those 3247 who chose to view at least one PGx result, 70 participants (2%; also see Figure 2) submitted at least 1 request for genetic counseling to a CPMC genetic counselor (62 participants submitted 1 request, 7 participants submitted 2 requests and 1 participant submitted 4 requests).

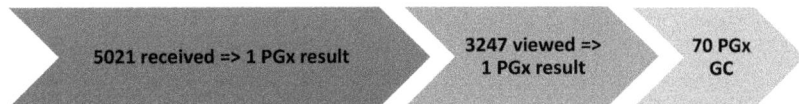

Figure 2. Participation in PGx genetic counseling.

Overall, 73% of the 5021 participants with available PGx results were taking at least 1 medication. On average, these participants were taking 3 medications. A smaller subset, 22% of participants, were taking at least 1 of the 7 drugs reported on in the study. A comparable proportion of the participants requesting genetic counseling for a PGx result were taking at least 1 medication (52/70; 74%). Compared to the 5021 participant pool, a higher proportion of participants requesting genetic counseling for a PGx result were taking at least 1 of the 7 drugs reported on in the study (30%; 21/70).

The 5021 participants who received at least one PGx result were primarily Caucasian (88%), middle-aged (mean: 47, range: 18–94), females (57%) with a Bachelor's degree or higher (69%); 35% were employed in a health or science occupation, and 18% reported a household income greater than USD 100,000 per year. Additional demographic characteristics of the 5021 CPMC participants and the subset of participants that requested genetic counseling are provided in Tables 1 and 2, respectively.

Table 1. Participant demographics.

	n (5021)	% | Range (SD)
Male	2142	43%
Female	2879	57%
Some high school	10	0%
High school graduate	255	5%
Vocational/trade school	28	1%
Some college	678	14%
Associate's degree	557	11%
Bachelor's degree	1335	27%
Graduate degree	2152	43%
Do not want to answer	6	0%
<USD 25,000	77	2%
USD 25,000–49,999	267	5%
USD 50,000–74,999	357	7%
USD 80,000–99,999	339	7%
equal or >USD 100,000	913	18%
Do not want to answer	3068	61%
Mean Age	47	18–94 (15)
Caucasian	4395	88%
African American	235	5%
Native American	9	0%
Asian	154	3%
Hawaiian/Pacific Islander	9	0%
Mixed Race	160	3%
Do not want to answer	59	1%

Table 2. Genetic counseling (GC) participant demographics.

	All Participants Requesting GC		Participants Requesting PGx GC		Participants Requesting Non-PGx GC	
	n (569)	% | Range (SD)	n (70)	% | Range (SD)	n (499)	% | Range (SD)
Male	201	35%	22	31%	179	36%
Female	368	65%	48	69%	320	64%
Some high school	3	1%	0	0%	3	1%
High school graduate	27	5%	9	13%	18	4%
Vocational/trade school	1	0%	0	0%	1	0%
Some college	67	12%	6	9%	61	12%
Associate's degree	54	9%	7	10%	47	9%
Bachelor's degree	147	26%	18	26%	129	26%
Graduate degree	268	47%	30	43%	238	48%
Do not want to answer	2	0%	0	0%	2	0%
<USD 25,000	25	4%	2	3%	23	5%
USD 25,000–49,999	72	13%	10	14%	62	12%
USD 50,000–74,999	92	16%	7	10%	85	17%
USD 80,000–99,999	111	20%	17	24%	94	19%
equal or > USD 100,000	262	46%	34	49%	228	46%
Do not want to answer	7	1%	0	0%	7	1%
Mean age	56	23–91 (13)	58	27–86 (12)	55	23–91 (13)
Caucasian	517	91%	64	91%	453	91%
African American	22	4%	1	1%	21	4%
Native American	3	1%	0	0%	3	1%
Asian	6	1%	3	4%	3	1%
Hawaiian/Pacific Islander	0	0%	0	0%	0	0%
Mixed Race	16	3%	2	3%	14	3%
Do not want to answer	5	1%	0	0%	5	1%

Eighty out of 690 (12%) total GC inquiries were focused on the discussion of PGx results. Qualitative analysis of these 80 GC session summaries revealed six main themes: (1) general help (2) issues with drugs (3) relevant disease experience (4) what do I do now? (5) sharing results, and (6) other drugs. Forty-three (54%) participants had general questions about their PGx results, while only 7 (9%) were looking for specific guidance on dosing or drug selection. Past issues with drug side effects ($n = 14$, 18%), dosing ($n = 2$, 3%), and efficacy ($n = 3$, 4%) were also mentioned; some alluded to a personal ($n = 12$, 15%) or family history ($n = 6$, 8%) of diseases treated by drugs reported on in the CPMC study. Seventeen participants (21%) were interested in the availability of PGx results for other non-study related drugs, while 28 (35%) asked about the impact of currently available PGx study results on other drugs. Some indicated sharing their PGx results with a doctor ($n = 5$, 6%), and some questioned the impact of their PGx results on family members ($n = 5$, 6%) (Figure 3).

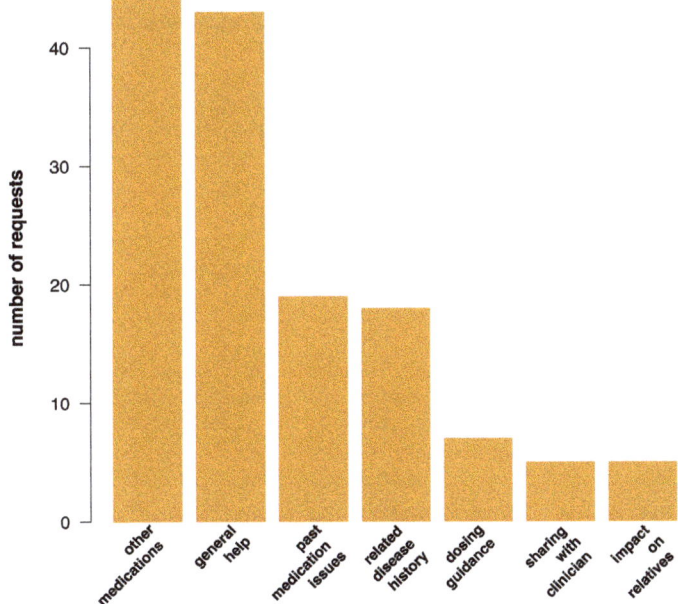

Figure 3. Broad PGx GC topical categories.

For the 569 unique participants that requested genetic counseling, recruitment cohort and age were the only demographic factors retained for the regression modeling (see Methods). The total number of CPMC risk reports viewed by a participant was marginally associated ($p = 0.02$) with a PGx counseling request, and the number of reported medications with a corresponding CPMC PGx risk report was significantly associated with PGx GC requests ($p = 0.007$) (Table 3). The following quotes illustrate key concepts and summaries of participant remarks representing each theme.

Table 3. Logistic regression results.

	Eta	Standard Error	z-Value	p-Value
Intercept	−4.504	0.824	−5.467	0.000
Number of Viewed Reports	0.047	0.020	2.341	0.019
Intercept	−6.296	1.980	−3.179	0.001
Number of PGx Report Medications	1.150	0.425	2.706	0.007

3.1. General Help

The majority of participants requesting genetic counseling for a PGx result (54%) were seeking general assistance with understanding their CPMC PGx result reports. Participants often alluded to uncertainty regarding whether they should or should not be taking a given medication based on their study result.

"I'm a little confused about the warfarin medication results. Currently I do not take warfarin. So, under (Your Result Interpretation) it states "Intermediate Dose of Warfarin MAY be Needed Based on Your Combined Genetic Result: CYP2C9*1/*1, VKORC1-AG, CYP4F2-GG". Is this advising me to start taking warfarin and seek a prescription...or simply like the other reports keep this in mind if the need arises that I need to start this drug?"

Some were confused by an "uncertain metabolizer" result, which was issued in instances of rare alleles, uncertain phase, or missing single nucleotide polymorphism (SNP) data on research-grade testing.

"In this test my result was referred to as "CYP2C19 *Uncertain (Clopidogrel Metabolizer Status Uncertain)" While I understand that my genetic combination is not known, that was stated directly in the results, I am just curious as to what about it is unknown. Does it not have a common singular response, or is this combination (7 out of 100 according to the "How Common" part of the result) not studied enough?"

Others were interested in gaining a better understanding of the details or terminology provided within their report:

"It is unclear what AA, GG, TT, etc. mean."

"You use the term -Clopidogrel Extensive Metabolizer- which offhand is meaningless to me, but after looking up the term on the web, it apparently means that if I took it, my body would use it well."

3.2. Issues with Drugs

A quarter of participants requesting genetic counseling for a PGx result did so because of a personal history of experiencing side effects of a drug ($n = 14$, 18%), dosing issues with a prescribed medication ($n = 2$, 3%), or of lack of efficacy of a prescribed medication ($n = 3$, 4%).

"I have high cholesterol and have had adverse effects with other statins. I have not used Simvastatin and would like to discuss if my results recommend trying this drug."

"I've been taking Nexium for weeks and it doesn't seem to be helping my GERD."

3.3. Relevant Disease Experience

About a quarter of participants (23%) referenced either a personal or family history of a disease being managed by one of the study drugs within their PGx genetic counseling inquiry.

"I am interested in more information regarding my warfarin results. I'm a physician and I'm fascinated by the results. During my residency, I suffered a significant superficial thrombosis is some large varicose veins. Due to the amount of venous dilation, I was treated with warfarin. If my memory serves me correctly, I required 10 days of lovenox therapy because of the difficulty getting my INR to a therapeutic level; I believe my final dose was 20 mg daily."

"I have a family history of stroke (mother) and she is currently on this medication. In the future, if this drug is offered, should I decline as it does not look effective in my case?"

3.4. What Do I Do Now?

Nine percent of PGx genetic counseling requests were seeking guidance on more concrete next steps that should be taken in light of the results. These included determining whether a dose change may be needed for a currently prescribed medication or whether a change in treatment approach to a different drug may be indicated by the results. These individuals were referred back to their prescribing healthcare provider or pharmacist for medication management guidance.

"I am taking Warfarin and would like to know what is a safe dosage for me and what range I should be in for protection against blood clots."

"My husband had a stroke and has been told to take Plavix. He is a ultra-rapid metabolizer. What should we do?"

3.5. Sharing Results

A few participants ($n = 10$, 12%) referenced a plan to share their PGx results, either with family members ($n = 5$, 6%) or with their doctor ($n = 5$, 6%). In some cases, participants were seeking guidance on which PGx results were worth sharing with family members or physicians. A few participants mentioned having already shared a PGx result with a physician who also did not know what to do with the information.

"I need info on my CYP2C9 results and how they are genetically carried to my children. I have a child in a critical care that may need this info."

"As an intermediate metabolizer of Plavix, I understand the implications of this finding if my medical care called for treatment in the future and I will inform my physician about this finding. I am less certain if the CPMC thinks it wise that I also talk to my physician about my current use of omeprazole for mild GERD for which, If I understand the findings correctly, I may currently be under-dosed."

"I took this result (Simvastatin) to my PCP and he did not know what to do with all this info, and I did not know either."

3.6. Other Drugs

Greater than half of all PGx result inquiries alluded to an interest in receiving additional PGx information. This included requests for future results on drugs not currently included in the CPMC study ($n = 17$, 21%) or interest in whether their PGx results impacted the metabolism of drugs that were not specifically referenced on their study result report ($n = 28$, 35%). CPMC genetic counselors responded to requests for additional PGx information by indicating whether the drug had been considered or approved by the study advisory board for eventual return to participants. CPMC genetic counselors did not attempt to independently interpret PGx results for drugs not included in the report interpretation but rather reminded participants of the report disclaimer stating that their result interpretation applied only to the drug(s) listed on the study report. Among the most common requests for future results were psychiatric medications (5/17, 29%). Additional medication types requested included antibiotics, bone health medications (Prolia, Xgeva), benzodiazepines (diazepam, valium), blood pressure medications (lisinopril), chemotherapeutic agents (Fulvestrant), pain medications (NSAIDs, Vioxx, codeine), insulin, other cholesterol lowering drugs (Lipitor, Zetia), prednisone, and tamoxifen. The impact of CPMC PGx results on other drugs was most commonly related to whether their SLCO1B1–simvastatin results also applied to other statin drugs. Others were interested in whether their CYP2C19–clopidogrel results also influenced the metabolism of other blood-thinning medications like aspirin.

"I was wondering if you are doing any work in the area of brain chemistry. I have been diagnosed with severe depression and we are searching for the optimal medication."

"I was wondering if the study will be doing tests for which antibiotics might not work with my genes?"

"Based on my reports I should not take Zocor (Simvastatin). Any information about Lipitor before I start taking it?"

4. Discussion

Through a qualitative exploration of genetic counseling interactions with participants in a large precision medicine biobank study, this study identified common questions that individuals have when receiving preemptive PGx test results. Most participants (54%) had general questions about how to interpret their PGx results, while only 9% were looking for specific guidance on dosing or drug selection that required referral to a healthcare provider or pharmacist. Other inquiries were related to past issues with drug side effects, dosing and efficacy, personal or family history of diseases treated by drugs reported on in the study, impact of study results on family members, and sharing results with healthcare providers. Several participants expressed interest in receiving additional PGx results for other drugs not included in the study. These results highlight for genetic counselors and other health care providers gaps in understanding of PGx test results, participant reaction to PGx results, as well as the desire that many expressed for additional PGx result information beyond what was offered through this study.

Consistent with existing literature on patient understanding of PGx test results, this study identified gaps in understanding of PGx test results even among a mostly highly educated study population [2–4,14]. Most participants requesting genetic counseling (54%) were seeking general assistance with understanding their PGx result reports, often alluding to uncertainty regarding whether they should or should not take a given medication in the future based on their results. The expectation for PGx test results to have the potential to inform physician prescribing decisions in a way that maximizes drug efficacy while limiting adverse reactions has been captured in several other studies, including studies of participants who have received PGx results [2,3,14–17].

Uncertain results, which were issued in instances of rare alleles, uncertain phase, or missing genetic data, were a source of confusion as was some of the terminology used on reports to describe metabolizer status. Others have also documented confusion with PGx test results and the metabolizer status terminology present in the interpretation of those PGx test results. Lee et al. [16] asked focus group participants with either prior PGx exposure or none to review educational handouts for clopidogrel and simvastatin PGx results. Participants expressed concern that only four categories were examined (poor metabolizer, intermediate metabolizer, extensive/normal metabolizer, ultra-rapid metabolizer) and wondered if that meant that the testing was either incomplete or too limited in scope to be useful. The Mayo Clinic Right Drug, Right Dose, Right Time (RIGHT) Protocol study surveyed 869 participants on their understanding of their *CYP2D6* PGx test results and accompanying educational materials [4]. They asked participants what would have made their results more helpful, and the most common suggestion was to use layperson's terms (e.g., extensive metabolizer is not as clear as "normal" metabolizer), followed by personalizing the result report (e.g., list the drugs that are impacted by the result) and simplifying the layout and content of the results report (e.g., add a graph showing where the result is in relation to a "normal" result). Current nomenclature that has replaced "extensive metabolizer" with "normal metabolizer" may reduce confusion.

As was expected, participants with either a personal or family history of a disease managed by one of the study drugs were among those placing a PGx genetic counseling request. Many participants requesting genetic counseling for a PGx result had a personal history of drug side effects, dosing issues, or lack of response to a medication and were curious if their PGx results validated or explained that experience.

About 70% of participants in a study that surveyed patients who had PGx testing in either a PGx clinic or via a direct access in-home test reported feeling validated about their history of previous drug side effects or lack of efficacy following receipt of PGx test results [2]. Participants in a focus group study on patient, physician, and pharmacist opinions on PGx conducted by Frigon et al. [15]

commented on the potential for PGx test results to limit the experience of having a physician discount a patient's report of a drug side-effect as a "psychosomatic" event rather than a real drug side effect. The notion of PGx results potentially leading people to conclude that any and all adverse events from a drug was due to their genetic make-up was noted by Lee et al. [16] in their focus group study comparing the attitudes and perceptions of individuals exposed to PGx-guided care versus those of individuals with traditional care. On the other hand, some studies have found that individuals receiving PGx test results may be more medication compliant and willing to tolerate some side effects if PGx testing was utilized to assist with drug and dose selection [2,16,18,19]. Results from a study by Haga et al. [14] lend further support to the hypothesis that PGx testing may improve patient adherence to medications. They studied participants who had pharmacist-assisted PGx testing and completed pre- and post-test surveys on their experiences and beliefs about prescription medicines and perceived risk and benefits of PGx testing. More than half of these participants post-test reported feeling confident that medications they were prescribed going forward would be safe and would improve their health condition compared with past prescriptions issued prior to their PGx testing. Similarly, Lemke et al. [2] found 73% of patients reporting greater confidence in medication efficacy and safety following PGx testing compared with prescriptions issued prior to testing.

Personal history of a drug side effect has been noted as a driver of PGx interest among individuals without prior PGx test exposure as well. In a 2012 telephone survey study looking at attitudes toward PGx testing in the United States [17], those who had experienced a side effect from a prescribed drug were more likely to have a strong interest in PGx testing, even after potential risks of PGx testing (e.g., privacy, confidentiality, blood draw) were reviewed.

More than half of all PGx genetic counseling inquiries mentioned an interest in receiving additional PGx information. These included requests for future results on drugs not yet included in the study (psychiatric medications), as well as interest in whether their PGx results impacted other drugs that were not specifically referenced on their result report (other statins, or other blood thinners). Other studies have also demonstrated that participants with exposure to PGx results have a strong receptiveness toward the use of pharmacogenomics and desire to see it used more routinely [3,14–16].

A few participants seeking genetic counseling were requesting guidance on which PGx results were worth sharing with family members or physicians. Awareness that PGx test results may have implications for family members has been noted by others [2,20], but participants without prior PGx exposure may confuse PGx testing for disease risk testing [16]. Haga et al. [14] also reported that about two-thirds of participants reported sharing their PGx test results with family members.

Among those who chose to share their PGx results with a physician, a few mentioned that their doctor did not know what to do with the information. In a survey study of patients who had had prior PGx testing conducted by Haga et al. [3], outcomes of PGx result sharing with either pharmacists (25% of participants) or physicians (61% of participants) were captured. About half who shared with a pharmacist felt the pharmacist responded positively and was helpful, while the other half reported either a negative response (no time to review) or no understanding of the result. For those who shared with doctors, 32% reported a positive or helpful response, 29% reported the doctor did not understand the result, and 14% were unsure of the doctor's response to their PGx result. Other studies capturing participant sharing of PGx test results with healthcare providers have also found that participants report that they are more likely to share results with their prescribing physician rather than a pharmacist [14–16]. The expectation among patients for prescribing physicians to be able to respond to PGx test results will have important implications for the broader implementation of PGx testing. A 2016 survey of pharmacy and medical students conducted by Yau and Haque [21] found that over 90% of pharmacy students had a course on PGx, while only 57% of medical students reported the same experience.

A small minority of PGx genetic counseling requests were from participants seeking guidance outside of the scope of genetic counseling practice (7 inquiries, 9%). These requests were regarding whether a dose change may be needed for a currently prescribed medication or whether a change to a different drug may be indicated by their PGx results. Study genetic counselors referred these participants to their prescribing physician or pharmacist to discuss any potential management changes related to their PGx results. As others have observed patients reporting discontinuing or changing medications following PGx testing without the advice of a physician [2], study participants were reminded both in the report text and by genetic counselors to not make any changes to medications without first discussing their results with their physician.

4.1. Study Limitations

This study has several limitations. The CPMC cohort is predominantly Caucasian, with relatively high education and income, and therefore not representative of the general public, but likely more representative of current consumers of PGx tests. This study included two methods of delivering genetic counseling—by telephone and e-mail—which could have influenced the type and number of questions asked. The analysis was conducted on written email exchanges between participants and genetic counselors when possible but, in part, relied on session notes taken by genetic counselors. While every effort was made to accurately capture participant questions expressed in telephone genetic counseling sessions, these notes do not capture the interactions verbatim. Ideally, transcripts of phone sessions would have been collected. This study only examines the informational needs of individuals who received preemptive PGx testing via participation in a research study; the needs of patients receiving clinically indicated PGx testing may be different. This study also only captured the questions of the participants who contacted us for genetic counseling and did not capture questions that participants asked other healthcare providers. Report design and content may have also influenced participant understanding of PGx test results. The PGx reports were designed by the CPMC study team, which consisted of several PhD-level genomic scientists and two genetic counselors. Iterative edits were made prior to releasing results to study participants based on feedback received from non-scientific administrative staff who viewed draft reports.

4.2. Practice Implications

Most participant questions in this study were able to be addressed by the study genetic counselors with only 7 inquiries (9%) seeking guidance on dosing or drug selection and therefore falling outside of genetic counselor scope of practice. These results lend further support for the partnership between genetic counselors and pharmacists proposed by Mills and Haga [22] to help clinicians in the multi-disciplinary team-based delivery of pharmacogenomics. Pharmacists can utilize their expertise in pharmacokinetics and pharmacodynamics to facilitate the appropriate application of PGx test results to medication selection and dosing, while genetic counselors who are well trained in genetics, risk communication, and patient education can facilitate pre-test discussion of risks, benefits and limitations of testing and post-test discussion of any familial implications, or incidental genomic findings impacting health. Both pharmacists and genetic counselors can lend their unique expertise to assist clinicians with the appropriate use and interpretation of PGx testing.

The data gathered in this study may also provide genetic counselors and other healthcare providers with insight into how to design test result reports and educational materials to better facilitate patient understanding of PGx test results. Use of lay terminology whenever possible, explicitly stating what medications the results apply to and what medications the results do not apply to, and clearly communicating the limitations of PGx testing for predicting drug dosing and response would likely reduce confusion. PGx reports and educational materials should also include more direction on which types of questions physicians, pharmacists, and genetic counselors can each address.

4.3. Research Recommendations

Further research should be performed to better understand the PGx informational needs of patients of more diverse racial, ethnic, educational, and socioeconomic status. More investigation is also needed to determine the informational needs of patients undergoing clinically-indicated PGx genetic testing.

Given that an estimated 97% of the population is expected to have an actionable PGx test result [23], further multi-disciplinary work to create scalable tools like online portals or chatbots to deliver PGx results and targeted education will help facilitate the broader clinical implementation of pharmacogenomics.

5. Conclusions

Our work illustrates a range of questions raised by study participants receiving PGx test results, most of which were addressed by a genetic counselor with few requiring input from prescribing providers or pharmacists. Genetic counselors may have a role to play in educating physicians and pharmacists on how to effectively communicate with patients about PGx as these are the providers that patients will seek out to manage and explain PGx test results. These results may also lend further support to a role for genetic counselors in a team-based approach to optimal PGx result delivery.

Author Contributions: Substantial contribution to conception/design of the work: T.S. and A.C.S.; Substantial contribution to the acquisition: T.S. and A.C.S.; Analysis and interpretation of data for the work: T.S., A.C.S., and L.B.S.; Drafting the work and/or revising it critically for important intellectual content: T.S., A.C.S., and L.B.S.; Final approval of the version to be published: T.S., A.C.S., and L.B.S.; Agreement to be accountable for all aspects of the work in ensuring that questions related to the accuracy or integrity of any part of the work are appropriately investigated and resolved: T.S. and L.B.S. All authors have read and agreed to the published version of the manuscript.

Funding: This study was funded by Applied Physics Laboratory Contract Number N00024-03-D-6606, Michael F. Christman, Principal Investigator, and by Cooperative Agreement FA8650-14-2-6533, Michael F. Christman, Principal Investigator. The content is solely the responsibility of the authors and does not necessarily represent the official views of the United States Air Force.

Acknowledgments: Special thanks to the participants of the Coriell Personalized Medicine Collaborative (CPMC) who made this work possible. The authors would also like to acknowledge the late Michael F. Christman for his leadership as Principal Investigator of the CPMC and President and Chief Executive Officer of the Coriell Institute for Medical Research.

Conflicts of Interest: The authors declare no conflict of interest.

Human Studies and Informed Consent: The Coriell Institute for Medical Research Institutional Review Board reviewed and approved this study. As a retrospective review of existing CPMC participant records, no additional participant consent was required.

Animal Studies: No non-human animal studies were carried out by the authors for this article.

References

1. Ellingrod, V.L. Pharmacogenomics testing: What the FDA says. *Curr. Psychiatry* **2019**, *18*, 29–33.
2. Lemke, A.A.; Hulick, P.J.; Wake, D.T.; Wang, C.; Sereika, A.W.; Yu, K.D.; Glaser, N.S.; Dunnenberger, H.M. Patient perspectives following pharmacogenomics results disclosure in an integrated health system. *Pharmacogenomics* **2018**, *19*, 321–331. [CrossRef]
3. Haga, S.B.; Liu, Y. Patient characteristics, experiences and perceived value of pharmacogenetic testing from a single testing laboratory. *Pharmacogenomics* **2019**, *20*, 581–587. [CrossRef]
4. Olson, J.E.; Rohrer Vitek, C.R.; Bell, E.J.; McGree, M.E.; Jacobson, D.J.; St Sauver, J.L.; Caraballo, P.J.; Griffin, J.M.; Roger, V.L.; Bielinski, S.J. Participant-perceived understanding and perspectives on pharmacogenomics: The Mayo Clinic RIGHT protocol (Right Drug, Right Dose, Right Time). *Genet. Med.* **2017**, *19*, 819–825. [CrossRef]

5. Keller, M.A.; Gordon, E.S.; Stack, C.B.; Gharani, N.; Sill, C.J.; Schmidlen, T.J.; Joseph, M.; Pallies, J.; Gerry, N.P.; Christman, M.F. Coriell Personalized Medicine Collaborative((R)): A prospective study of the utility of personalized medicine. *Pers. Med.* **2010**, *7*, 301–317. [CrossRef]
6. Gharani, N.; Keller, M.A.; Stack, C.B.; Hodges, L.M.; Schmidlen, T.J.; Lynch, D.E.; Gordon, E.S.; Christman, M.F. The Coriell personalized medicine collaborative pharmacogenomics appraisal, evidence scoring and interpretation system. *Genome Med.* **2013**, *5*, 93. [CrossRef] [PubMed]
7. Burmester, J.K.; Sedova, M.; Shapero, M.H.; Mansfield, E. DMET microarray technology for pharmacogenomics-based personalized medicine. *Methods Mol. Biol.* **2010**, *632*, 99–124. [CrossRef] [PubMed]
8. Schmidlen, T.J.; Wawak, L.; Kasper, R.; Garcia-Espana, J.F.; Christman, M.F.; Gordon, E.S. Personalized genomic results: Analysis of informational needs. *J. Genet. Couns.* **2014**, *23*, 578–587. [CrossRef] [PubMed]
9. Sweet, K.; Gordon, E.S.; Sturm, A.C.; Schmidlen, T.J.; Manickam, K.; Toland, A.E.; Keller, M.A.; Stack, C.B.; Garcia-Espana, J.F.; Bellafante, M.; et al. Design and implementation of a randomized controlled trial of genomic counseling for patients with chronic disease. *J. Pers. Med.* **2014**, *4*, 1–19. [CrossRef] [PubMed]
10. Diseati, L.; Scheinfeldt, L.B.; Kasper, R.S.; Zhaoyang, R.; Gharani, N.; Schmidlen, T.J.; Gordon, E.S.; Sessions, C.K.; Delaney, S.K.; Jarvis, J.P.; et al. Common genetic risk for melanoma encourages preventive behavior change. *J. Pers. Med.* **2015**, *5*, 36–49. [CrossRef]
11. Scheinfeldt, L.B.; Gharani, N.; Kasper, R.S.; Schmidlen, T.J.; Gordon, E.S.; Jarvis, J.P.; Delaney, S.; Kronenthal, C.J.; Gerry, N.P.; Christman, M.F. Using the Coriell Personalized Medicine Collaborative Data to conduct a genome-wide association study of sleep duration. *Am. J. Med. Genet. B Neuropsychiatr. Genet.* **2015**, *168*, 697–705. [CrossRef] [PubMed]
12. Scheinfeldt, L.B.; Schmidlen, T.J.; Gharani, N.; MacKnight, M.; Jarvis, J.P.; Delaney, S.K.; Gordon, E.S.; Kronenthal, C.J.; Gerry, N.P.; Christman, M.F. Coronary artery disease genetic risk awareness motivates heart health behaviors in the Coriell Personalized Medicine Collaborative. *Expert Rev. Precis. Med. Drug Dev.* **2016**, *1*, 407–413. [CrossRef]
13. Schmidlen, T.J.; Scheinfeldt, L.; Zhaoyang, R.; Kasper, R.; Sweet, K.; Gordon, E.S.; Keller, M.; Stack, C.; Gharani, N.; Daly, M.B.; et al. Genetic Knowledge Among Participants in the Coriell Personalized Medicine Collaborative. *J. Genet. Couns.* **2016**, *25*, 385–394. [CrossRef] [PubMed]
14. Haga, S.B.; Mills, R.; Moaddeb, J.; Allen Lapointe, N.; Cho, A.; Ginsburg, G.S. Patient experiences with pharmacogenetic testing in a primary care setting. *Pharmacogenomics* **2016**, *17*, 1629–1636. [CrossRef] [PubMed]
15. Frigon, M.P.; Blackburn, M.E.; Dubois-Bouchard, C.; Gagnon, A.L.; Tardif, S.; Tremblay, K. Pharmacogenetic testing in primary care practice: Opinions of physicians, pharmacists and patients. *Pharmacogenomics* **2019**, *20*, 589–598. [CrossRef] [PubMed]
16. Lee, Y.M.; McKillip, R.P.; Borden, B.A.; Klammer, C.E.; Ratain, M.J.; O'Donnell, P.H. Assessment of patient perceptions of genomic testing to inform pharmacogenomic implementation. *Pharm. Genom.* **2017**, *27*, 179–189. [CrossRef]
17. Haga, S.B.; O'Daniel, J.M.; Tindall, G.M.; Lipkus, I.R.; Agans, R. Survey of US public attitudes toward pharmacogenetic testing. *Pharm. J.* **2012**, *12*, 197–204. [CrossRef]
18. Charland, S.L.; Agatep, B.C.; Herrera, V.; Schrader, B.; Frueh, F.W.; Ryvkin, M.; Shabbeer, J.; Devlin, J.J.; Superko, H.R.; Stanek, E.J. Providing patients with pharmacogenetic test results affects adherence to statin therapy: Results of the Additional KIF6 Risk Offers Better Adherence to Statins (AKROBATS) trial. *Pharm. J.* **2014**, *14*, 272–280. [CrossRef]
19. Li, J.H.; Joy, S.V.; Haga, S.B.; Orlando, L.A.; Kraus, W.E.; Ginsburg, G.S.; Voora, D. Genetically guided statin therapy on statin perceptions, adherence, and cholesterol lowering: A pilot implementation study in primary care patients. *J. Pers. Med.* **2014**, *4*, 147–162. [CrossRef]
20. Bloss, C.S.; Schork, N.J.; Topol, E.J. Direct-to-consumer pharmacogenomic testing is associated with increased physician utilisation. *J. Med. Genet.* **2014**, *51*, 83–89. [CrossRef]
21. Yau, A.; Haque, M. Pharmacogenomics: Knowledge, Attitude and Practice among Future Doctors and Pharmacists-A Pilot Study. *J. Appl. Pharm. Sci.* **2016**, *6*, 141–145. [CrossRef]

22. Mills, R.; Haga, S.B. Clinical delivery of pharmacogenetic testing services: A proposed partnership between genetic counselors and pharmacists. *Pharmacogenomics* **2013**, *14*, 957–968. [CrossRef] [PubMed]
23. Dunnenberger, H.M.; Crews, K.R.; Hoffman, J.M.; Caudle, K.E.; Broeckel, U.; Howard, S.C.; Hunkler, R.J.; Klein, T.E.; Evans, W.E.; Relling, M.V. Preemptive clinical pharmacogenetics implementation: Current programs in five US medical centers. *Annu. Rev. Pharmacol. Toxicol.* **2015**, *55*, 89–106. [CrossRef] [PubMed]

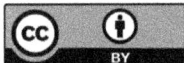

© 2020 by the authors. Licensee MDPI, Basel, Switzerland. This article is an open access article distributed under the terms and conditions of the Creative Commons Attribution (CC BY) license (http://creativecommons.org/licenses/by/4.0/).

MDPI
St. Alban-Anlage 66
4052 Basel
Switzerland
Tel. +41 61 683 77 34
Fax +41 61 302 89 18
www.mdpi.com

Journal of Personalized Medicine Editorial Office
E-mail: jpm@mdpi.com
www.mdpi.com/journal/jpm

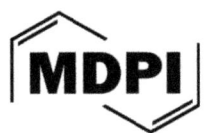

www.ingramcontent.com/pod-product-compliance
Lightning Source LLC
LaVergne TN
LVHW070625100526
838202LV00012B/724

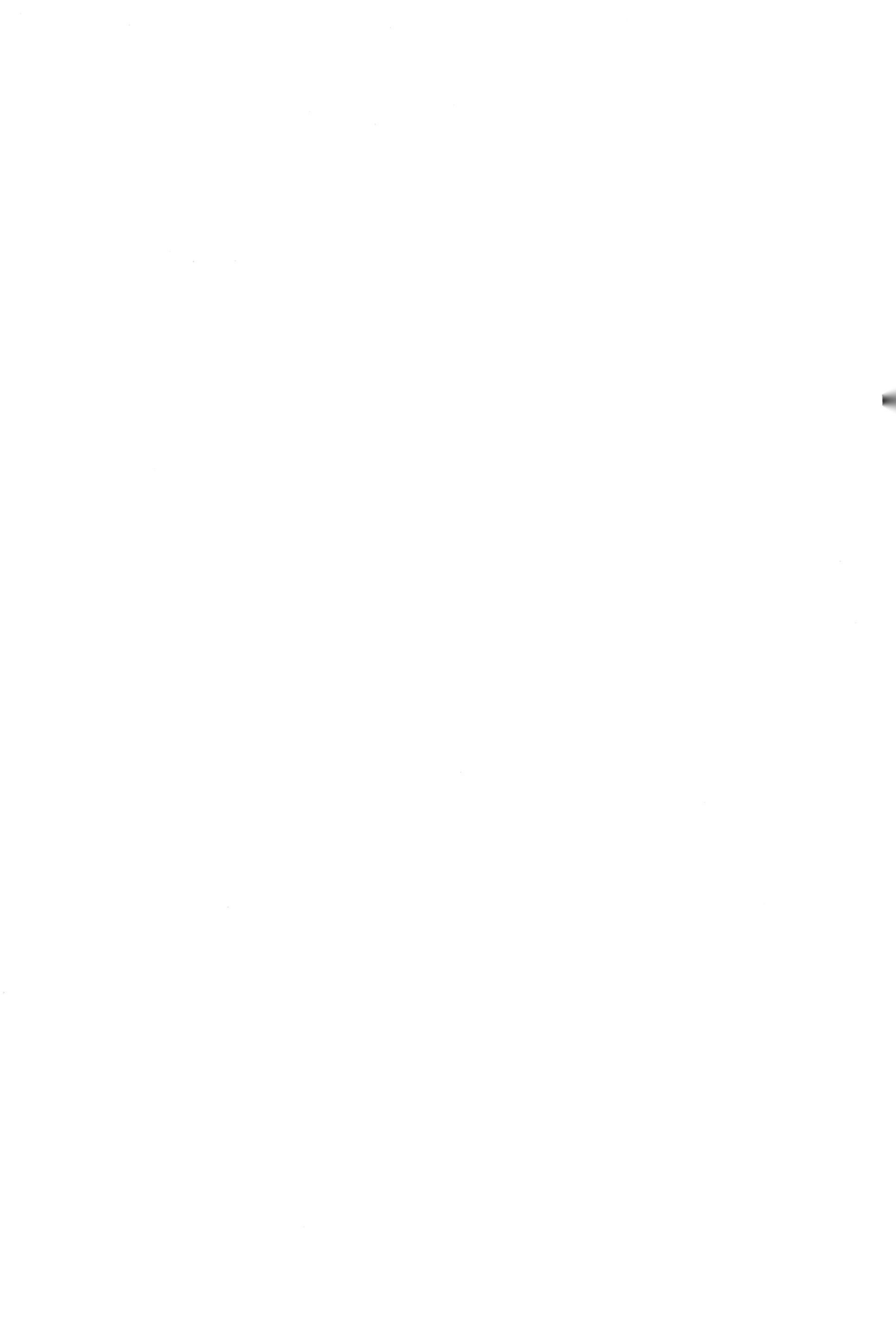